# Emergencies in the Outpatient Setting

*Editor*

JOSEPH F. SZOT

# MEDICAL CLINICS
# OF NORTH AMERICA

www.medical.theclinics.com

*Consulting Editor*
BIMAL H. ASHAR

May 2017 • Volume 101 • Number 3

# ELSEVIER

1600 John F. Kennedy Boulevard • Suite 1800 • Philadelphia, Pennsylvania, 19103-2899

http://www.theclinics.com

**MEDICAL CLINICS OF NORTH AMERICA Volume 101, Number 3**
**May 2017 ISSN 0025-7125, ISBN-13: 978-0-323-52846-7**

Editor: Jessica McCool
Developmental Editor: Alison Swety

Medical Clinics of North America (ISSN 0025-7125) is published bimonthly by Elsevier Inc., 360 Park Avenue South, New York, NY 10010-1710. Months of publication are January, March, May, July, September, and November. Business and editorial offices: 1600 John F. Kennedy Boulevard, Suite 1800, Philadelphia, PA 19103-2899. Periodicals postage paid at New York, NY, and additional mailing offices. Subscription prices are USD $268.00 per year (US individuals), $563.00 per year (US institutions), $100.00 per year (US Students), $330.00 per year (Canadian individuals), $731.00 per year (Canadian institutions), $200.00 per year (Canadian and foreign students), $402.00 per year (foreign individuals), and $731.00 per year (foreign institutions). To receive student/resident rate, orders must be accompanied by name of affiliated institution, date of term, and the signature of program/residency coordinator on institution letterhead. Orders will be billed at individual rate until proof of status is received. Foreign air speed delivery is included in all Clinics' subscription prices. All prices are subject to change without notice. **POSTMASTER:** Send address changes to *Medical Clinics of North America*, Elsevier Health Sciences Division, Subscription Customer Service, 3251 Riverport Lane, Maryland Heights, MO 63043. **Customer Service: Telephone: 1-800-654-2452** (U.S. and Canada); **1-314-447-8871** (outside U.S. and Canada). **Fax: 314-447-8029. E-mail: journalscustomerserviceusa@elsevier.com** (for print support); **journalsonlinesupport-usa@elsevier.com** (for online support).

*Reprints.* For copies of 100 or more of articles in this publication, please contact the Commercial Reprints Department, Elsevier Inc., 360 Park Avenue South, New York, NY 10010-1710. Tel.: 212-633-3874; Fax: 212-633-3820; E-mail: reprints@elsevier.com.

*Medical Clinics of North America* is also published in Spanish by McGraw-Hill Interamericana Editores S. A., P.O. Box 5-237, 06500 Mexico, D.F., Mexico.

*Medical Clinics of North America* is covered in *MEDLINE/PubMed (Index Medicus), Current Contents, ASCA, Excerpta Medica, Science Citation Index, and ISI/BIOMED.*

## PROGRAM OBJECTIVE
The goal of the *Medical Clinics of North America* is to keep practicing physicians up to date with current clinical practice by providing timely articles reviewing the state of the art in patient care.

## TARGET AUDIENCE
All practicing physicians and other healthcare professionals.

## LEARNING OBJECTIVES
Upon completion of this activity, participants will be able to:
1. Review cardiac outpatient emergencies such as arrhythmias and acute heart failure, among others.
2. Discuss the management of psychiatric emergencies.
3. Recognize trends in emergency outpatient care for pulmonary, neurological, and otolaryngolic emergencies, among others.

## ACCREDITATION
The Elsevier Office of Continuing Medical Education (EOCME) is accredited by the Accreditation Council for Continuing Medical Education (ACCME) to provide continuing medical education for physicians.

The EOCME designates this enduring material for a maximum of 15 *AMA PRA Category 1 Credit*(s)™. Physicians should claim only the credit commensurate with the extent of their participation in the activity.

All other healthcare professionals requesting continuing education credit for this enduring material will be issued a certificate of participation.

## DISCLOSURE OF CONFLICTS OF INTEREST
The EOCME assesses conflict of interest with its instructors, faculty, planners, and other individuals who are in a position to control the content of CME activities. All relevant conflicts of interest that are identified are thoroughly vetted by EOCME for fair balance, scientific objectivity, and patient care recommendations. EOCME is committed to providing its learners with CME activities that promote improvements or quality in healthcare and not a specific proprietary business or a commercial interest.

**The planning committee, staff, authors and editors listed below have identified no financial relationships or relationships to products or devices they or their spouse/life partner have with commercial interest related to the content of this CME activity:**
Bimal H. Ashar, MD, MBA, FACP; Ashley Behrens, MD; Raphael E. Bonita, MD, ScM; Timothy Joseph Byrnes, DO; Kristi E. Chang, MD; Otto Costantini, MD; Salvador Cruz-Flores, MD, MPH; Joseph H. Donroe, MD, MPH; Matthew G. Drake, MD; Maya Fayfman, MD; Jess G. Fiedorowicz, MD, PhD; Anjali Fortna; Brenda Marsh, MD, PhD; Jessica McCool; Maria Michail, PhD; Malgorzata Mysliwiec, MD; Premkumar Nandhakumar; M. Lee Sanders, MD, PhD; Namrata Singh, MD; Manish Suneja, MD, FASN, FACP; Joseph F. Szot, MD, FACP; Andreina Tarff, MD; Kendall K. Tasche, MD; Jeanette M. Tetrault, MD; Scott A. Vogelgesang, MD; Andrea N. Weber, MD, MME; Katie Widmeier.

**The planning committee, staff, authors and editors listed below have identified financial relationships or relationships to products or devices they or their spouse/life partner have with commercial interest related to the content of this CME activity:**
**Scott P. Commins, MD, PhD** is on the speakers' bureau for Genentech, a member of the Roche Group, has research support from National Institutes of Health - National Institutes of Allergy and Infectious Disease, and receives royalties/patents from Wolters Kluwer.
**Francisco J. Pasquel, MD, MPH** is a consultant/advisor for Merck & Co., Inc and Boehringer Ingelheim GmbH.
**Alex Thompson, MD, MBA, MPH** is on the speakers' bureau for the American Psychiatric Association and the American Academy of Clinical Psychiatrists, and is a consultant/advisor for MCG, Inc. and Decker Intellectual Properties inc.
**Guillermo E. Umpierrez, MD, CDE, FACE, FACP** is a consultant/advisor for Sanofi; Merck & Co., Inc.; and Johnson & Johnson Services, Inc, and has research support from Sanofi; Merck & Co., Inc; Boehringer Ingelheim GmbH; AstraZeneca; and Novo Nordisk A/S.

## UNAPPROVED/OFF-LABEL USE DISCLOSURE
The EOCME requires CME faculty to disclose to the participants:
1. When products or procedures being discussed are off-label, unlabelled, experimental, and/or investigational (not US Food and Drug Administration [FDA] approved); and

2. Any limitations on the information presented, such as data that are preliminary or that represent ongoing research, interim analyses, and/or unsupported opinions. Faculty may discuss information about pharmaceutical agents that is outside of FDA-approved labelling. This information is intended solely for CME and is not intended to promote off-label use of these medications. If you have any questions, contact the medical affairs department of the manufacturer for the most recent prescribing information.

## TO ENROLL
To enroll in the *Medical Clinics of North America* Continuing Medical Education program, call customer service at 1-800-654-2452 or sign up online at http://www.theclinics.com/home/cme. The CME program is available to subscribers for an additional annual fee of USD $295.

## METHOD OF PARTICIPATION
In order to claim credit, participants must complete the following:
1. Complete enrolment as indicated above.
2. Read the activity.
3. Complete the CME Test and Evaluation. Participants must achieve a score of 70% on the test. All CME Tests and Evaluations must be completed online.

## CME INQUIRIES/SPECIAL NEEDS
For all CME inquiries or special needs, please contact elsevierCME@elsevier.com.

# MEDICAL CLINICS OF NORTH AMERICA

**FORTHCOMING ISSUES**

*July 2017*
**Disease Prevention**
Michael P. Pignone and
Kirsten Bibbins-Domingo, *Editors*

*September 2017*
**Complementary and Integrative Medicine**
Robert B. Saper, *Editor*

*November 2017*
**Care of Cancer Survivors**
Kimberly S. Peairs, *Editor*

**RECENT ISSUES**

*March 2017*
**Anemia**
Thomas G. DeLoughery, *Editor*

*January 2017*
**Hypertension**
Edward D. Frohlich, *Editor*

*November 2016*
**Practice-Based Nutrition Care**
Scott Kahan and Robert F. Kushner, *Editors*

**RELATED INTEREST**

*Immunology and Allergy Clinics of North America*, August 2016 (Vol. 36, Issue 3)
**Severe Asthma**
Rohit K. Katial, *Editor*
http://www.immunology.theclinics.com/

# MEDICAL CLINICS OF NORTH AMERICA

## Contents

# Contributors

## CONSULTING EDITOR

**BIMAL H. ASHAR, MD, MBA, FACP**
Associate Professor of Medicine, Division of General Internal Medicine, Johns Hopkins University School of Medicine, Baltimore, Maryland

## EDITOR

**JOSEPH F. SZOT, MD, FACP**
Clinical Professor, Division of General Internal Medicine, Department of Internal Medicine, University of Iowa Carver College of Medicine, Iowa City, Iowa

## AUTHORS

**ASHLEY BEHRENS, MD**
Chief, Division of Comprehensive Eye Care, KKESH/WEI Professor of International Ophthalmology, The Wilmer Eye Institute, Johns Hopkins University School of Medicine, Baltimore, Maryland

**RAPHAEL E. BONITA, MD, ScM**
Department of Medicine, Jefferson Heart Institute, Sidney Kimmel Medical College of Thomas Jefferson University, Philadelphia, Pennsylvania

**TIMOTHY JOSEPH BYRNES, DO**
Cardiology Fellow, SummaHealth Heart and Vascular Institute, North East Ohio Medical University, Akron, Ohio

**KRISTI E. CHANG, MD**
University of Iowa, Iowa City, Iowa

**SCOTT P. COMMINS, MD, PhD**
Associate Professor, Division of Rheumatology, Allergy and Immunology, Departments of Medicine and Pediatrics, Thurston Research Center, University of North Carolina, Chapel Hill, North Carolina

**OTTO COSTANTINI, MD**
Director of Clinical Research, Associate Director of Cardiology Fellowship, SummaHealth Heart and Vascular Institute, North East Ohio Medical University, Akron, Ohio

**SALVADOR CRUZ-FLORES, MD, MPH**
Professor and Founding Chair, Department of Neurology, Paul L Foster School of Medicine, Texas Tech University Health Sciences Center El Paso, El Paso, Texas

**JOSEPH H. DONROE, MD, MPH**
Yale New Haven Hospital, St. Raphael Campus, Assistant Professor of Medicine, Yale University School of Medicine, New Haven, Connecticut

**MATTHEW G. DRAKE, MD**
Division of Pulmonary and Critical Care Medicine, Oregon Health and Science University, Portland, Oregon

**MAYA FAYFMAN, MD**
Division of Endocrinology and Metabolism, Department of Medicine, Emory University School of Medicine, Atlanta, Georgia

**JESS G. FIEDOROWICZ, MD, PhD**
Associate Professor, Department of Psychiatry, University of Iowa; Department of Internal Medicine, Carver College of Medicine, University of Iowa; Department of Epidemiology, College of Public Health, University of Iowa; Abboud Cardiovascular Research Center, University of Iowa, Iowa City, Iowa

**BRENDA MARSH, MD, PhD**
Division of Pulmonary and Critical Care Medicine, Oregon Health and Science University, Portland, Oregon

**MARIA MICHAIL, PhD**
Senior Research Fellow/Interim Director of Postgraduate Research, Faculty of Medicine & Health Sciences, School of Health Sciences, University of Nottingham, Nottingham, United Kingdom

**MALGORZATA MYSLIWIEC, MD**
Department of Medicine, Jefferson Heart Institute, Sidney Kimmel Medical College of Thomas Jefferson University, Philadelphia, Pennsylvania

**FRANCISCO J. PASQUEL, MD, MPH**
Division of Endocrinology and Metabolism, Department of Medicine, Emory University School of Medicine, Atlanta, Georgia

**M. LEE SANDERS, MD, PhD**
Division of Nephrology and Hypertension, Department of Medicine, University of Iowa Hospitals and Clinics, Iowa City, Iowa

**NAMRATA SINGH, MD**
Division of Immunology: Rheumatology and Allergy, Department of Internal Medicine, University of Iowa Carver College of Medicine, Iowa City, Iowa

**MANISH SUNEJA, MD, FASN, FACP**
Division of Nephrology and Hypertension, Department of Medicine, University of Iowa Hospitals and Clinics, Iowa City, Iowa

**ANDREINA TARFF, MD**
Ophthalmology Postdoctoral Research Fellow, The Wilmer Eye Institute, Johns Hopkins University School of Medicine, Baltimore, Maryland

**KENDALL K. TASCHE, MD**
University of Iowa, Iowa City, Iowa

**JEANETTE M. TETRAULT, MD**
Associate Professor of Medicine, Department of Internal Medicine, Yale University School of Medicine, New Haven, Connecticut

**ALEX THOMPSON, MD, MBA, MPH**
Clinical Associate Professor, Department of Psychiatry, Carver College of Medicine, University of Iowa, Iowa City, Iowa

**GUILLERMO E. UMPIERREZ, MD, CDE, FACE, FACP**
Professor of Medicine, Division of Endocrinology and Metabolism, Department of Medicine, Emory University School of Medicine, Atlanta, Georgia

**SCOTT A. VOGELGESANG, MD**
Division of Immunology: Rheumatology and Allergy, Department of Internal Medicine, University of Iowa Carver College of Medicine, Iowa City, Iowa

**ANDREA N. WEBER, MD, MME**
Resident Physician, Department of Internal Medicine, University of Iowa; Department of Psychiatry, Carver College of Medicine, University of Iowa, Iowa City, Iowa

# Contents

A rapid and severe increase in blood pressure resulting in new or progressive end-organ damage is defined as hypertensive emergency. Clinicians should effectively use the patient interview, physical examination, and additional testing to differentiate hypertensive emergency from nonemergent hypertension. Patients with evidence or high suspicion for end-organ damage should be expediently referred from the outpatient setting to a higher level of care. Knowledge of appropriate hypertensive emergency management and the ability to initiate this care in the clinic could help reduce patient morbidity in certain situations. Patients presenting with nonemergent hypertension can continue to be safely managed in the clinic.

Ischemic stroke is cause of substantial death and disability in the United States. Transient ischemic attack, a precursor to ischemic stroke, conveys a high risk of recurrent stroke within 90 days from event. These conditions are highly preventable and treatable. The cause is heterogenous and includes atherothrombosis, cardioembolism, lacunar disease, or cryptogenic, and some uncommon causes, such as arterial dissection and prothrombotic states. The emergent evaluation includes establishing time of onset, vital signs, glucose level, and severity of the deficit.

Tachyarrhythmias and bradyarrhythmias are often seen in the outpatient setting. Patients can present minimally symptomatic or in extremis. Accurate diagnosis of the rhythm, plus a detailed clinical history, are critical for best management and optimal outcome. A 12-lead electrocardiogram is the cornerstone for diagnosis. Practitioners must identify patients who need immediate transport to an emergency department versus those who can safely wait for an outpatient specialty referral. This article reviews how to accurately diagnose and differentiate the most common tachyarrhythmias and bradyarrhythmias, the associated symptoms, and important concepts for the initial steps in the office management of such arrhythmias.

Heart failure is an epidemic in the United States and a major health problem worldwide. The syndrome of acute heart failure is marked by a recent onset of symptoms usually in terms of days to a few weeks of worsening fatigue, shortness of breath, orthopnea, swelling, and sudden onset of weight gain. Physicians caring for patients with heart failure must know the risk factors for this disease, pathophysiology, symptomatology, important examination findings, key diagnostic tests, and management approach so as to improve symptoms and reduce mortality.

Anaphylactic fatalities are rare; however, mild reactions can rapidly progress to cardiovascular and respiratory arrest. The clinical course of anaphylaxis can be unpredictable. Prompt and early use of epinephrine should be considered. Most anaphylaxis episodes have an immunologic mechanism involving immunoglobulin E (IgE). Foods are the most common cause in children; medications and insect stings are more common in adults. When the cause is not completely avoidable or cannot be determined, a patient should be supplied with autoinjectable epinephrine and be instructed its use. They should keep the device with them at all times and taught the signs and symptoms of anaphylaxis.

Primary care providers tasked with treating acute exacerbations of asthma and chronic obstructive pulmonary disease must be able to recognize exacerbation of symptoms and triage patients based on exacerbation severity to the appropriate level of care. Early treatment with bronchodilators and corticosteroids should be followed by repeated assessments of treatment efficacy. Primary care providers should also provide symptom-guided action plans to empower patients to manage their disease.

The assessment of suicide risk is a daunting, but increasingly frequent task for outpatient practitioners. Guidelines for depression screening identify more individuals at risk for treatment and mental health resources are not always easily accessible. For those patients identified as in need of a formal suicide risk assessment, this article reviews established risk and protective factors for suicide and provides a framework for the assessment and management of individuals at risk of suicide. The assessment should be explicitly documented with a summary of the most relevant risk/protective factors for that individual with a focus on interventions that may mitigate risk.

Recognizing an acute intoxication syndrome in patients presenting to an outpatient clinical practice with behavior or mental status changes requires initial consideration of a broad differential diagnosis. After a thorough evaluation, early management may include triage to a higher level of care, treatment of the presenting concern, and consideration of treatment of potential substance withdrawal. Additionally, there are medicolegal aspects of caring for intoxicated patients related to privacy, informed consent, and risk of harm to self and others after leaving the clinic with which practitioners should become familiar.

Diabetic ketoacidosis (DKA) and hyperglycemic hyperosmolar state (HHS) are the most serious and life-threatening hyperglycemic emergencies in diabetes. DKA is more common in young people with type 1 diabetes and HHS in adult and elderly patients with type 2 diabetes. Features of the 2 disorders with ketoacidosis and hyperosmolality may coexist. Both are characterized by insulinopenia and severe hyperglycemia. Early diagnosis and management are paramount. Treatment is aggressive rehydration, insulin therapy, electrolyte replacement, and treatment of underlying precipitating events. This article reviews the epidemiology, pathogenesis, diagnosis, and management of hyperglycemic emergencies.

Monoarticular arthritis is inflammation characterized by joint pain, swelling, and sometimes periarticular erythema. Although chronic causes are seen, the onset is often acute. An infected joint can quickly lead to permanent damage, making it a medical emergency. However, acute gout presenting as monoarticular arthritis is often so uncomfortable it requires urgent attention. Monoarticular crystalline arthritis is common and a septic joint is a medical emergency so it is no surprise that these diagnoses come to mind with complaint of inflammation in 1 joint. However, there are many causes of monoarticular arthritis that clinicians must consider.

"Red eye" is used as a general term to describe irritated or bloodshot eyes. It is a recognizable sign of an acute/chronic, localized/systemic underlying inflammatory condition. Conjunctival injection is most commonly caused by dryness, allergy, visual fatigue, contact lens overwear, and local infections. In some instances, red eye can represent a true ocular emergency that should be treated by an ophthalmologist. A comprehensive assessment of red eye conditions is required to preserve the patients visual function. Severe ocular pain, significant photophobia, decreased vision, and

# Foreword

# Recognize, Assess, and Treat

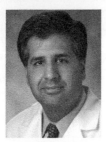

Bimal H. Ashar, MD, MBA, FACP
*Consulting Editor*

Acute medical problems account for a large proportion of visits to primary care providers. Yet, only a small proportion of these visits can be classified as true emergencies—conditions that carry an immediate risk of mortality or significant morbidity. Despite their limited incidence, misdiagnosis or improper treatment of patients with medical emergencies can be catastrophic.

Over the last decade, emphasis has been placed on reducing the number of emergency room (ER) visits due to their high cost. The Affordable Care Act specifically underscored the need to shift care from the ER into medical offices (preferentially primary care offices). Medical practices have been encouraged to become Patient-Centered Medical Homes that have the ability and availability to prevent their patients from needing to go to ERs. Similarly, Accountable Care Organizations have tried to unify hospitals, their ERs, and medical practices in working together to reduce ER visits and hospital admissions.

This increased emphasis on shifting care from the ER to the office has expanded the need for acute care access in office settings. Although most of these visits will likely not be emergent, logic would suggest that the overall number of emergencies in office settings will increase. As a result, it is imperative for providers and their staff to be knowledgeable in the diagnosis and management of such events: The need to recognize, assess, and treat efficiently. In this issue of the *Medical Clinics of North America*, Dr Szot has enlisted experts from around the country to provide an overview of the

Med Clin N Am 101 (2017) xv–xvi
http://dx.doi.org/10.1016/j.mcna.2017.02.002
0025-7125/17/© 2017 Published by Elsevier Inc.

most common and important emergencies that office-based providers may face. I am confident that it will serve as a valuable reference.

Bimal H. Ashar, MD, MBA, FACP
Division of General Internal Medicine
Johns Hopkins University School of Medicine
601 North Caroline Street
#7143
Baltimore, MD 21287, USA

E-mail address:
Bashar1@jhmi.edu

# Preface

# Emergencies in the Outpatient Setting

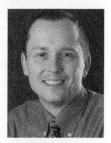

Joseph F. Szot, MD, FACP
*Editor*

Ambulatory clinical practice is becoming increasingly challenging with more and more demands placed on clinicians' time. In addition, because the patient population is aging and is more likely to have multiple comorbidities, the complexity and acuity of outpatients are significantly increasing. In light of the ever-changing landscape of health care delivery, recognition and management of emergent and urgent conditions in outpatient venues are paramount. It is therefore critical that clinicians have the knowledge and skills to diagnose, triage, and manage these situations in an efficient, high-quality, and cost-effective manner.

This issue of *Medical Clinics of North America* focuses on the most common urgencies/emergencies encountered in the outpatient setting. These topics were chosen by polling seasoned general internists who had experience in both academic and private practice environments. It is not meant to be an exhaustive review of all emergencies encountered in the outpatient setting but rather a compilation of the more common urgencies/emergencies that may present. The authors were tasked with focusing on the recognition of the emergency and its diagnosis, and on the evidence-based treatment of the condition when appropriate on an outpatient basis, and triage to a higher level of care when needed.

It has been my privilege to serve as guest editor for this issue of *Medical Clinics of North America*. The topics covered in this issue span a wide breadth of medicine, with the unifying theme being the need to rapidly and accurately diagnose and treat the condition to prevent patient suffering and even mortality. It is my hope that the articles contained within this issue will enhance and improve the clinician's ability to

Med Clin N Am 101 (2017) xvii–xviii
http://dx.doi.org/10.1016/j.mcna.2017.02.001
0025-7125/17/© 2017 Published by Elsevier Inc.

medical.theclinics.com

manage urgencies/emergencies that present in the outpatient setting and advance their ability to provide efficient, high-quality, cost-effective care.

Joseph F. Szot, MD, FACP
Clinical Professor
Division of General Internal Medicine
Department of Internal Medicine
University of Iowa Carver College of Medicine
200 Hawkins Drive
Iowa City, IA 52242, USA

E-mail address:
joseph-szot@uiowa.edu

# Hypertensive Emergency

Manish Suneja, MD, FASN*, M. Lee Sanders, MD, PhD

## KEYWORDS

- Hypertensive emergency • Hypertensive urgency • Hypertensive crisis
- Autoregulation

## KEY POINTS

- The distinguishing clinical characteristic of hypertensive emergency is an acute increase in blood pressure that is associated with new or progressive end-organ damage.
- Autoregulation is intended to maintain adequate and stable blood flow to the brain, heart, and kidneys during fluctuations in blood pressure. The lower pressure threshold of autoregulation also corresponds with the threshold of hypoperfusion and is approximately 20% to 25% lower than the existing blood pressure. This physiologic observation is the rationale behind the clinical recommendation to limit the initial blood pressure reduction to 20% to 25% of pretreatment values.
- The management of hypertension should always begin with an accurate assessment of blood pressure.
- The patient-physician interaction following a confirmed measurement of severely increased blood pressure should focus on determining whether end-organ damage is present, paying particular attention to the neurologic, cardiovascular, and renal systems.
- Evidence for end-organ damage dictates urgent transfer to an emergency department or inpatient setting, whereas hypertensive patients without end-organ damage can be safely managed in the outpatient setting, which includes an appropriate follow-up plan.

## INTRODUCTION

Hypertension is the most common disorder seen in the primary care setting and management of this disorder has become a cornerstone of outpatient clinical practice. It is estimated that at least 30% of the adult population in the United States has hypertension, defined as a systolic blood pressure (SBP) greater than 140 mm Hg, a diastolic blood pressure (DBP) greater than 90 mm Hg, or anyone taking antihypertensive medication. Patients at times present to the clinic with a severely increased blood pressure (BP), known as a hypertensive crisis. Hypertensive crises have historically been further

Disclosure: The authors have nothing to disclose.
Division of Nephrology and Hypertension, Department of Medicine, University of Iowa Hospitals and Clinics, 200 Hawkins Drive, Iowa City, IA 52242, USA
* Corresponding author.
E-mail address: manish-suneja@uiowa.edu

Med Clin N Am 101 (2017) 465–478
http://dx.doi.org/10.1016/j.mcna.2016.12.007
medical.theclinics.com

subdivided into hypertensive urgencies and emergencies.[1] This subdivision is clinically significant because it should ultimately determine acute BP management.

## TERMINOLOGY

Outpatient management decisions can often be delayed or unnecessarily deferred to an emergency room by not having a clear understanding of how to differentiate hypertensive emergency from urgency.

- Hypertensive crisis: usually defined as an acute and severe increase in SBP greater than or equal to 180 mm Hg or a DBP greater than or equal to 120 mm Hg and can occur in both a hypertensive emergency and urgency situation.
- Hypertensive emergency: the severe increase in BP is associated with new or progressive end-organ damage (**Table 1**) and is a true emergency requiring immediate BP control usually over the course of minutes to hours.
- Hypertensive urgency: the severe increase in BP is not associated with end-organ damage, although non–life threatening symptoms, such as anxiety, headache, epistaxis, palpitations, or mild dyspnea, may be present. It is not an emergency, and, contrary to its name, the BP does not require urgent reduction most of the time but instead can be reduced over the course of hours to days.
- Hypertensive emergency in pregnancy: acute-onset, severe hypertension of greater than or equal to 160/110 mm Hg persisting more than 15 minutes. End-organ damage includes severe preeclampsia, HELLP (hemolysis, elevated liver enzymes, low platelet count) syndrome, and eclampsia.[2]

It is important to remember that, during the clinical assessment, regardless of the BP measurement, the emphasis remains on determining whether end-organ damage is present. Hypertensive emergency can present in patients with an acute increase in BP with or without a preexisting history of hypertension. Although the incidence of hypertensive emergency is low at less than 2% of all hypertension presentations annually,[3] knowledge of how to recognize key signs and symptoms as well as an understanding of immediate medical management could help reduce patient morbidity and mortality.

## HEMODYNAMIC DETERMINANTS OF BLOOD PRESSURE

An overall understanding of the hemodynamic determinants of BP is important in order to effectively manage hypertension.

| Table 1 New or progressive end-organ damage associated with hypertensive emergency | |
|---|---|
| **End Organ** | **Damage Type** |
| Brain | Seizure, transient ischemic attack, cerebral infarction, intracerebral or subarachnoid bleed, hypertensive encephalopathy, posterior reversible leukoencephalopathy |
| Heart | Acute pulmonary edema, acute congestive heart failure, acute coronary syndrome |
| Blood vessels | Acute aortic dissection, microangiopathic hemolytic anemia |
| Kidney | Acute kidney injury |
| Retina | Papilledema, hemorrhages, retinal edema |
| Uterus | Eclampsia |

## Mean Arterial Pressure

A pressure is generated when the heart contracts against the resistance of the blood vessels according to the formula: MAP = CO × SVR, where:

- *MAP* is mean arterial pressure, estimated by DBP + (SBP − DBP)/3 or ([2 × DBP] + SBP)/3
- *CO* is cardiac output, which is the product of stroke volume × heart rate (HR)
- *SVR* is systemic vascular resistance, estimated by [80(MAP − MVP)]/CO, where *MVP* is the mean venous pressure, which equals the mean right atrial pressure or central venous pressure (CVP).

Systemic hypertension therefore necessitates an increase in CO and/or SVR. Hypertension most typically results from an increase in SVR because even pathologic conditions that initially increase CO eventually have a normalization of CO over time with a resultant increase in SVR to sustain the hypertension.[4]

## Blood Volume

Blood volume is an important physical factor that helps determine BP. Approximately two-thirds to three-quarters of the blood volume is contained within the venous capacitance vessels; the remaining one-third to one-quarter is contained within the arterial side. Arterial blood volume is determined by the difference in the blood volume ejected by the heart per unit time (CO) and the outflow through the arterial resistance vessels into the venous capacitance vessels (peripheral runoff). When CO and peripheral runoff are balanced, arterial blood volume and arterial pressure remain constant. If CO increases but peripheral runoff does not increase, then arterial blood volume increases and BP also increases.[4]

## Arterial Elasticity and Compliance

Both arterial elasticity and compliance are important determinants of the increase in SBP that occurs for any given increase in blood volume. Arterial elasticity is generally inversely related to age in that younger persons have greater arterial elasticity and arterial elasticity declines with increasing age. Arterial compliance is determined by elastic properties of the large vessels and is reflective of the change in pressure that occurs with a given change in arterial volume. The greater the arterial elasticity, the smaller the increase in systolic pressure during the systolic ejection phase of the cardiac cycle; conversely, a decrease in arterial elasticity, as occurs during atherosclerotic disease, causes a greater increase in SBP during the systolic ejection phase.[4]

## Autoregulation

Autoregulation is an important process that works to maintain adequate and stable blood flow during changes in BP (**Fig. 1**). Under normal conditions, tissue perfusion in the brain, heart, and kidneys remains fairly constant. In the presence of severe hypertension, especially chronic hypertension, the baseline MAP is increased and this ability to autoregulate shifts upward to protect the exposed organ from excessive pressure. Under normal circumstances, cerebral blood flow (CBF) is roughly 50 mL/100 g/min. The cerebral circulation has a physiologic protective mechanism, cerebral autoregulation, that maintains fairly constant CBF across a broad range of systemic perfusion pressures. In normal, nonhypertensive persons, cerebral autoregulation keeps CBF constant between MAPs of 60 to 120 mm Hg (see **Fig. 1**). This autoregulation is accomplished by dilatation and constriction of cerebral resistance

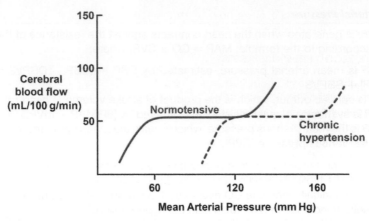

**Fig. 1.** Cerebral autoregulation.

vessels in response to reductions and increases in systemic BP. In chronic hypertension, when BP is poorly controlled, the entire autoregulatory curve is shifted to the right (see **Fig. 1**). The curve is shifted rightward, in part, because of the pressure-related hypertrophy of the cerebral resistance vessels, which diminishes their capacity for maximum dilation (necessary to maintain blood flow when systemic pressure decreases). The lower pressure threshold of autoregulation in both the normal and upward-shifted situations also corresponds with the threshold for hypoperfusion and this threshold is approximately 20% to 25% lower than the existing BP.[5] This physiologic observation is the rationale behind the clinical recommendation to limit the initial BP reduction to 20% to 25% of pretreatment values. If the initial BP reduction exceeded this 20% to 25% threshold, the marked reduction in organ blood flow would lead to organ ischemia and infarction.[1]

### Pathophysiology Leading to a Hypertensive Crisis

The factors leading to the severe and rapid increase of BP in patients presenting with hypertensive urgency and emergency have been investigated but remain poorly understood. The events that explain the transition from hypertensive urgency to emergency resulting in abrupt end-organ damage are even less well understood. The overall acute increase in BP is thought to result from an abrupt increase in SVR that occurs from an acute increase in humoral vasoconstrictors in conjunction with a failure of the normal autoregulatory function. This abrupt increase in SVR causes an increase in mechanical stress on the vascular wall resulting in endothelial injury and vascular permeability. This vascular injury leads to the activation of platelets and the coagulation cascade, fibrin deposition, and the induction of oxidative stress and inflammatory cytokines, which result in tissue ischemia and the characteristic vascular lesion of fibrinoid necrosis of arterioles and small arteries. This cascade of events results in the propagation of an ongoing cycle of tissue ischemia, further release of vasoactive substances, and continued worsening of hypertension, which accelerates the clinical deterioration of the patient.[6–8]

Note that the rate of BP change influences the degree of end-organ damage as well as the clinical symptoms associated with a given BP increase. Chronic hypertension can, to an extent, protect end organs from abrupt increases in transmitted pressure during acute increases in BP because of arteriolar hypertrophy induced by chronic hypertension. In contrast, far smaller increases of BP can result in true hypertensive emergencies in the setting of de novo hypertension, such as that seen during pre-eclampsia or acute drug toxicity.[6–8]

## ACCURATE BLOOD PRESSURE ASSESSMENT

The physical examination is of utmost importance for the diagnosis of hypertensive emergency and should start with an accurate assessment of BP. Although hypertensive emergency presents a different diagnostic and treatment dilemma for clinicians compared with chronic hypertension, the BP measurement technique should essentially remain consistent for all patients to ensure accuracy. To ensure an accurate BP measurement, the following steps should be considered[4]:

- Preparing the equipment
  - Use equipment that has been validated as accurate against a mercury sphygmomanometer
  - Use equipment that has been checked for disrepair (eg, cracks or leaks in tubing, breaks in stitching, tears in fabric)
  - Use equipment that has been checked for an intact gauge (the mercury meniscus or aneroid needle is at zero)
  - Obtain appropriate cuff size by measuring circumference of the patient's arm and choosing the cuff size that corresponds with that measurement (the inflatable part of the cuff should cover 80% of the circumference of the upper arm and the cuff length should be greater than two-thirds the distance between the shoulder and elbow)
- Preparing the patient
  - Confirm that the patient has not recently consumed nicotine or caffeine
  - Have the patient sit quietly for 5 minutes before measuring BP
  - Use a sitting or semireclining position with the back supported
  - The arm should be at heart level (middle of the cuff should be at midsternum level)
  - Legs should be uncrossed with feet flat and supported on the floor or on a foot rest and not dangling from the examination table or bed
  - Clear the upper arm of any constrictive clothing (should be able to get at least 1 finger under a rolled-up sleeve)
  - Palpate the brachial artery and position center of cuff bladder over the brachial artery
- Making the BP measurement
  - Support the arm of the patient at heart level
  - For auscultation measurements:
    - Obtain an estimated systolic pressure by palpation before auscultation
    - Inflate the cuff as rapidly as possible to a maximum inflation level (20 mm Hg greater than the estimated SBP)
    - Deflate the cuff slowly at a rate of 2 to 3 mm Hg per second
    - Note the first of 2 regular beats as the SBP (simultaneous palpation helps avoid underestimating systolic pressure caused by an auscultatory gap)
    - Use the last sound heard as the DBP
    - Continue deflation for 10 mm Hg past the last sound to ensure that the sound is not a skipped beat
    - The measurement should be recorded as an even number and to the nearest 2 mm Hg (round upward)
  - Neither the patient nor observer should talk during the measurement
  - If 2 readings are measured, record the average of the readings

- Additional considerations:
  - Additional consideration should be given to assessment of BP in both upper extremities and in the lower limbs. These additional measurements could assist with the diagnosis of additional disorder: (1) thoracic aortic dissection, in which there may be a wide BP variation between arms; (2) abdominal aortic dissection, in which there may be a wide BP variation between the upper and lower extremities; and (3) coarctation of the aorta, in which there may be a difference in the SBP between the upper and lower extremities while the DBP is similar.

## MAKING THE DIAGNOSIS OF HYPERTENSIVE EMERGENCY

The clinician should efficiently perform a history and physical examination and also strongly consider additional work-up if available to thoroughly evaluate the patient for evidence of end-organ damage after ensuring an accurate BP measurement has been obtained. The main areas of focus should be the neurologic, cardiovascular, and renal systems (**Fig. 2**). In addition, the patient should be asked about recent or chronic use of medications that can produce a hyperadrenergic state (eg, cocaine, amphetamines, phencyclidine) followed by a urine toxicology assessment if indicated.[9] The patient should also be questioned about recent discontinuation of medications known to cause a rebound hypertension effect (eg, clonidine and minoxidil) and also asked about compliance with any prescribed antihypertensive regimen.[10,11] Ingesting tyramine-rich foods in the setting of monoamine oxidase inhibitor use[12] or the abrupt withdrawal from alcohol[13] could also lead to a hypertensive emergency. A diagnosis of preeclampsia and eclampsia should also be considered in pregnant patients.[2,14] A future work-up for resistant hypertension including secondary causes of hypertension (**Table 2**) should also be considered if clinically indicated.

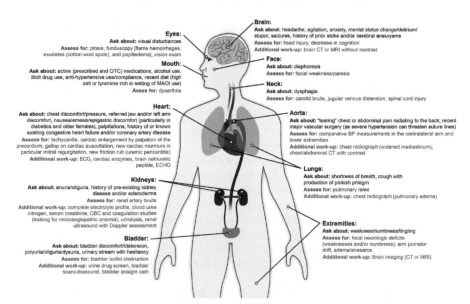

**Fig. 2.** Clinical assessment for end-organ damage in patients with hypertensive crisis. CBC, complete blood count; CT, computed tomography; ECG, electrocardiogram; ECHO, echocardiogram; MAOI, monoamine oxidase inhibitor; OTC, over the counter.

**Table 2**
**Causes of secondary and resistant hypertension**

| System | Possible Cause |
|---|---|
| Neurologic | Head trauma, spinal cord injury, autonomic dysfunction |
| Cardiac/respiratory | Obstructive sleep apnea |
| Renal | Chronic kidney disease, renovascular hypertension |
| Immunologic | Scleroderma, vasculitis |
| Endocrine | Primary aldosteronism, pheochromocytoma, hyperthyroidism, hypothyroidism, Cushing syndrome, acromegaly, hyperparathyroidism, carcinoid tumor, congenital adrenal hyperplasia, renin-secreting tumor |
| Drugs inducing or exacerbating hypertension | NSAIDs, oral contraceptives, sympathomimetics, illicit drugs, glucocorticoids, mineralocorticoids, calcineurin inhibitors, erythropoietin, herbal supplements, VEGF inhibitors |
| Lifestyle | Excessive dietary salt intake, obesity, alcohol consumption |
| Pregnancy | Preeclampsia, HELLP syndrome, Eclampsia |

*Abbreviations:* NSAIDs; nonsteroidal antiinflammatory drugs, VEGF; vascular endothelial growth factor.

## Clues for Previously Uncontrolled Hypertension

Clinicians often encounter patients in the clinic or acute care setting in whom they do not have prior medical records that document important historical trends in BP. Patients are also often unaware of their prior level of BP control. However, there are clinically available clues that can be detected and that could indicate the prior level of BP control (**Box 1**). Documentation of any or all of these findings could suggest that

**Box 1**
**Clinically available clues that indicate poorly controlled hypertension**

*Retinopathy*

- Arteriolar narrowing, AV nicking
- Focal and general arteriolar narrowing, arteriolar silver wiring
- Hemorrhages, exudates, cotton-wool spots, papilledema, and/or microaneurysms

*Cardiac examination*

- Laterally displaced and/or enlarged point of maximal impulse
- S4 gallop
- Other signs of heart failure (eg, JVP, edema and rales)

*Electrocardiogram*

- Voltage criteria for LVH
- Inverted or biphasic P wave in precordial lead V1

*Volume examination/renal (heart failure or kidney dysfunction)*

- Evidence of volume overload (eg, JVP, edema, crackles)
- Increased creatinine level and proteinuria

*Abbreviations:* AV, arteriovenous; JVP, jugular venous pressure; LVH, left ventricular hypertrophy; PMI, point of maximal impulse; S4, fourth heart sound.

previous BP control has been less than optimal and the current increased reading may not indicate an emergency.[4]

### Neurologic End-organ Damage

Severe hypertension with acute neurologic signs and/or symptoms is usually the most complicated and difficult clinical scenario because the differential diagnosis includes varied conditions, such as ischemic stroke, hemorrhagic stroke, and hypertensive encephalopathy, that have different treatments. The patient should be asked about a prior stroke and/or cerebral aneurysm as well as any existing neurologic complaints, to include headache, nausea, emesis, dysphagia, agitation, delirium, stupor, seizures, visual disturbances, focal weaknesses, or numbness/tingling. The physical examination should include looking for obvious signs of recent head injury, an assessment of cognition and speech, carotid artery auscultation, and an assessment for strength and/or sensation deficits. Facial paresis, arm drift/weakness, and abnormal speech are the three most predictive examination findings for the diagnosis of acute stroke.[15] The neurologic examination should also include a direct funduscopic examination to look for flame hemorrhages, exudates, cotton-wool spots, or papilledema. Severe autonomic dysfunction[16–18] is occasionally associated with hypertensive emergency so, if a history of conditions such as Guillain-Barré and Shy-Drager syndrome is present or there is evidence of acute spinal cord injury on examination, severe autonomic dysfunction should be considered. Additional work-up includes checking glucose level to rule out hypoglycemia and obtaining a brain computed tomography (CT) or MRI scan if readily available.

### Cardiovascular End-organ Damage

The evolution of several cardiac emergencies, including acute heart failure, acute coronary syndrome, and aortic dissection, could be initiated by severe hypertension.[19–21] The patient should be asked about a prior heart disease history, to include existing congestive heart failure or coronary artery disease as well as any potential cardiac-related complaints such as shortness of breath, weakness/fatigue, irregular heartbeat, coughing with production of pinkish phlegm, chest discomfort/pressure, referred jaw/ear/arm/epigastric discomfort, nausea/emesis, or a tearing chest or abdominal pain radiating to the back. The patient should also be questioned about any recent vascular surgeries because severe hypertension can threaten suture lines. The physical examination should include looking for the presence of jugular venous distension, palpation of the precordium to assess for cardiac enlargement, pulmonary rales, gallop on cardiac auscultation, new cardiac murmurs (in particular mitral regurgitation), ascites, congestive hepatomegaly, or anasarca. Comparative BP measurements in the contralateral arm and lower extremities can also be considered if aortic dissection or coarctation is a diagnostic possibility, as described earlier. If cardiac ischemia is suspected, cardiac enzymes should be checked in addition to an electrocardiogram. Additional work-up to consider includes checking a brain natriuretic peptide level; a chest radiograph to look for cardiomegaly or pulmonary edema in addition to evidence for a widened mediastinum in aortic dissection or rib notching in aortic coarctation; and, if available, a contrasted CT could be obtained if aortic dissection is suspected.

### Renal End-organ Damage

Renal damage from severe hypertension may present as acute oliguria or as any of the typical features of renal failure, including nausea/emesis, anorexia, mental status changes, uremic pericarditis, or edema. It may be difficult to determine initially whether the renal failure is an acute or a chronic process if the patient is new to the practice; therefore, establishing the timeline for the onset of these symptoms is important to help determine whether the patient had preexisting kidney disease. Renal artery stenosis secondary to fibromuscular dysplasia in younger patients or atherosclerosis in older patients can lead to severe hypertension and renal dysfunction.[22,23] Systemic scleroderma can involve the kidneys and present with severe hypertension, hyperreninemia, azotemia, and microangiopathic anemia.[24] The physical examination should determine whether a cardiac friction rub or renal bruits are present on auscultation. If unexplained hardening or scarring of the skin is present in the setting of a history of gastroesophageal reflux, dysphasia, and attacks of discoloration of the hands and feet in response to cold, then scleroderma renal crisis can be included in the differential. Work-up to assess renal manifestations of severe hypertension should include a complete electrolyte profile, blood urea nitrogen level, serum creatinine level, coagulation studies, and a urinalysis. Doppler ultrasonography assessment to look for renal artery stenosis should also be considered if readily available.

### Hormonal Causes of Hypertensive Emergency

Excess hormonal causes, such as pheochromocytoma, renin-secreting tumors, and aldosterone-secreting tumors, can result in a hypertensive emergency. In these cases, the hypertension is treated and a more thorough evaluation follows later, but these conditions are briefly discussed here for completeness. Pheochromocytomas can be familial or present as part of a multiple endocrine neoplasia syndrome so a family history of refractory hypertension or the presence of other endocrine organ cancers could provide a diagnostic clue. Recurring episodes of headache, diaphoresis, palpitations, tachycardia, and anxiety are suggestive symptoms of pheochromocytoma. The work-up should include measurement of plasma and/or urine catecholamine and metanephrine levels in addition to imaging.[25] Severe hypertension from an excess of aldosterone, whether from primary hyperaldosteronism or from a secondary cause like excess renin secretion, occasionally results in muscle weakness, spasms, and cramps from the resultant hypokalemia but most of the time is fairly asymptomatic. Secondary hyperaldosteronism can contribute to a decreased CO so there may be heart failure symptoms. An aldosterone/renin ratio is used for differentiation of primary and secondary causes and additional testing and imaging needs to be performed.[26]

## TREATMENT APPROACH AND CONSIDERATIONS

The differentiation between hypertensive urgency and emergency using the encounter history, physical examination, and additional work-up options as described earlier is vital because it determines the goals of treatment, including whether or not the patient should be expediently transferred to the emergency department (ED). BP reduction for a nonemergency (increased BP with no evidence for end-organ damage) can be done over hours to days without need for a visit to the ED. Patel and colleagues[27] recently showed that the rate of major adverse cardiovascular events was low in patients who presented to an outpatient setting with hypertensive urgency and, although referral of these patients to the ED did result in more hospitalizations, ED referral was not associated with improved outcomes. There are limited definitive data with regard to hypertensive urgency and emergency management. The recent Eighth Joint National Committee (JNC 8) guidelines do not address hypertensive crisis management[28]; however, by using JNC 7 guidelines and other consensus statements, some general principles can safely be applied.

### Hypertensive Urgency

Patients with nonemergent hypertension are not likely to benefit from aggressive normalization of BP and there could even be increased morbidity if rapid correction is attempted. Rapid correction potentially results in hypotension, further contributing to ischemic complications such as stroke or myocardial infarction. The goal after the exclusion of end-organ damage is to gradually reduce the BP over the next 24 to 48 hours to a more pathophysiologic safe level, generally defined as less than or equal to 160/95 mm Hg. There is rarely a compelling reason to treat hypertensive urgency with intravenous medications because safe and effective treatment can usually be accomplished using common oral medications. The JNC 7 guidelines specifically comment that, "Unfortunately, the term 'urgency' has led to overly aggressive management of many patients with severe, uncomplicated hypertension."[1]

Therapy can be initiated with fast and short-acting oral medications such as clonidine, captopril, labetalol, or nicardipine with a definitive plan to transition to longer-acting antihypertensives that are more suitable for chronic therapy.[28] Multiple dosage adjustments are likely to be needed over the following weeks to months. Hospital observation should still be considered in those patients with hypertensive urgency who remain symptomatic, those who fail to show any improvement in BP despite initial therapy, those with extreme increases of BP, and those very unlikely to obtain follow-up care. The risks of starting an angiotensin-converting enzyme (ACE) inhibitor or an angiotensin receptor blocker (ARB) acutely in patients with chronic kidney disease need to be carefully considered if the likelihood of the patient obtaining appropriate follow-up care seems low. A notable exception is in scleredema renal crisis, which is a hypertensive emergency and the initiation of an ACE inhibitor is the recommended therapy regardless of the serum creatinine measurement.[24]

### Hypertensive Emergency

Patients with evidence or high suspicion for end-organ damage should be expediently referred from the outpatient setting to the ED because a rapid BP reduction over minutes to hours is often indicated to prevent additional end-organ damage. This need for immediate but controlled BP management usually indicates the requirement for monitoring in a critical care setting; however, the initiation of goal-directed therapy in the clinic should be strongly considered because delay could result in end-organ damage progression. Several rapid-acting intravenous antihypertensive agents are available for the treatment of hypertensive emergencies and the choice of which agent to use is mainly related to the clinical manifestations of end-organ damage. Clinicians should be knowledgeable of frequently used medications, potential clinical scenarios in which these medications can be used most effectively, and the side effect profiles/risks for each of these medications in order to successfully initiate therapy (**Table 3**). No large clinical trials have been conducted to define specific treatment goals or to compare the efficacy of the various medications available to treat hypertensive emergency. In general, the BP should be reduced no more than 25% within the first hour and then to 160/100 to 110 mm Hg within 2 to 6 hours.[1] An alternative and more conservative approach is to reduce the BP approximately 10% in the first few hours and then by no more than 25% during the first 24 hours.

Two notable exceptions to this general approach are patients with an aortic dissection and those with an ischemic stroke. The estimated acute mortality for an aortic dissection is approximately 40%. The SBP goal for an aortic dissection is less than 120 mm Hg in addition to a heart rate goal of less than 60 beats per minute. These goals should be obtained quickly and then BP should ideally be titrated as low as

**Table 3**
Common presenting scenarios of hypertensive emergency with treatment considerations

| Clinical Scenario | BP Reduction[a] | IV Drug Options | Additional Considerations |
|---|---|---|---|
| Acute ischemic stroke | tPA candidate: ≤185/110 mm Hg tPA not planned: lower if BP ≥220/120 mm Hg | Labetalol, esmolol, nicardipine | Avoid nitroprusside; can lead to intracranial edema |
| Acute hemorrhagic stroke | Reduce to <180/105 mm Hg to avoid hematoma expansion and edema | Labetalol, esmolol, nicardipine | Avoid nitroprusside; can lead to intracranial edema |
| Hypertensive encephalopathy | Reduce BP 20%–25% to reduce intracranial pressure | Labetalol, esmolol, nicardipine | Avoid nitroprusside; can lead to intracranial edema |
| Acute heart failure | Reduce BP until resolution of acute pulmonary edema | Nitroglycerine, nitroprusside, furosemide | β-Blocker or calcium-channel blocker use could cause exacerbation of symptoms |
| Acute coronary syndrome | Reduce BP to reduce cardiac workload and improve coronary perfusion | Nitroglycerine, nitroprusside, labetalol, metoprolol, esmolol, nicardipine | Consider type A dissection as cause of acute coronary syndrome; avoid selective β-blockers if cocaine abuse suspected |
| Acute aortic dissection | Reduce BP to <120/80 mm Hg (lower if tolerable) and HR to <60 bpm in order to reduce wall shear stress | Labetalol, nitroprusside, nicardipine | Avoid β-blockers if severe aortic regurgitation is noted |
| Acute renal failure | Reduce pressure in the kidney | Nitroprusside, nicardipine | Caution with ACE inhibitors and ARBs unless scleredema renal crisis suspected; monitor for cyanide toxicity if nitroprusside is used |
| Eclampsia | Reduce intracranial pressure and maintain placental perfusion | Labetalol, hydralazine, magnesium | Definitive treatment is delivery of fetus |
| Sympathetic crisis | Reduce BP until symptom resolution | Phentolamine, nitroglycerine, nicardipine, labetalol | Avoid β-blocker monotherapy (except for labetalol) |
| Pheochromocytoma | Reduce BP until symptom resolution | Labetalol, phentolamine | Avoid β-blocker monotherapy (except for labetalol) |

*Abbreviations:* ACE, angiotensin-converting enzyme; ARB, angiotensin receptor blocker; IV, intravenous; tPA, tissue plasminogen activator.
[a] General rule: BP should be reduced no more than 25% within the first hour and then to 160/100 to 110 mm Hg within 2 to 6 hours.

end organs allow, with attention to measuring BP in both arms.[20] Ischemic strokes represent approximately 85% of total stroke events. The initial assessment for patients suspected of having an ischemic stroke is to determine whether or not the patient is a candidate for tissue plasminogen activator (tPA), because this decision determines the most appropriate BP management. If the patient is a tPA candidate, the BP should be promptly reduced to less than or equal to 185/110 mm Hg before administration of tPA and maintained at less than or equal to 180/105 mm Hg for at least 24 hours after administration. If the patient is not a tPA candidate, a BP greater than or equal to 220/120 mm Hg should be safely decreased; however, for an SBP between 140 and 220 mm Hg, there is no definitive proof that reducing the BP is beneficial unless the patient has another clear indication to decrease the BP.[29]

Hypertensive emergencies can also arise from states of catecholamine excess such as a pheochromocytoma,[25] interactions between monoamine oxidase inhibitors and sympathomimetic drugs,[12] or cocaine use.[9] The sole use of β-blockers in these situations could result in unopposed alpha-adrenergic stimulation and additional peripheral vasoconstriction worsening the hypertension. The use of a ganglion blocking agent such as intravenous phentolamine (or in less urgent situations oral phenoxybenzamine) must therefore precede the use of a pure β-blocker in these situations. Alternatively, labetalol, which has combined alpha-adrenergic and beta-adrenergic blocking properties, is safe and effective in these situations.[26] Rebound hypertension following sudden discontinuation of high-dose clonidine (>1.2 mg/d) is also a state of catecholamine excess, and although this situation also responds quickly to combined alpha-adrenergic and beta-adrenergic blockade, resumption of clonidine is another simple alternative.[10]

Other supplemental treatment options, in addition to reducing the BP, should also be considered while awaiting patient transfer to the ED. Intravenous loop diuretics (furosemide, bumetanide, or torsemide) should be considered if volume overload is suspected. Oxygen should be administered to treat hypoxemia. Morphine has vasodilator properties and may reduce preload and the sensation of air hunger if needed. Noninvasive ventilation may be used to relieve symptoms in patients with pulmonary edema and severe respiratory distress or in those patients who fail to improve with initial pharmacologic therapy.

## SUMMARY

Hypertensive emergency results from an increased BP (generally greater than 180 mm Hg systolic and/or 120 mm Hg diastolic) that is associated with acute and/or evolving end-organ damage primarily to the neurologic, cardiovascular, and renal systems. Properly diagnosing hypertensive emergency and differentiating it from hypertensive urgency and/or uncontrolled chronic hypertension using accurate BP measurement techniques, a pertinent patient interview, physical examination, and additional work-up if available is essential to appropriate patient triage and initial treatment. A diagnosis of hypertensive emergency requires urgent transfer to an ED or inpatient setting but initiation of goal-directed therapy in the clinic should not be delayed because delay could result in end-organ damage progression. Several antihypertensive agents are available and the choice of which agent to use is mainly dictated by the type of end-organ damage present, although no large clinical trials have been conducted to compare efficacy or define specific treatment goals. The most efficient way to prevent further episodes of hypertensive emergency in each patient is to ensure that the patient has close follow-up on discharge with the primary care provider.

## REFERENCES

1. Chobanian A, Bakris G, Black H, et al. The seventh report of the Joint National Committee on Prevention, Detection, Evaluation, and Treatment of High Blood Pressure: the JNC 7 report. JAMA 2003;289:2560–72.
2. Committee on Obstetric Practice. Committee opinion no. 623: emergent therapy for acute-onset, severe hypertension during pregnancy and the postpartum period. Obstet Gynecol 2015;125:521–5.
3. Zampaglione B, Pascale C, Marchisio M, et al. Hypertensive urgencies and emergencies. prevalence and clinical presentation. Hypertension 1996;27:144–7.
4. Suneja M, Maliske S. Hypertension. In: Chatterjee K, Vandenberg B, editors. Common problems in cardiology. 1st edition. New Delhi (India): Jaypee Brothers Medical Pub; 2015. p. 84–101.
5. Strandgaard S, Paulson O. Cerebral autoregulation. Stroke 1984;15:413–6.
6. Ault M, Ellrodt A. Pathophysiologic events leading to the end-organ effects of acute hypertension. Am J Emerg Med 1985;3:10–5.
7. Luft F, Mervaala E, Muller D, et al. Hypertension-induced end-organ damage: a new transgenic approach to an old problem. Hypertension 1999;33:212–8.
8. Taylor D. Hypertensive crisis: a review of pathophysiology and treatment. Crit Care Nurs Clin North Am 2015;27:439–47.
9. Grossman E, Messerli F. Drug-induced hypertension: an unappreciated cause of secondary hypertension. Am J Med 2012;125:14–22.
10. Karachalios G, Charalabopoulos A, Papalimneou V, et al. Withdrawal syndrome following cessation of antihypertensive drug therapy. Int J Clin Pract 2005;59: 562–70.
11. Makker S, Moorthy B. Rebound hypertension following minoxidil withdrawal. J Pediatr 1980;96:762–6.
12. Rao T, Yeragani V. Hypertensive crisis and cheese. Indian J Psychiatry 2009;51: 65–6.
13. Kawano Y. Physio-pathological effects of alcohol on the cardiovascular system: its role in hypertension and cardiovascular disease. Hypertens Res 2010;33: 181–91.
14. Olson-Chen C, Seligman N. Hypertensive emergencies in pregnancy. Crit Care Clin 2016;32:29–41.
15. Goldstein L, Simel D. Is this patient having a stroke? JAMA 2005;293:2391–402.
16. Ropper A, Wijdicks E. Blood pressure fluctuations in the dysautonomia of Guillain Barre syndrome. Arch Neurol 1990;47:706–8.
17. Shannon J, Jordan J, Costa F, et al. The hypertension of autonomic failure and its treatment. Hypertension 1997;30:1062–7.
18. Shannon J, Jordan J, Diedrich A, et al. Sympathetically mediated hypertension in autonomic failure. Circulation 2000;101:2710–5.
19. Gandhi S, Powers J, Nomeir A, et al. The pathogenesis of acute pulmonary edema associated with hypertension. N Engl J Med 2001;344:17–22.
20. Hiratzka L, Bakris G, Beckman J, et al. 2010 ACCF/AHA/AATS/ACR/ASA/SCA/ SCAI/SIR/STS/SVM guidelines for the diagnosis and management of patients with Thoracic Aortic Disease: a report of the American College of Cardiology Foundation/American Heart Association Task Force on Practice Guidelines, American Association for Thoracic Surgery, American College of Radiology, American Stroke Association, Society of Cardiovascular Anesthesiologists, Society for Cardiovascular Angiography and Interventions, Society of Interventional

Radiology, Society of Thoracic Surgeons, and Society for vascular medicine. Circulation 2010;122:e270–410.

21. Peacock F, Amin A, Granger C, et al. Hypertensive heart failure: patient characteristics, treatment, and outcomes. Am J Emerg Med 2011;29:855–62.

22. Giavarini A, Savard S, Sapoval M, et al. Clinical management of renal artery fibromuscular dysplasia: temporal trends and outcomes. J Hypertens 2014;32:2433–8.

23. Bavishi C, de Leeuw P, Messerli F. Atherosclerotic renal artery stenosis and hypertension: pragmatism, pitfalls, and perspectives. Am J Med 2016;129:635.e5-14.

24. Bussone G, Noel L, Mouthon L. Renal involvement in patients with systemic sclerosis. Nephrol Ther 2011;7:192–9.

25. Werbel S, Ober KP. Update on diagnosis, localization and management. Med Clin North Am 1995;79:131–53.

26. Acelajado M, Calhoun D. Resistant hypertension, secondary hypertension, and hypertensive crisis: diagnostic evaluation and treatment. Cardiol Clin 2010;28:639–54.

27. Patel K, Young L, Howell E, et al. Characteristics and outcomes of patients presenting with hypertensive urgency in the office setting. JAMA Intern Med 2016;176:981–8.

28. James P, Oparil S, Carter B, et al. 2014 evidence-based guidelines for the management of high blood pressure in adults: report from the panel members appointed to the Eighth Joint National Committee (JNC 8). JAMA 2014;311:507–20.

29. Jauch E, Saver J, Adams H, et al. Guidelines for the early management of patients with acute ischemic stroke: a guideline for healthcare professionals from the American Heart Association/American Stroke Association. Stroke 2013;44:870–947.

# Acute Stroke and Transient Ischemic Attack in the Outpatient Clinic

Salvador Cruz-Flores, MD, MPH

## KEYWORDS

- Stroke • TIA • Transient ischemic attack • Emergent evaluation • Risk stratification
- Treatment

## KEY POINTS

- Stroke and transient ischemic attack are time-critical, treatable, and preventable medical emergencies.
- Decisions on hospital admission and acute management require the establishment of accurate time of onset and/or time when the patient was last seen normal.
- A thorough workup aimed at establishing the cause is required to guide secondary prevention.
- Stroke patients must be cared for at centers with stroke expertise.
- Secondary stroke prevention targets the management of vascular risk factors, appropriate antithrombotic therapy including anticoagulation for those with absolute indication for anticoagulation (ie, atrial fibrillation), and carotid endarterectomy or carotid artery stenting for symptomatic significant carotid artery stenosis.

## INTRODUCTION

Cerebrovascular disease is fourth leading cause of death and the leading cause of disability in the United States. In recent years, the incidence and mortality have declined. Stroke is categorized as ischemic (87%) and hemorrhagic (13%).[1,2] Ischemic stroke and transient ischemic attack (TIA) are 2 clinical ends of a common pathophysiologic mechanism, the occlusion of a cerebral artery. As in cardiovascular disease in general, vascular risk factors, such as diabetes mellitus, hypertension, smoking, and hyperlipidemia, play an important role. Compared with acute coronary syndromes in which the vascular occlusion in most cases is local atherothrombosis, ischemic stroke and TIA have a heterogeneous cause, with 4 main subtypes explaining most cases, namely, large vessel atherothrombosis, cardioembolic, lacuna, and cryptogenic.[1,2] In addition, there is a smaller group of uncommon causes such as

Department of Neurology, Paul L. Foster School of Medicine, Texas Tech University Health Sciences Center El Paso, 4800 Alberta Avenue, Room 108, El Paso, TX 79905, USA
*E-mail address:* Salvador.cruz-flores@ttuhsc.edu

Med Clin N Am 101 (2017) 479–494
http://dx.doi.org/10.1016/j.mcna.2017.01.001
0025-7125/17/© 2017 Elsevier Inc. All rights reserved.

arterial dissection or prothrombotic states that should be considered in specific circumstances such as in stroke in young patients or after trauma. The causal heterogeneity is an important consideration in deciding diagnostic workup, and therapy for vascular studies is necessary to find carotid stenosis amenable to revascularization; in contrast, a patient with atrial fibrillation may need anticoagulation. Two or more potential causes of stroke may coexist in a patient and all will require treatment.[3]

In recent years, the definitions of ischemic stroke and TIA have changed from a time-based diagnosis (symptom duration >24 vs <24 hours duration for stroke vs TIA) to a diagnosis based on the sine qua non criterion: the presence of an infarct pathologically or by imaging in stroke and its absence in a TIA, regardless of the duration of the symptoms.[4,5] Recent decades have seen an accumulation of knowledge on the natural history and treatment of ischemic stroke and TIA enough to impact the diagnostic and therapeutic paradigm, making these time-critical conditions highly preventable and treatable, and therefore, true medical emergencies that require an expedited approach. This article reviews current concepts on pathophysiology, clinical presentation, diagnosis, and treatment of TIA and ischemic stroke that present in the office.

## CLINICAL HISTORY AND EXAMINATION

The patient history of stroke or TIA will include symptoms that indicate a focal neurologic deficit of sudden onset. Focal deficit implies the dysfunction of a discrete area of the brain leading to symptoms and signs that can be located to the area affected (**Box 1**).

Typical symptoms include speech impairment referred by patients as either slurred speech and/or word finding impairment, visual loss in one side, double vision, facial weakness or facial droop, altered mental status, limb weakness, sensory symptoms, and incoordination. Seizures and headache may occur in less than 10% to 15% of patients.[6]

Tips for the bedside evaluation:

- Dysarthria is a frequent sign of stroke, although it has poor localization value.
- Dizziness in isolation is not a common symptom of stroke.
- The combination of headache, dizziness, nausea/vomiting, and difficulty walking is a common presentation of cerebellar infarct even in absence of focal neurologic findings.
- Aphasia and neglect/inattention indicate a cortical lesion in the dominant versus nondominant hemisphere, respectively
- Gaze deviation away from the hemiparesis indicates a large hemispheric infarct in the side toward where the eyes are looking to.
- Gaze deviation toward the hemiparesis indicates a brainstem lesion.
- In trying to localize the lesion, consider that cortical hemispheric lesions will have a gradient in the weakness depending on the vascular distribution affected such that:
  ○ Middle cerebral artery territory infarcts result in greater weakness in the face and arm compared with the leg.
  ○ Anterior cerebral artery territory infarcts result in greater weakness in the leg.
- Weakness with no gradient (similar degree in arm and leg) indicates a subcortical lesion (ie, internal capsule as in lacunar infarcts).
- The more posterior the lesion is in the hemisphere, the more sensory and visual symptoms.
- Changes in the level of consciousness, gaze deviation, aphasia, neglect, and weakness (hemiparesis or quadriparesis) indicate the presence of large vessel

| Box 1 |
| --- |
| **Clinical signs by location** |

*Left hemisphere*

Aphasia

Left gaze deviation

Right facial weakness

Right hemiparesis

Right hemiataxia

Right hemisensory loss

Right homonymous hemianopia

*Right hemisphere*

Right gaze deviation

Left neglect, extinction, or inattention

Left facial weakness

Left hemiparesis

Left hemiataxia

Left hemisensory loss

Left homonymous hemianopia

*Thalamus*

Drowsiness

Confusion

Amnestic syndrome

Hemisensory loss

Hemiataxia

*Midbrain*

Confusion

Amnestic syndrome

Stupor/coma

Ophthalmoparesis/eye movement disturbance

Skew deviation

Ptosis

Chorea/ataxia

Hemiparesis or quadriparesis

*Pons*

Stupor/coma

Ophthalmoparesis

Pinpoint pupils

Internuclear ophthalmoplegia

Gaze palsy, ipsilateral or bilateral

Facial weakness, unilateral or bilateral

| |
|---|
| Hemiparesis/quadriparesis |
| Hemiataxia |
| *Medulla* |
| Hemisensory loss |
| Hemiataxia |
| Horner syndrome |
| *Cerebellum* |
| Hemiataxia |
| Inability to stand or walk |

occlusion. These signs pose important triaging significance for a highest level of care when the patient is otherwise eligible for endovascular therapy.

Considering the potential patient eligibility for intravenous thrombolysis and/or mechanical thrombectomy, the initial evaluation and triage of a stroke patient requires answers to key questions.[7]

Key questions in the evaluation of acute stroke.

- What was the time of symptom onset or time when the patient was last seen normal? A common source of confusion is when symptoms are present upon waking up versus developing shortly after waking up. If symptoms were present upon waking up, then time of onset must be set at the time went to bed.
- Is the patient taking anticoagulants? If so, what anticoagulant and when was the last dose?
- What is the patient's blood pressure?
- Does the patient have hypoglycemia?
- What is the National Institutes of Health Stroke Scale (NIHSS) score? The NIHSS was adopted as a standard measure of the neurologic deficit; although it does not replace a neurologic examination, it is useful in the triage and facilitates communication among physicians and other health care providers. NIHSS standard training and certification can be obtained through organizations like the American Heart Association (**Table 1**).
- What is the international normalized ratio (INR) or activated partial thromboplastin timeaPTT? (for those patients taking anticoagulants)

In contrast to patients with ischemic stroke, patients with TIA usually have resolving symptoms within minutes to hours.[5] The natural history of TIA is not benign because a substantial proportion of patients will have a recurrent stroke or other vascular events within the following 90 days.[5,8–14] In fact, the risk of recurrent stroke may be as high as 20% in the first 90 days after the event; more importantly, half of the recurrent events occur in the first 2 days.[8–12,15] In addition, about 25% of strokes are preceded by TIA.[15]

The high rate of early stroke recurrence raises some questions:

- Should patients with TIA be admitted to the hospital for diagnostic investigation and/or treatment with thrombolysis if the symptoms recur?
  - Admitting all patients with a TIA to the hospital seems intuitively reasonable. A Canadian cohort study based on the Ontario Stroke Registry including 8540 patients showed that patients admitted to the hospital were more likely to receive

**Table 1**
**National Institutes of Health Stroke Scale**

| | |
|---|---|
| 1a. Level of consciousness (LOC) | 0 = Alert; keenly responsive<br>1 = Not alert; but arousable by minor stimulation to obey, answer, or respond<br>2 = Not alert; requires repeated stimulation to attend, or is obtunded and requires strong or painful stimulation to make movements (not stereotyped)<br>3 = Responds only with reflex motor or autonomic effects or totally unresponsive, flaccid, and areflexic |
| 1b. LOC questions | 0 = Answers both questions correctly<br>1 = Answers one question correctly<br>2 = Answers neither question correctly |
| 1c. LOC commands | 0 = Performs both tasks correctly<br>1 = Performs one task correctly<br>2 = Performs neither task correctly |
| 2. Best gaze | 0 = Normal. Able to move both eyes left to right across midline<br>1 = Partial gaze palsy. Gaze is abnormal in one or both eyes, but forced deviation or total gaze paresis is not present. Able to move one or both eyes, but may not be able to cross midline<br>2 = Forced deviation. Total gaze paresis is not overcome by the oculocephalic maneuver |
| 3. Best visual | 0 = No visual loss<br>1 = Partial hemianopia. Includes loss in only one quadrant<br>2 = Complete hemianopia. Loss of vision in both top and bottom quadrants on the right or left side of a patient's visual field<br>3 = Bilateral hemianopia. Blindness of any cause, including cortical blindness, or if visual loss is noted on both right and left sides of the visual fields |
| 4. Facial palsy | 0 = Normal. Symmetric movements<br>1 = Minor paralysis. Flattened nasolabial fold, asymmetry on smiling<br>2 = Partial paralysis. Total or near-total paralysis of lower face<br>3 = Complete paralysis of one or both sides of face. Absence of movement in the upper and lower face |
| 5. Motor arm<br>a. Left | 0 = No drift. Limb holds 90° (or 45°) for a full 10 s<br>1 = Drift. Limb holds 90° (or 45°), but then drifts down before full 10 s; does not hit bed or other support<br>2 = Some effort against gravity. Limb cannot get to or maintain 90° (or 45°), drifts down to bed, but has some effort against gravity<br>3 = No effort against gravity. Limb falls<br>4 = No movements. Flaccid extremities with no effort noted |
| b. Right | 0 = no drift. Limb holds 90 degrees (or 45 degrees) for full 10 s<br>1 = Drift. Limb holds 90 degrees (or 45 degrees) but then drifts down before full 10 s: does not hit bed or other support<br>2 = Some effort against gravity. Limb cannot get to or maintain 90 degrees) of 45 degrees), drifts down to bed<br>3 = no effort against gravity. Limb falls<br>4 = No movements. Flaccid extremities with no effort noted |
| 6. Motor leg<br>a. Left | 0 = No drift. Leg holds 30° position for full 5 s<br>1 = Drift. Leg falls by the end of the 5-s period, but does not hit bed<br>2 = Some effort against gravity. Leg falls to bed by 5 s, but has some effort against gravity<br>3 = No effort against gravity. Leg falls to bed immediately<br>4 = No movement. Flaccid extremities with no effort noted |

*(continued on next page)*

| Table 1 (*continued*) | |
|---|---|
| b. Right | 1 = Drift. Leg falls by the end of the 5-s period, but does not hit bed<br>2 = Some effort against gravity. Leg falls to bed by 5 s, but has some effort against gravity<br>3 = No effort against gravity. Leg falls to bed immediately<br>4 = No movement. Flaccid extremities with no effort noted |
| 7. Limb ataxia | 0 = Absent<br>1 = Present in 1 limb<br>2 = Present in 2 limbs |
| 8. Sensory | 0 = Normal. No sensory loss<br>1 = Mild to moderate sensory loss. Patient feels pin prick is less sharp or is dull on the affected side or there is a loss of superficial pain with pin prick, but patient is aware of being touched<br>2 = Severe to total sensory loss. Patient is not aware of being touched on the face, arm, and leg |
| 9. Best language | 0 = No aphasia. Normal fluent speech<br>1 = Mild to moderate aphasia. Some obvious loss of fluency or facility of comprehension without significant limitation on ideas expressed or form of expression. Reduction of speech and/or comprehension, however, makes conversation about provided materials difficult or impossible. For example, in conversation about provided materials, examiner can identify picture or naming card content from patient's response<br>2 = Severe aphasia. All communication is through fragmentary expression; great need for inference, questioning, and guessing by the listener. Often limited to one-word answers. Range of information that can be exchanged is limited; listener carries burden of communication. Examiner cannot identify materials provided from patient response<br>3 = Mute. Global aphasia. No usable speech or auditory comprehension |
| 10. Dysarthria | 0 = Normal<br>1 = Mild to moderate dysarthria. Patient slurs at least some words, and at worst, can be understood with some difficulty<br>2 = Severe dysarthria. Patient's speech is so slurred as to be unintelligible in the absence of or out of proportion to any dysphasia or is mute |
| 11. Extinction and inattention | 0 = Normal<br>1 = Visual, tactile, auditory, special, or personal inattention or extinction to bilateral simultaneous stimulation in one of the sensory modalities<br>2 = Profound hemi-inattention or extinction to more than one modality. Patient does not recognize own hand or orients to only one side of space |

the diagnostic testing, antithrombotic, antihypertensive, and lipid-lowering therapy than those not admitted; in addition, the 1-year mortality was lower among those admitted.[16] Another cohort study from the Australian Stroke Clinical Registry showed that even among patients admitted to the hospital with TIA, those admitted to a stroke unit had a lower mortality than patients admitted to a regular medical ward; the stroke recurrence rate was not different.[17]

○ However, there is evidence of a high false-positive rate in the initial diagnosis of TIA by nonexperts, which can potentially lead to a substantial increase in the

admission of non-TIA patients and an inefficient use of resources.[18–22] Furthermore, cost-effectiveness and decision analyses have indicated that admission may not be justified if the risk of stroke is less than 4%.[22,23] Therefore, although it seems clear that early urgent evaluation is necessary, it remains debatable if admission to the hospital is necessary in every patient with TIA.
  ○ At present, there are several potential models to allow the fast evaluation and treatment of these patients, and the basic approach involves admission to the hospital.[19] Other approaches involve the complete evaluation in the emergency department with or without the involvement of a vascular neurologist and a follow-up telephone call by a nurse, evaluation in outpatient urgent TIA clinic, and evaluation by general practitioner using an electronic TIA decision support, all of which have shown better outcome and adherence to diagnostic and therapeutic recommendations than the old delayed approach.[19,24]
• How soon should treatment be started to decrease the early recurrence of stroke?
  ○ Several studies with different observational methodologies and one cluster randomized controlled trial showed lower-risk 90-day risk of stroke, thus suggesting that diagnostic evaluation and initiation of secondary prevention are indeed required within the first 24 hours from the event.[17,19,25–31]

Therefore, identifying those patients at higher early stroke risk seems to be the best strategy to maximize better outcomes and improve system efficiency. It is now possible to stratify patients at high risk using the validated ABCD2 score (**Tables 2 and 3**).[8,12,32–35] In a recent systematic review, the ABCD2 scoring system showed limitations in reliably identifying patients at high risk and those with carotid stenosis and atrial fibrillation.[36] The limitations are due to the fact that most studies included patients that were confirmed to have a TIA by a specialist, which then questions the usefulness of such scoring system in the primary care setting. Acknowledging the limitation, it might be still possible to use the score to stratify patients with TIA.[36]

Current guidelines address the concern of the early risk of stroke by recommending that patients with TIA undergo a rapid workup to[37]

a. Identify and treat vascular risk factors such as hypertension, diabetes mellitus, hyperlipidemia, and atrial fibrillation;

| Table 2 ABCD2 score | |
| --- | --- |
| **Risk Factor** | **Points** |
| Age ≥60 y | 1 |
| Blood pressure | |
|   Systolic ≥140 mm Hg or diastolic ≥90 mm Hg | 1 |
| Clinical features | |
|   Unilateral weakness with or without speech impairment | 2 |
|   Speech impairment without weakness | 1 |
| Duration | |
|   ≥60 min | 2 |
|   10–59 min | 1 |
| Diabetes | 1 |
| Total score | 0–7 |

**Table 3**
**Risk stratification**

| ABCD2 Score | 2 d (%) | 7 d (%) | 90 d (%) |
|---|---|---|---|
| Low risk | | | |
| 0–3 | 1 | 1.2 | 3.1 |
| High risk | | | |
| 4–5 | 4.1 | 5.9 | 9.8 |
| 6–7 | 8.1 | 11.7 | 17.8 |

b. Initiate the appropriate antithrombotic therapy;
c. Search for symptomatic carotid artery stenosis amenable to either carotid endarterectomy (CEA) or carotid artery stenting (CAS).

## DIFFERENTIAL DIAGNOSIS

The differential diagnosis of stroke includes stroke mimics, which refer to conditions that present with strokelike symptoms. Stroke mimics represent about 25% of patients presenting with strokelike symptoms.[6,38] The most common stroke mimics are included in **Table 4** and **Box 2**. In considering the differential diagnosis, is important to remember that there are also stroke chameleons that refer to stroke presentations that can mimic another medical or neurologic condition and therefore may cause delay in identification.[38] Stroke chameleons include limb-shaking TIA, which may resemble seizures when in fact they represent unilateral transient shaking movements usually associated with critical carotid artery stenosis; occipital infarcts that may present as acute delirium with no apparent focal neurologic deficits; and small cortical infarcts that may present with wrist drop mimicking a radial nerve palsy, among other conditions.[38]

**Table 4**
**Differential diagnosis and stroke mimics**

| Condition | Percent | Clues |
|---|---|---|
| Seizure | 20 | History of seizures, witnessed event, loss of consciousness |
| Syncope | 15 | Loss of consciousness, hypotension, arrhythmias |
| Sepsis | 12 | Fever, changes in level of consciousness |
| Functional | 9 | Recent stressor, not anatomic deficit, changing examination |
| Primary headache disorder | 9 | History of migraine |
| Brain tumor | 7 | Slow symptom onset, seizure at onset |
| Metabolic | 6 | Hypoglycemia changes in level of consciousness, asterixis |
| Neuropathy | 4 | Sensory pattern stocking/glove distribution, absent reflexes |
| Peripheral vestibular disorder | 4 | Positional vertigo, fatigable nystagmus, head thrust positive |
| Dementia | 3 | Progressive cognitive decline history |
| Subdural hematoma | 2 | Trauma, antithrombotic therapy |
| Drugs and alcohol | 2 | Changes in level of consciousness, myoclonus, asterixis |
| Transient global amnesia | 2 | Isolated and reversible memory impairment |
| Other | 6 | — |

---

**Box 2**
**Diagnostic studies in acute stroke**

*All patients*

Noncontrast brain CT or brain MRI

Blood electrolytes and renal function

Blood glucose

Oxygen saturation

CBC

Troponin and/or CK-MB

Prothrombin time/INR

aPTT

ECG

*Selected patients*

Thrombin time/Ecarin clotting time for patients suspected to be taking direct thrombin inhibitors or direct factor Xa inhibitors

Liver function tests

Toxicology screen

Blood alcohol level

Pregnancy test

Arterial blood gas among those with hypoxemia or suspected to have $CO_2$ narcosis

Chest radiograph

Electroencephalogram when seizures are suspected

---

## IMAGING AND ADDITIONAL TESTING

The current diagnostic recommendations for patients with a TIA or stroke include a complete blood count (CBC), glucose level, chemistry including electrolytes and renal function, lipid panel, hemoglobin A1c, oxygen saturation; aPTT and INR should be checked, in addition to markers of cardiac ischemia and electrocardiogram (ECG).[38] In selected patients taking direct thrombin or factor Xa inhibitors, the thrombin time should be checked. Other special considerations for selected patients include liver function tests, toxicology screen, alcohol level, pregnancy test, chest radiograph, and electroencephalography. Some patients will require an echocardiogram and a Holter monitor. Recent studies suggest that the rate of paroxysmal atrial fibrillation in stroke patients presenting in normal sinus rhythm may be as high as 15%, which suggest that some patients will require prolonged ECG monitoring because the presence of atrial fibrillation may require treatment with anticoagulation.[7]

Brain imaging is absolutely necessary, and a nonenhanced CT scan of the brain provides enough initial information to make decisions with regards to thrombolysis and/or thrombectomy.[7] Computed tomographic (CT) angiography and MRI brain scan with MR angiography are indicated and recommended urgently with the provision that in those patients eligible for intravenous thrombolysis, the performance of these tests should not delay the administration of the treatment.[7] At present, the use of perfusion imaging by CT or MRI in making decisions is still debatable;

however, these technologies may be useful in selecting patients for acute intervention when they present beyond the approved window for treatment.[7]

## TREATMENT

This article addresses the diagnosis and treatment of patients with TIA or acute ischemic stroke in the clinic or office; as such, the first step in the approach of these patients is to activate the 911 system to allow immediate transportation to the emergency department because acute interventions like intravenous thrombolysis or endovascular thrombectomy may be an option.[7]

Once the 911 system has been activated for an acute stroke and while waiting their arrival, it is appropriate to

- Check the vital signs
- Maintain airway, breathing, and circulation
- Ask the key questions addressed earlier in this article
- Establish and document if the patient takes anticoagulants
- Establish severity of deficits with the examination, and if possible, the NIHSS
- Review eligibility for intravenous thrombolysis and endovascular thrombectomy (**Table 5**).

Patients with symptom onset within the past 6 hours must be prioritized for stroke center transportation and consideration for intravenous thrombolysis and/or endovascular thrombectomy.[7,39]

### General Medical for all Patients

- *Oxygen:* Supplemental oxygen should be administered to the patient with hypoxemia to maintain oxygen saturation greater than 94%.
- *Temperature:* Patients should be kept euthermic, and fever should be treated.
- *Blood pressure:* For patients eligible for thrombolysis, blood pressure should be treated to maintain it at or less than 185/105 mm Hg. Importantly, the blood pressure of patients not eligible for thrombolysis should not be treated unless is >220/120 mm Hg or in presence of acute end organ damage, such as decompensated congestive heart failure, aortic dissection, pulmonary edema, or acute renal failure. Hypotension must be avoided.
- *Glucose:* Hypoglycemia must be corrected and avoided. Although the correction of hyperglycemia has not been shown to improve outcome, hyperglycemia continues to impact functional outcome; therefore, it is reasonable to treat hyperglycemia to maintain glucose level less than 180 mg.

Ischemic stroke patients beyond the window for intervention will still need transportation to the emergency department for full evaluation. Patients with TIA must be stratified according to the ABCD2 score; those at high risk will require a complete evaluation within 24 hours.[5,37] The best course of action for high-risk patients in terms of admission to the hospital versus outpatient evaluation will depend on the available model or resources from those described before and that allow the complete evaluation within 24 hours. For patients at low risk, the evaluation, while urgent, one can allow a few more days.[5,19,37,40,41]

Secondary prevention must be started as soon as possible, and that includes initiating or optimizing antihypertensive therapy, diabetes control, and lipid-lowering therapy. In addition, smoking cessation must be offered to all patients. Antithrombotic treatment with antiplatelet agents for patients with non-cardioembolic TIA or stroke must be initiated.[37] The options include aspirin or the combination of aspirin/

**Table 5**
Eligibility criteria for intravenous thrombolysis and endovascular thrombectomy

| Intravenous (IV) Thrombolysis ≤3 h from Onset | IV Thrombolysis 3–4.5 h from Onset | Endovascular Thrombectomy Recommendations |
|---|---|---|
| Inclusion criteria<br>1. Diagnosis of ischemic stroke causing measurable neurologic deficit<br>2. Onset of symptoms <3 h before beginning treatment<br>3. Aged ≥18 y<br><br>Exclusion criteria<br>1. Significant head trauma or prior stroke in previous 3 mo<br>2. Symptoms suggest subarachnoid hemorrhage<br>3. Arterial puncture at noncompressible site in previous 7 d<br>4. History of previous intracranial hemorrhage<br>5. Intracranial neoplasm, arteriovenous malformation, or aneurysm<br>6. Recent intracranial or intraspinal surgery<br>7. Elevated blood pressure (systolic >185 mm Hg or diastolic >110 mm Hg)<br>8. Active internal bleeding<br>9. Acute bleeding diathesis, including but not limited to<br>10. Platelet count <100,000/mm$^3$<br>11. Heparin received within 48 h, resulting in abnormally elevated aPTT<br>12. Greater than the upper limit of normal<br>13. Current use of anticoagulant with INR >1.7 or prothrombin time >15 s<br>14. Current use of direct thrombin inhibitors or direct factor Xa inhibitors with<br>15. Elevated sensitive laboratory tests (such as aPTT, INR, platelet count, and | Inclusion criteria<br>1. Diagnosis of ischemic stroke causing measurable neurologic deficit<br>2. Onset of symptoms within 3–4.5 h before beginning treatment<br><br>Relative exclusion criteria<br>1. Aged >80 y<br>2. Severe stroke (NIHSS >25)<br>3. Taking an oral anticoagulant regardless of INR<br>4. History of both diabetes and prior ischemic stroke | 1. Prestroke mRS score 0–1<br>2. Acute ischemic stroke receiving intravenous r-tPA within 4.5 h of onset<br>3. Causative occlusion of the ICA or proximal MCA (M1)<br>4. Age ≥18 y<br>5. NIHSS score of ≥6<br>6. ASPECTS of ≥6<br>7. Treatment can be initiated within 6 h of symptom onset<br>8. Reperfusion should be achieved as early as possible and within 6 h of stroke onset<br>9. The effectiveness of endovascular therapy is uncertain beyond 6 h of symptom onset<br>10. In selected patients with anterior circulation occlusion who have contraindications to intravenous r-tPA, endovascular therapy with stent retrievers completed within 6 h of stroke onset is reasonable<br>11. The clinical efficacy of endovascular therapy with stent retrievers for those patients whose contraindications are time based or not time based (eg, prior stroke, serious head trauma, hemorrhagic coagulopathy, or receiving anticoagulant medications) is uncertain. More data are needed<br>12. Endovascular therapy with stent retrievers may be reasonable for carefully selected patients within 6 h of symptom onset and occlusion of the M2 or M3 portion of the MCAs, anterior cerebral arteries, vertebral arteries, basilar artery, or posterior cerebral arteries |

(continued on next page)

**Table 5**
*(continued)*

| Intravenous (IV) Thrombolysis ≤3 h from Onset | IV Thrombolysis 3–4.5 h from Onset | Endovasacular Thrombectomy Recommendations |
|---|---|---|
| 16. ECT, TT, or appropriate factor Xa activity assays)<br>17. Blood glucose concentration <50 mg/dL (2.7 mmol/L)<br>18. CT demonstrates multilobar infarction (hypodensity >1/3 cerebral hemisphere)<br>19. Relative exclusion criteria<br>20. Recent experience suggests that under some circum-stances—with careful<br>21. consideration and weighting of risk to benefit—patients may receive<br>22. Fibrinolytic therapy despite 1 or more relative contrain-dications. Consider<br>23. Risk to benefit of IV r-tPA administration carefully if any of these relative<br>24. Contraindications are present:<br>25. Only minor or rapidly improving stroke symptoms (clearing spontaneously)<br>26. Pregnancy<br>27. Seizure at onset with postictal residual neurologic impairments<br>28. Major surgery or serious trauma within previous 14 d<br>29. Recent gastrointestinal or urinary tract hemorrhage (within previous 21 d)<br>30. Recent acute myocardial infarction (within previous 3 mo) | | 13. Endovascular therapy with stent retrievers may be reasonable for some patients <18 y of age with a large-vessel occlusion with treatment initiated within 6 h of symptom onset. Benefits in this age group are not established |

*Abbreviations:* ASPECTS, Alberta Stroke Program Early CT Score; ECT, Ecarin Clotting Time; ICA, internal carotid artery; MCA, Middle cerebral artery; mRS, Modified Rankin Score; r-tPA, recombinant tissue Plasminogen activator; TT, Thrombin time.

| Table 6 | |
|---|---|
| **CHADS2 score risk stratification for atrial fibrillation** | |
| Congestive heart failure | 1 |
| Hypertension | 1 |
| Age >75 y | 1 |
| Diabetes mellitus | 1 |
| Stroke/TIA | 2 |
| Total score | 0–6 |
| **CHADS2 Score** | **Annual Stroke Risk (%)** |
| 0 | 1.9 |
| 1 | 2.8 |
| 2 | 4 |
| 3 | 5.9 |
| 4 | 8.5 |
| 5 | 12.5 |
| 6 | 18.2 |

dipyridamole as first option with clopidogrel as a reasonable alternative.[37] A recent trial from China suggests that treatment with the combination of aspirin and clopidogrel for a minor stroke or TIA decreases the risk of recurrent stroke in the first 90 days and could be considered an alternative.[42,43] At the present time, there is an ongoing American randomized controlled trial testing the same hypothesis.[44]

Anticoagulation with warfarin or one of the new oral anticoagulants (NOAC), such as dabigatran, apixaban, or rivaroxaban, must be considered in patients with atrial fibrillation at high risk or re-embolization with a CHADS2 ≥3 (**Table 6**); if on warfarin, the target INR must be 2 to 3.[37] Other high-risk cardiac sources of embolism that require anticoagulation with warfarin include rheumatic valve disease, mechanical prosthetic valves, myocardial infarction complicated with a left ventricular thrombus, and anterior wall STEMI (ST-elevation myocardial infarction).[37] NOAC are not recommended in any of these conditions.

For patients with symptomatic carotid artery stenosis greater than 70%, CEA is recommended provided the operator has a 6% or less perioperative complication rate; CAS is an alternative for patients at high operative risk as estimated by cardiac or pulmonary conditions or local vascular anatomy or specific circumstances such a neck radiation.[37] The benefit of revascularization by either of these methods is more marginal for patients with stenosis 50% to 69% and more dependent on specific patient variables such as age and gender.[37] When the decision has been made to proceed with CEA or CAS, it is safe and advisable to perform the procedure within 2 weeks from symptom onset to maximize efficacy.[37]

## SUMMARY

- TIA and ischemic stroke are treatable medical emergencies.
- Identifying stroke patients within the window eligible for interventions such as thrombolysis or thrombectomy and high-risk TIA patients is a priority because it requires emergent brain imaging.
- From the clinic, the first step is activating the 911 EMS system for emergent transportation to the hospital.

- Workup to identify patients with carotid stenosis and atrial fibrillation is paramount.
- Secondary prevention must be started very early and that includes appropriate antithrombotic therapy according to the cause.
- In those with symptomatic carotid stenosis, CEA or CAS must be offered and ideally completed within 2 weeks from symptom onset.

## REFERENCES

1. Moulin T, Tatu L, Vuillier F, et al. Role of a stroke data bank in evaluating cerebral infarction subtypes: patterns and outcome of 1,776 consecutive patients from the Besancon stroke registry. Cerebrovasc Dis 2000;10(4):261–71.
2. Grau AJ, Weimar C, Buggle F, et al. Risk factors, outcome, and treatment in subtypes of ischemic stroke: the German stroke data bank. Stroke 2001; 32(11):2559–66.
3. Yamamoto H, Bogousslavsky J. Mechanisms of second and further strokes. J Neurol Neurosurg Psychiatry 1998;64(6):771–6.
4. Sacco RL, Kasner SE, Broderick JP, et al. An updated definition of stroke for the 21st century: a statement for healthcare professionals from the American Heart Association/American Stroke Association. Stroke 2013;44(7):2064–89.
5. Easton JD, Saver JL, Albers GW, et al. Definition and evaluation of transient ischemic attack: a scientific statement for healthcare professionals from the American Heart Association/American Stroke Association Stroke Council; Council on Cardiovascular Surgery and Anesthesia; Council on Cardiovascular Radiology and Intervention; Council on Cardiovascular Nursing; and the Interdisciplinary Council on Peripheral Vascular Disease. The American Academy of Neurology affirms the value of this statement as an educational tool for neurologists. Stroke 2009;40(6):2276–93.
6. Cordonnier C, Leys D. Stroke: the bare essentials. Pract Neurol 2008;8(4): 263–72.
7. Jauch EC, Saver JL, Adams HP Jr, et al. Guidelines for the early management of patients with acute ischemic stroke: a guideline for healthcare professionals from the American Heart Association/American Stroke Association. Stroke 2013;44(3): 870–947.
8. Giles MF, Albers GW, Amarenco P, et al. Early stroke risk and ABCD2 score performance in tissue- vs time-defined TIA: a multicenter study. Neurology 2011; 77(13):1222–8.
9. Giles MF, Rothwell PM. Prognosis and management in the first few days after a transient ischemic attack or minor ischaemic stroke. Int J Stroke 2006;1(2):65–73.
10. Giles MF, Rothwell PM. Risk of stroke early after transient ischaemic attack: a systematic review and meta-analysis. Lancet Neurol 2007;6(12):1063–72.
11. Johnston SC, Gress DR, Browner WS, et al. Short-term prognosis after emergency department diagnosis of TIA. JAMA 2000;284(22):2901–6.
12. Rothwell PM, Giles MF, Flossmann E, et al. A simple score (ABCD) to identify individuals at high early risk of stroke after transient ischaemic attack. Lancet 2005; 366(9479):29–36.
13. Writing Group M, Mozaffarian D, Benjamin EJ, et al. Heart disease and stroke statistics-2016 update: a report from the American Heart Association. Circulation 2016;133(4):e38–360.
14. Sangha RS, Caprio FZ, Askew R, et al. Quality of life in patients with TIA and minor ischemic stroke. Neurology 2015;85(22):1957–63.

15. Bogousslavsky J, Van Melle G, Regli F. The Lausanne Stroke Registry: analysis of 1,000 consecutive patients with first stroke. Stroke 1988;19(9):1083–92.

16. Kapral MK, Hall R, Fang J, et al. Association between hospitalization and care after transient ischemic attack or minor stroke. Neurology 2016;86(17):1582–9.

17. Cadilhac DA, Kim J, Lannin NA, et al. Better outcomes for hospitalized patients with TIA when in stroke units: an observational study. Neurology 2016;86(22):2042–8.

18. Ferro JM, Pinto AN, Falcao I, et al. Diagnosis of stroke by the nonneurologist. A validation study. Stroke 1998;29(6):1106–9.

19. Ranta A, Barber PA. Transient ischemic attack service provision: a review of available service models. Neurology 2016;86(10):947–53.

20. Ranta A, Cariga P. Who should manage transient ischemic attacks? A comparison between stroke experts, generalists, and electronic decision support. N Z Med J 2013;126(1372):25–31.

21. Rizos T, Ringleb PA, Huttner HB, et al. Evolution of stroke diagnosis in the emergency room–a prospective observational study. Cerebrovasc Dis 2009;28(5):448–53.

22. Nguyen-Huynh MN, Johnston SC. Is hospitalization after TIA cost-effective on the basis of treatment with tPA? Neurology 2005;65(11):1799–801.

23. Joshi JK, Ouyang B, Prabhakaran S. Should TIA patients be hospitalized or referred to a same-day clinic? A decision analysis. Neurology 2011;77(24):2082–8.

24. Giles MF, Rothwell PM. Substantial underestimation of the need for outpatient services for TIA and minor stroke. Age Ageing 2007;36(6):676–80.

25. Rothwell PM, Giles MF, Chandratheva A, et al. Effect of urgent treatment of transient ischaemic attack and minor stroke on early recurrent stroke (EXPRESS study): a prospective population-based sequential comparison. Lancet 2007;370(9596):1432–42.

26. Ranta A, Yang CF, Funnell M, et al. Utility of a primary care based transient ischaemic attack electronic decision support tool: a prospective sequential comparison. BMC Fam Pract 2014;15:86.

27. Ranta A, Dovey S, Weatherall M, et al. Cluster randomized controlled trial of TIA electronic decision support in primary care. Neurology 2015;84(15):1545–51.

28. Ranta A. Transient ischaemic attack and stroke risk: pilot of a primary care electronic decision support tool. J Prim Health Care 2013;5(2):138–40.

29. Olivot JM, Wolford C, Castle J, et al. Two aces: transient ischemic attack work-up as outpatient assessment of clinical evaluation and safety. Stroke 2011;42(7):1839–43.

30. Lavallee PC, Meseguer E, Abboud H, et al. A transient ischaemic attack clinic with round-the-clock access (SOS-TIA): feasibility and effects. Lancet Neurol 2007;6(11):953–60.

31. Gladstone DJ, Kapral MK, Fang J, et al. Management and outcomes of transient ischemic attacks in Ontario. CMAJ 2004;170(7):1099–104.

32. Chandratheva A, Geraghty OC, Luengo-Fernandez R, et al, Oxford Vascular Study. ABCD2 score predicts severity rather than risk of early recurrent events after transient ischemic attack. Stroke 2010;41(5):851–6.

33. Merwick A, Albers GW, Amarenco P, et al. Addition of brain and carotid imaging to the ABCD(2) score to identify patients at early risk of stroke after transient ischaemic attack: a multicentre observational study. Lancet Neurol 2010;9(11):1060–9.

34. Giles MF, Albers GW, Amarenco P, et al. Addition of brain infarction to the ABCD2 Score (ABCD2I): a collaborative analysis of unpublished data on 4574 patients. Stroke 2010;41(9):1907–13.
35. Johnston SC, Rothwell PM, Nguyen-Huynh MN, et al. Validation and refinement of scores to predict very early stroke risk after transient ischaemic attack. Lancet 2007;369(9558):283–92.
36. Wardlaw JM, Brazzelli M, Chappell FM, et al. ABCD2 score and secondary stroke prevention: meta-analysis and effect per 1,000 patients triaged. Neurology 2015; 85(4):373–80.
37. Kernan WN, Ovbiagele B, Black HR, et al. Guidelines for the prevention of stroke in patients with stroke and transient ischemic attack: a guideline for healthcare professionals from the American Heart Association/American Stroke Association. Stroke 2014;45(7):2160–236.
38. Fernandes PM, Whiteley WN, Hart SR, et al. Strokes: mimics and chameleons. Pract Neurol 2013;13(1):21–8.
39. Powers WJ, Derdeyn CP, Biller J, et al. 2015 American Heart Association/American Stroke Association Focused Update of the 2013 Guidelines for the Early Management of Patients With Acute Ischemic Stroke Regarding Endovascular Treatment: a Guideline for Healthcare Professionals From the American Heart Association/American Stroke Association. Stroke 2015;46(10):3020–35.
40. Luengo-Fernandez R, Gray AM, Rothwell PM. Effect of urgent treatment for transient ischaemic attack and minor stroke on disability and hospital costs (EX-PRESS study): a prospective population-based sequential comparison. Lancet Neurol 2009;8(3):235–43.
41. Ranta A, Bonning J, Fink J, et al. Emergency and stroke physician combined consensus statement on thrombolysis for acute stroke. N Z Med J 2014; 127(1392):113–4.
42. Wang Y, Pan Y, Zhao X, et al. Clopidogrel with aspirin in acute minor stroke or transient ischemic attack (CHANCE) trial: one-year outcomes. Circulation 2015; 132(1):40–6.
43. Wang Y, Wang Y, Zhao X, et al. Clopidogrel with aspirin in acute minor stroke or transient ischemic attack. N Engl J Med 2013;369(1):11–9.
44. Johnston SC, Easton JD, Farrant M, et al. Platelet-oriented inhibition in new TIA and minor ischemic stroke (POINT) trial: rationale and design. Int J Stroke 2013;8(6):479–83.

# Tachyarrhythmias and Bradyarrhythmias

## Differential Diagnosis and Initial Management in the Primary Care Office

Timothy Joseph Byrnes, DO[a], Otto Costantini, MD[b],*

**KEYWORDS**

- Arrhythmias • Atrial fibrillation • Supraventricular tachycardia
- Ventricular tachycardia • Sinus node dysfunction • Atrioventricular block

**KEY POINTS**

- Symptoms of tachyarrhythmias and bradyarrhythmias can vary from absent or subtle to urgent or emergent.
- In conjunction with a detailed clinical history, a 12-lead electrocardiogram is the cornerstone for accurate arrhythmia diagnosis and appropriate treatment.
- Because outpatient clinics are often ill-equipped to handle the treatment of patients with arrhythmias, the main task of providers is to identify patients who are critically ill (or potentially unstable) and should be transported to the nearest emergency department versus those who can safely be referred to a cardiologist for an outpatient appointment.
- For the more stable patients, certain diagnostic testing and therapeutic maneuvers should be initiated before the referral to a cardiologist.

## INTRODUCTION

Cardiac arrhythmias are common among patients who present in the outpatient setting.[1] In particular, with an aging population, the frequency of cardiac arrhythmias, such as atrial fibrillation or atrioventricular (AV) block, is projected to increase and greatly affect health care use in the future.[2] This article reviews the most common presentations, differential diagnosis, and initial management of patients presenting to the outpatient clinic with tachyarrhythmia or bradyarrhythmia. Emphasis is placed on whether and when to immediately refer the patient to an emergency department or

---

Disclosure: The authors have nothing to disclose.
<sup>a</sup> SummaHealth Heart and Vascular Institute, North East Ohio Medical University, 95 Arch Street, Suite 300, Akron, OH 44304, USA; <sup>b</sup> SummaHealth Heart and Vascular Institute, North East Ohio Medical University, 95 Arch Street, Suite 350, Akron, OH 44304, USA
* Corresponding author.
*E-mail address:* costantinio@summahealth.org

Med Clin N Am 101 (2017) 495–506
http://dx.doi.org/10.1016/j.mcna.2016.12.005

whether to refer the patient to an outpatient cardiology visit. Fortunately, true emergencies are rare.

## Tachyarrhythmias

### Symptoms

The symptoms of tachyarrhythmias are heterogeneous and can be subtle, especially in elderly patients.[1] Palpitation is a common symptom and clinicians should focus on the length, the onset and offset, the frequency, and precipitating factors. Often associated with palpitation is shortness of breath at rest or dyspnea on exertion. Dizziness and lightheadedness are also often part of the symptom complex, because the blood pressure is often decreased by the arrhythmia. However, syncope is much less common, particularly in a young population or even an elderly population with structurally normal hearts.[3,4] Typically, patients are more symptomatic with faster heart rates (HRs). However, it should be emphasized that elderly patients presenting with seemingly rate-controlled atrial fibrillation or atrial flutter can be symptomatic from diastolic dysfunction and the loss of atrial kick. In contrast, it is common to see elderly patients present to the office without any symptoms at all. Most patients with a supraventricular tachycardia tolerate very fast HRs fairly well for several hours in the setting of a structurally normal heart. However, sustained HRs faster than 100 beats/min (bpm) for several weeks can lead even a structurally normal heart to a dilated cardiomyopathy and florid heart failure symptoms.[5] Elderly patients with underlying coronary artery disease or baseline left ventricular dysfunction tolerate any tachyarrhythmia poorly and often need more urgent or emergent care. It is common for such patients to present with florid heart failure or typical angina caused by the increased demand placed on the ventricular myocardium.

### Differential diagnosis and acute management

In the outpatient setting, a 12-lead electrocardiogram (ECG) is the cornerstone needed to initially diagnose a tachyarrhythmia and thereby develop the most appropriate treatment plan. It is beyond the scope of this article to delve into the mechanisms, cause, and pathophysiology of each of these rhythms, but many excellent reviews exist.[1,6] The electrocardiographic features helpful in the differential diagnosis of a SVT are covered in many excellent reviews and in the guidelines for the management of supraventricular tachycardia in adults.[1,7] **Fig. 1** offers a simple algorithm for the differential diagnosis of a tachyarrhythmia. The initial, and most important, question is whether the rhythm has a narrow QRS complex ($\leq$120 milliseconds) or a wide one (>120 milliseconds). This distinction immediately differentiates between a supraventricular rhythm versus the possibility of a more dangerous ventricular tachycardia. However, not every wide complex tachycardia is ventricular in origin. Many supraventricular rhythms have a wide QRS if the rate is fast enough that the electrical signal is conducted slowly (ie, aberrantly) down the normal conduction system. Once the rhythm is identified as a narrow complex tachycardia, the next step is to determine whether it is regular or irregular based on the R-R intervals (see **Fig. 1**). Based on these 2 simple steps the differential diagnosis can be simplified as follows.

#### Narrow and regular tachycardia

**Sinus tachycardia** Although clearly not an abnormal rhythm, this tachycardia may be the most often seen in the primary care office and is typically driven by an underlying physiologic, psychological, or pharmacologic stimulus. Young, healthy patients can have HRs of 150 bpm or more. Infections, anemia, hyperthyroidism, chronic obstructive pulmonary disease (COPD), and heart failure exacerbations are some of the most frequent clinical stimuli. Illicit stimulants and beta-agonist use should be inquired

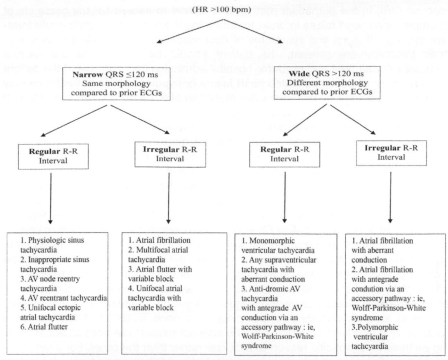

**Fig. 1.** Two-step differential of a tachyarrhythmia.

about. Treatment should focus on treating the underlying cause. Note that patients with baseline poor cardiac function are tachycardic as a compensatory mechanism in order to maintain an adequate cardiac output. In this setting, sinus tachycardia is a poor prognostic sign, indicating the potential need for admission for advanced heart failure therapy. Rarely is consultation with a cardiologist or electrophysiologist needed in this setting other than in the case of patients with suspected inappropriate sinus tachycardia and symptoms of dizziness, palpitation, and syncope suggestive of the postural orthostatic tachycardia syndrome.[8]

**Atrial flutter** Atrial flutter and atrial fibrillation are by far the most common supraventricular tachyarrhythmias seen in practice. Typical atrial flutter is caused by a macroreentrant circuit in the right atrium, initiated, as are all reentrant rhythms, by a premature atrial contraction.[9] On the ECG, the atrial rate is ~300 bpm and flutter waves are seen in the classic saw-tooth pattern; that is, very negative atrial waves in the inferior leads as the left atrium is depolarized from bottom to top. Atrial rates in atrial flutter can be as slow as 240 bpm, especially in patients with large or structurally very abnormal atria, or in patients on antiarrhythmic drugs. The ventricular rate depends on the atrial rate and on the conduction properties of the AV node. Most commonly patients present with 2:1 AV conduction and a ventricular rate of ~150 bpm. However, AV conduction can be 1:1, especially when the atrial rate is slow or in young patients. Although less common types of atrial flutter are seen, a detailed discussion of different types of atrial flutter is beyond the scope of this article. Suffice it to say that atrial flutter can be clockwise or counterclockwise, typical or atypical, and left or right atrial.[10] Patients with atrial flutter with 2:1 AV conduction often present with palpitation and shortness of breath because of the rapid ventricular response (VR). In the outpatient setting, it is critical to assess for the presence of decompensated heart failure in order to determine the most appropriate acute treatment strategy. If signs and symptoms of decompensated heart failure or hemodynamic instability are present, the patient should be referred to the nearest emergency department and probable hospital admission for treatment. If the patient shows no signs of decompensated heart failure or hypotension, then treatment may be tailored depending on the ventricular response and the duration of symptoms. If the ventricular response is rapid (>130 bpm), then it still may be prudent to refer the patient to the emergency department, because the ventricular rate may be difficult to control and the patient's medications may be more easily titrated in an inpatient setting. If the patient's ventricular response is less than 130 bpm and the patient is only minimally symptomatic, then an outpatient treatment strategy, with an early referral to a cardiologist or electrophysiologist, may be reasonable. In this scenario, regardless of the CHA2DS2-VASC score (C- Congestive Heart Failure History, H- Hypertension History, A- Age, D- Diabetes History, S- Prior Stroke, VA -Peripheral Vascular Disease History, Sc- Sex Category), and unless there is any absolute contraindication, the authors recommend starting anticoagulation, because the most pressing decision facing the cardiologist is whether the patient should eventually be electrically cardioverted. Starting anticoagulation at this juncture, before referral to a cardiologist, decreases the amount of time needed for elective cardioversion, because the patient needs to be anticoagulated for least 3 weeks before that procedure, unless a transesophageal echocardiogram is done. In terms of rate control, a β-blocker or a nondihydropyridine calcium channel blocker are both acceptable, as long as there is no specific reason to pick one rather than the other. For example, a prior history of coronary artery disease or systolic heart failure would favor a β-blocker. All patients should get routine blood work, including a complete blood count, metabolic panel, magnesium, and thyroid stimulating hormone. An echocardiogram should be ordered, if not previously done for other reasons, to assess left ventricular function and to rule out significant valvular disease as a possible cause.

**Atrioventricular node reentrant tachycardia** Other than atrial fibrillation and atrial flutter, this is the most common supraventricular tachycardia seen in practice.[11] A large minority of adults (up to 40% in some cohorts) are born with 2 pathways that can conduct electricity in the AV node, rather than 1. Under the right conditions, AV node reentrant tachycardia (AVNRT) can be initiated by a premature atrial or ventricular beat. If the 2 pathways are able to sustain a stable circuit, the atrium and the ventricle are depolarized almost simultaneously. As a result, on the ECG, the P wave is not seen, buried in the QRS complex, or is seen at the terminal portion of the QRS, typically as a pseudo-s (negative) wave in the inferior leads or a pseudo-r′ in lead V1. Because this tachyarrhythmia depends on the AV node, both vagal maneuvers and adenosine are potential acute treatment options. In the outpatient setting, if the patient is in a sustained supraventricular tachycardia, attempting vagal maneuvers is reasonable. These maneuvers should include bearing down, isometric contractions, and carotid sinus massage. Importantly, elderly patients should have their carotids auscultated first. If a bruit is present a carotid sinus massage should not be performed. If the supraventricular tachycardia does not terminate with vagal maneuvers, the authors recommend sending the patient to the emergency room. Most offices are not equipped to administer intravenous (IV) adenosine, but, even if they are, the authors do not recommend doing so without having placed defibrillator patches on the patient. Although small, there is a chance that adenosine may precipitate atrial fibrillation. If the patient has unrecognized Wolff-Parkinson-White syndrome, the patient could go from atrial fibrillation to ventricular fibrillation and require emergent cardioversion. If the supraventricular tachycardia terminates with vagal maneuvers, the patient can be referred electively to an electrophysiologist unless other symptoms persist. Prescribing an AV nodal blocking agent is reasonable at that time to make future episodes less likely to occur.

**Atrioventricular reentrant tachycardia** Similarly to AVNRT, AV reentrant tachycardia (AVRT) is a reentrant tachyarrhythmia dependent on the AV node, initiated by a premature atrial contraction or premature ventricular contraction. However, the reentrant circuit in this case uses a congenital accessory pathway located between the atrium and the ventricle, anywhere on the right or left side. Wolff-Parkinson-White syndrome is only one type of such an arrhythmia. The finding of a delta wave on an ECG, whether the patient is symptomatic or not, should be a reason for referral to an electrophysiologist, because the management of these patients is complicated and controversial, and a small number of these patients are at risk of sudden cardiac death. In the office, treatment of AVRT is the same as that of AVNRT, because the arrhythmias are difficult to discern from each other. On the ECG, the P wave is slightly removed from the preceding QRS, usually in the ST segment.[1]

**Ectopic (unifocal) atrial tachycardia** Atrial tachycardia can be caused by increased automaticity of atrial tissue or by a reentrant circuit within the atrial tissue. Typically, the atrial rate is slower than in atrial flutter, usually less than 240 bpm.[12] The ECG shows discrete P waves in front of a narrow QRS.[1] The P-wave morphology depends on the location of the atrial focus. Often it is significantly different than the sinus rhythm P wave, but, occasionally, if the focus is near the sinus node, the P-wave morphology may be very similar to sinus rhythm. In the acute setting, treatment includes rate control with AV node blockers. Long-term treatment may include antiarrhythmic drug therapy and, potentially, radiofrequency ablation.

**Junctional tachycardia** This rhythm is extremely rare in adults, but more common in children. In adults it is caused by inflammation near the AV node. Endocarditis is one possible cause. The rate of a junctional tachycardia is usually no faster than 110 to 120 bpm. Similar to AVNRT, the P wave is buried in the QRS complex on the ECG. If no P wave is visible, AVNRT is much more likely than a junctional tachycardia in adult patients. Treatment options include AV node blockers and treatment of the underlying illness.

### Narrow and irregular

**Atrial fibrillation** This atrial tachyarrhythmia is by far the most common encountered in the office. Atrial fibrillation appears as an irregular rhythm on the ECG with a narrow QRS and without clear atrial activity. The QRS may be wide in cases in which an underlying bundle branch block already exists or when the ventricular rate is fast enough to cause aberrant conduction through the bundles. The classification of atrial fibrillation and its long-term management are the focus of many publications and are not be covered in this article.[10,13] Very little has been written about the initial management of atrial fibrillation encountered in the office. From an acute management standpoint, clinicians have to assess several issues. First, secondary causes of atrial fibrillation or atrial flutter, such as pulmonary emboli, myocardial infarction, decompensated heart failure, or acute asthma or COPD exacerbations, need to be ruled out. These causes are usually absent without significant associated symptoms. Second, the severity of symptoms should be assessed. If the symptoms are subtle or absent, elective referral to a cardiologist can be considered as long as anticoagulation and rate control with AV nodal blockers are initiated. Third, if symptoms are present but myocardial ischemia, hypotension, angina, or heart failure are absent, the clinician must attempt to determine the duration of atrial fibrillation or atrial flutter. In the office, the duration of the arrhythmia, in conjunction with the severity of symptoms, determines whether the patient should be referred to the emergency department or for an elective, outpatient cardiology visit. If secondary causes are excluded, but the patient is very symptomatic, and the onset can reliably be determined to be less than 48 hours, the patient should be referred to the emergency room so that anticoagulation can be started immediately and cardioversion can be considered without the need for a transesophageal echocardiogram.[10] If the patient is very symptomatic but the onset of symptoms is unknown or longer than 48 hours, the clinician must determine whether anticoagulation and rate control can be achieved in an outpatient setting or whether an inpatient stay is needed. Studies have shown that if symptoms can be treated and the ventricular response can be controlled, a strategy of a minimum of 3 weeks of anticoagulation followed by a direct current (DC) cardioversion is equivalent to an immediate transesophageal echo followed by a DC cardioversion.[14] For patients who present to the office asymptomatic or minimally symptomatic, the long-term management decision to adopt a rate-control strategy versus a rhythm-control strategy has been made easier by the Atrial Fibrillation Follow-Up Investigation of Rhythm Management (AFFIRM) trial.[15] Long-term mortality, risk of stroke, and quality of life are similar with both strategies. However, it should be emphasized that the symptoms of atrial fibrillation can be subtle and a careful history is needed to elicit them. Quality of life can often be improved significantly by a rhythm-control strategy in patients even if the symptoms are subtle.

**Multifocal atrial tachycardia** This tachyarrhythmia arises from multiple foci of increased automaticity within the atria and typically presents in the elderly with a severe pulmonary disorder such as COPD or pulmonary hypertension, and in patients with acutely decompensated heart failure.[16] Such patients are often at an increased risk of developing atrial fibrillation or atrial flutter. The ECG shows an irregular rhythm with 3 or more distinct P-wave morphologies and 1:1 AV conduction. Treatment is targeted toward the underlying disorder (ie, COPD, heart failure, or respiratory infection). Patients who present in the office with this rhythm often need to be admitted because of the underlying illness. Calcium channel blockers are usually preferred to β-blockers in this setting.[17]

### Wide and regular

**Monomorphic ventricular tachycardia** The most common wide complex tachycardia is monomorphic ventricular tachycardia (MMVT). MMVT is not always hemodynamically unstable and patients may present to the primary care office with shortness of breath, palpitation, and dizziness. Almost uniformly, this occurs in the setting of known coronary disease and a low left ventricular ejection fraction. However, other forms of MMVT in structurally normal hearts can be seen.[18]

**Supraventricular tachycardia with aberrant conduction** A supraventricular tachycardia can have a wide complex QRS, while still using the normal conduction system (ie, the right or left bundle branch). Such an instance is termed aberrant or slow conduction. It can occur for a variety of reasons, including a fast ventricular rate, electrolyte imbalances, and preexisting bundle branch blocks. The ECG in this setting should have a typical right or left bundle branch block appearance. A typical example of this tachyarrhythmia is atrial flutter with 1:1 AV conduction.

**Supraventricular tachycardia with atrioventricular conduction via an accessory pathway** This entity is only (and rarely) seen in patients with Wolff-Parkinson-White syndrome. It involves conduction of the atrial signal antegrade down the accessory pathway and retrograde up the AV node. Because ventricular depolarization occurs cell to cell, rather than via the normal conduction system, the QRS is wide and mimics monomorphic ventricular tachycardia. This tachycardia is also known as antidromic AVRT.[1] A prior ECG with a delta wave typical of Wolff-Parkinson-White syndrome is helpful for this diagnosis.

If the ECG shows a regular wide complex tachycardia, our recommendation is that all patients should be referred to the emergency department. Although the differential diagnosis includes benign arrhythmias, the differentiation of a benign versus malignant rhythm is best conducted in an emergency setting, even when the patient is hemodynamically stable or minimally symptomatic. These patients should be connected to defibrillator patches and transported urgently to the nearest emergency department by emergency medical services. For discussion purposes, a simple medical history differentiates patients 80% to 90% of the time (**Table 1**). MMVT is more common in patients with prior myocardial infarction, coronary artery disease, or any type of structural heart disease. Supraventricular tachycardia with aberrant conduction (SVT-A) and antidromic AVRT are more common in young patients without known structural heart disease. Several algorithms based on QRS morphology also exist to differentiate

**Table 1**
**Differential Diagnosis of Regular Wide Complex Tachycardia**

| Factors | Favor MMVT | Favor SVT with Aberrancy |
|---|---|---|
| Medical history | • History of structural heart disease<br>• History of prior myocardial infarction<br>• History of ischemic heart disease<br>• History of systolic heart failure<br>• History of dilated cardiomyopathy<br>• Family history of sudden cardiac death | • No history of structural heart disease<br>• Prior ECGs with a right or left bundle branch block pattern<br>• Prior ECGs with WPW syndrome<br>• Prior history of paroxysmal atrial tachyarrhythmias |
| ECG characteristics | • Absence of typical bundle branch block morphology<br>• RSR' complexes in V1 (R taller than R')<br>• Extreme right axis deviation (+180° to −90°)<br>• QRS >160 ms<br>• AV dissociation (P and QRS complexes at different rates)<br>• Capture beats (sinus QRS beat during runs of ventricular beats)<br>• Fusion beats (fusion of sinus and ventricular beat)<br>• Precordial concordance (positive or negative in leads V1–V6) or absence of RS complex<br>• QRS onset to nadir of S wave >100 ms in septal leads<br>• Josephson sign (notch in downslope of S wave in septal leads)<br>• R-wave peak time ≥50 ms in lead II<br>• Amplitude of initial 40 ms of QRS ≤amplitude change in terminal 40 ms of QRS | • Typical bundle branch block morphology<br>• RS complex in precordial leads with onset of R to nadir of S <100 ms<br>• Absence of AV dissociation (independent P and QRS rates, capture beat, fusion beat) |

*Abbreviations:* SVT, supraventricular tachycardia; WPW, Wolff-Parkinson-White syndrome.

MMVT from SVT-A.[19] These algorithms are difficult to remember, not always reliable, and probably beyond the scope of acute management in a primary care outpatient setting. Once again, if patients present to the office with a wide complex tachycardia, the authors believe that the best and safest course of action is to transfer them to the nearest emergency department.

### Irregular and wide

**Atrial fibrillation with aberrancy versus atrial fibrillation with preexcitation** Most patients have atrial fibrillation conducting rapidly and aberrantly via the normal conduction system. Occasionally young patients present with atrial fibrillation with a rapid ventricular rate caused by antegrade conduction down a Wolff-Parkinson-White pathway.[20] Typically, these patients are symptomatic, present to an emergency room rather than to the office, and need to be urgently cardioverted.

**Polymorphic ventricular tachycardia or torsades de pointes** For the sake of completeness, rarely patients present to the office complaining of palpitation or near syncope. A 12-lead ECG may show a wide complex rhythm, typically nonsustained, consistent with polymorphic ventricular tachycardia or torsades de pointes. This finding may occur in the setting of hyperkalemia and acute renal insufficiency or with initiation of QT-prolonging drugs. This is a true medical emergency and the patient needs to be referred to the emergency department immediately for further care.

### Treatment and management

Throughout this article a common-sense approach to the acute management of supraventricular and ventricular tachyarrhythmias is highlighted. Given the lack of

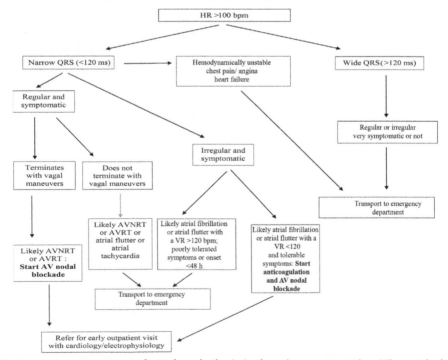

**Fig. 2.** Acute management of a tachyarrhythmia in the primary care setting. VR, ventricular response.

literature published in this regard, **Fig. 2** presents an algorithm to guide clinicians further. Patients who present with a wide complex tachycardia, regular or irregular, regardless of the severity of symptoms, should be referred to an emergency department. Simple interventions such as AV nodal blockers in these patients may worsen symptoms and cause true emergencies depending on the underlying rhythm. Patients presenting with a narrow QRS and hemodynamic instability manifested by hypotension, acute mental status change, respiratory distress, ischemic chest pain, or acute heart failure should also be immediately referred to the emergency department, unless the office is equipped to deliver synchronized electrical cardioversion via an external defibrillator. Patients with a narrow QRS and no evidence of hemodynamic compromise can be managed depending on the severity of their symptoms. If the symptoms are poorly tolerated, and especially if the ventricular response is faster than ~ 120 bpm, the patients should be referred to the emergency department. If the rhythm is regular and cannot be terminated with vagal maneuvers, it may be terminated in the emergency department with IV adenosine. If it is irregular, and consistent with either atrial fibrillation or atrial flutter, rate control or rhythm control can be achieved quicker as an inpatient. If the tachycardia terminates with vagal maneuvers or if it is thought to be atrial fibrillation or atrial flutter with a fairly well-controlled ventricular response and minimal symptoms, then an early referral to a cardiologist can be considered rather than transport to the emergency department. In the latter scenario, AV nodal blockade should be initiated for both regular and irregular narrow complex tachycardia. In addition, if the rhythm is thought to be atrial fibrillation or atrial flutter, anticoagulation should also be initiated in order to expedite electrical cardioversion in case a rhythm-controlling strategy is adopted.

### Bradyarrhythmias

Bradycardia is defined as a HR less than 60 bpm, but generally a HR less than 50 bpm is needed to cause significant symptoms. Young patients and athletes tolerate very slow HRs without symptoms. In contrast, older patients complain of fatigue, exercise intolerance, and transient dizziness with HRs in the 40s. The symptoms of bradycardias are often subtle and difficult to document. In the office, a 12-lead ECG may show sinus rhythm in the range of 40 to 50 bpm. Symptoms of brief, transient dizziness not related to change in position and occurring while sitting should alert primary care physicians to possible bradyarrhythmias. In the office, other than a 12-lead ECG, other diagnostic tests should include a 24-hour Holter monitor or a 30-day event recorder if the symptoms do not occur daily. In addition, an exercise treadmill test, if the patient is able to exercise, is often helpful in determining the chronotropic competence of the sinus node and to rule out exercise-related AV block. Routine blood work, including a complete blood count, complete metabolic panel, magnesium level, thyroid function studies, and an echocardiogram, are indicated to rule out secondary causes of bradyarrhythmias.

### Differential diagnosis

The differential diagnosis of bradycardia involves abnormalities of the sinus node or abnormalities of the AV node.[21,22] Note that syncope and near syncope in the elderly are overwhelmingly likely to be either hypotensive or bradycardic, not neurologic. A neurologic work-up or referral to a neurologist is often unnecessary.

**Sinus node dysfunction** In general, this is a disease of the elderly. Although rare instances of congenital sinus node dysfunction have been reported to run in some families, almost all patients with symptomatic sinus bradycardia are elderly. The patients present to the office with sinus rhythm and HRs of 40 to 50 bpm. Symptoms are subtle, and include fatigue, exertional dyspnea, dizziness, near syncope, or syncope. Often the patients also complain of palpitation, either sustained or nonsustained. These patients often have atrial tachyarrhythmias such as atrial fibrillation, atrial flutter, or atrial tachycardia. This syndrome is named sick sinus syndrome or tachy-brady syndrome. Although a 12-lead ECG is helpful in the diagnosis, a 24-hour Holter monitor or a 30-day event recorder is necessary to correlate the slow rhythm with symptoms. These patients should be referred to an electrophysiologist because a pacemaker is necessary to alleviate symptoms and prevent syncope. There are no medications that can help in improving the sinus node function. Indications for pacing are well described in the literature.[22]

**Atrioventricular dysfunction** Elderly patients also often develop AV node and His-Purkinje disease. It is common for patients to present to the office with symptoms of fatigue, exercise intolerance, dizziness, near syncope, or syncope. First-degree AV block is defined as a prolongation of the PR interval, but with maintenance of a 1:1 P:QRS ratio. This condition is generally benign. Second-degree AV block, type I (Wenckebach), is characterized by progressive PR prolongation until a QRS is missing. In this case, the conduction abnormality is typically in the AV node, and the QRS morphology is usually narrow. Second-degree AV block, type II, is characterized by missing QRS complexes in the absence of PR prolongation. In this case the conduction disease is typically below the AV node, within the His-Purkinje system. The QRS morphology is therefore often wide. This type of block is more likely to progress to third-degree AV block. Finally, third-degree AV block is present when no P waves are conducted. The atrial rate is dissociated from the ventricular rate. This condition is a true medical emergency because the patient's escape rhythm may be unstable and result in a cardiac arrest.

### Treatment and management
If a 12-lead ECG in the office shows second-degree AV block, type I or type II, or third-degree AV block, the patient should be referred to the emergency department, especially if the patient has had a syncopal episode in the recent past. Once in the emergency department, secondary causes should be ruled out, including hypoxemia, electrolytes abnormalities, hypothyroidism, or drug toxicity. However, these causes rarely explain sinus node dysfunction or AV block in the elderly. This disease process is typically a primary electrical system process related to aging and fibrosis of the conduction system.[23] If the patient is on digoxin, a level should be taken, especially if the renal function has recently worsened. A high digoxin level can clearly be a cause of bradycardia in the elderly.

If the 12-lead ECG shows a first-degree AV block alone or a first-degree AV block with evidence of His-Purkinje disease (either a right bundle branch block or left bundle branch block) the patient should have a 30-day event recorder to try to document a higher degree of AV block and to correlate it with symptoms. First-degree AV block alone, bifascicular block, and trifascicular block by themselves are not an indication for pacing. In select circumstances, when symptoms seem related to possible bradycardias, but a 30-day event recorder is nondiagnostic, referral to an electrophysiologist to consider implanting a subcutaneous loop recorder or even a permanent pacemaker is appropriate. Importantly, many elderly patients are on AV nodal blockers for the treatment of hypertension, coronary artery disease, heart failure, or atrial tachyarrhythmias. Although these medications may be contributors, especially if the dose has recently been increased, it is unusual that these medications are solely responsible for sinus node dysfunction or AV block. Although it is reasonable to decrease them, or even stop them, if they are not absolutely indicated, they are rarely enough to explain the bradyarrhythmia.

## SUMMARY

Tachyarrhythmias and bradyarrhythmias are often seen in the primary care office setting because patients can present with intermittent and frequently subtle symptoms. Most patients present as fairly symptomatic but typically are hemodynamically stable. True emergencies are rare. The initial management of such patients depends on the type and duration of the arrhythmia, the initial 12-lead ECG, and the severity of symptoms.

## REFERENCES

1. Page RL, Joglar JA, Caldwell MA, et al. 2015 ACC/AHA/HRS guideline for the management of adult patients with supraventricular tachycardia. Heart Rhythm 2016;13:e136–221.
2. Bengston LG, Lutsey PL, Loehr LR, et al. Impact of atrial fibrillation on healthcare utilization in the community: the Atherosclerosis Risk in Communities Study. J Am Heart Assoc 2014;3:e001006.
3. Orejarena LA, Vidaillet H, Destefano F, et al. Paroxysmal supraventricular tachycardia in the general population. J Am Coll Cardiol 1998;31:150–7.
4. Kalusche D, Ott P, Arentz T, et al. AV nodal reentry tachycardia in elderly patients: clinical presentation and results of radiofrequency ablation. Coron Artery Dis 1998;9:359–63.
5. Gupta S, Figueredo VM. Tachycardia mediated cardiomyopathy: pathophysiology, mechanisms, clinical features and management. Int J Cardiol 2014;172:40–6.
6. Mirza M, Strunets A, Shen WK, et al. Mechanisms of arrhythmias and conduction disorders in older adults. Clin Geriatr Med 2012;28:555–73.
7. Link MS. Evaluation and initial treatment of supraventricular tachycardia. N Engl J Med 2012;367:1438–48.
8. Olshansky B, Sullivan RM. Inappropriate sinus tachycardia. J Am Coll Cardiol 2013;61:793–801.
9. Dhar S, Lidhoo P, Koul D, et al. Current concepts and management strategies in atrial flutter. South Med J 2009;102:917–22.
10. January CT, Wann LS, Alpert JS, et al. 2014 AHA/ACC/HRS guideline for the management of patients with atrial fibrillation. J Am Coll Cardiol 2014;64:e1–76.
11. Porter MJ, Morton JB, Denman R, et al. Influence of age and gender on the mechanism of supraventricular tachycardia. Heart Rhythm 2004;1:393–6.
12. Steinbeck G, Hoffmann E. True atrial tachycardia. Eur Heart J 1998;19:E48–9.
13. Moukabary T, Gonzalez MD. Management of atrial fibrillation. Med Clin North Am 2015;99:781–94.
14. Klein AL, Grimm RA, Murray RD, et al. Use of transesophageal echocardiography to guide cardioversion in patients with atrial fibrillation. N Engl J Med 2001;344:1411–20.
15. Wyse DG, Waldo AL, DiMarco JP, et al, The Atrial Fibrillation Follow-Up Investigation of Rhythm Management (AFFIRM) Investigators. A comparison of rate control and rhythm control in patients with atrial fibrillation. N Engl J Med 2002;347:1825–33.
16. Kastor JA. Multifocal atrial tachycardia. N Engl J Med 1990;322:1713–7.

17. Levine JH, Michael JR, Guarnieri T. Treatment of multifocal atrial tachycardia with verapamil. N Engl J Med 1985;312:21–5.
18. Moss JD, Tung R. Sustained ventricular tachycardia in apparently normal hearts. Card Electrophysiol Clin 2016;8:623–30.
19. Vereckei A, Duray G, Szenasi G, et al. New algorithm using only lead aVR for differential diagnosis of wide complex tachycardia. Heart Rhythm 2008;5:89–98.
20. Beck H, See VY. Acute management of atrial fibrillation. from emergency department to cardiac care unit. Cardiol Clin 2012;30:567–89.
21. Samii SM. Indications for pacemakers, implantable cardioverter-defibrillator and cardiac resynchronization devices. Med Clin North Am 2015;99:795–804.
22. Tracy CM, Epstein AE, Darbar D, et al. 2012 ACCF/AHA/HRS focused update of the 2008 guidelines for device–based therapy of cardiac rhythm abnormalities. J Am Coll Cardiol 2012;60:1297–313.
23. Sanders P, Morton JB, Kistler PM, et al. Electrophysiological and electroanatomic characterization of the atria in sinus node disease: evidence of diffuse atrial remodeling. Circulation 2004;109:1514–22.

# Outpatient Emergencies
## Acute Heart Failure

Malgorzata Mysliwiec, MD, Raphael E. Bonita, MD, ScM*

## KEYWORDS

- Acute heart failure • Cardiomyopathy • BNP • Heart failure hospitalization
- Volume overload

## KEY POINTS

- Heart failure is a growing health care crisis given the aging population.
- Volume overload manifested by symptoms of congestion is the most common clinical presentation of acute heart failure.
- Consider a broad differential diagnosis when evaluating patients with shortness of breath.
- Treatment of acute heart failure must address precipitating factors, identification of etiology, and should be tailored to the degree of volume overload and adequacy of end-organ perfusion.

## INTRODUCTION AND DEFINITIONS

Heart failure is a major health care problem in the United States and internationally. For Americans, the lifetime risk of developing heart failure is 20% after the age of 40 years.[1] The prevalence of heart failure has been well documented to increase with age, and is higher in men and African American individuals.[2] The diagnosis of heart failure is associated with a significant degree of overall morbidity, recurrent hospitalizations leading to tremendous health care expenditures, and readmissions, and is marked with a strikingly high rate of mortality estimated to be 50% at 5 years.[3] Heart failure is a complex syndrome in which patients manifest symptoms from either impaired contractility of the heart to eject blood forward to vital tissues or in the setting of normal cardiac function at the expense of elevated filling pressures. Symptomatic heart failure results from volume overload due to reduced left ventricular systolic function or secondary to preserved cardiac contractility with impaired relaxation and increased diastolic stiffness. The left ventricular ejection fraction (EF) is used to classify the type of heart failure. According to the 2013 American College of Cardiology (ACC)/American Heart Association

Disclosure Statement: Authors have nothing to disclose.
Department of Medicine, Jefferson Heart Institute, Sidney Kimmel Medical College of Thomas Jefferson University, 925 Chestnut Street, Suite 323A, Philadelphia, PA 19107, USA
* Corresponding author.
E-mail address: Raphael.Bonita@jefferson.edu

Med Clin N Am 101 (2017) 507–519
http://dx.doi.org/10.1016/j.mcna.2016.12.010
medical.theclinics.com

(AHA) Heart Failure Guideline, heart failure with reduced EF (HFrEF) is defined by an EF ≤40% with heart failure with preserved EF (HFpEF) defined by an EF ≥50%.[4]

## PATHOPHYSIOLOGY

The pathophysiology of heart failure is a highly complex process that can involve a multitude of factors. Some are extrinsic to the myocardium, others result from cardiac structural abnormalities that activate well-defined neurohormonal pathways in the circulatory system that become dysregulated, culminating in reduced pump function or a stiffened left ventricle with impaired relaxation[5] (**Fig. 1**). The neurohormonal model of renin-angiotensin-aldosterone and sympathetic nervous system activation of heart failure play a paramount role in the progressive cardiac remodeling that occurs with heart failure and is the target of current guideline-directed medical therapy (ie, angiotensin-converting enzyme [ACE] inhibitors, angiotensin receptor blockers, aldosterone antagonists, and beta-blockade, respectively).

The natriuretic peptides (NPs) are a well-known family of hormones that play a major role in the body's response to fluid and sodium retention. Atrial natriuretic peptide (ANP) and B-type (BNP) are secreted from atrial and ventricular tissue, respectively, in response to stretch secondary to volume or pressure overload.[6] The mechanisms of action of these hormones include natriuresis, diuresis, and vasodilation via activation of guanylyl cyclase causing increase in intracellular cyclic guanosine monophosphate.[7] NPs are degraded and cleared from the circulation by the neutral endopeptidase neprilysin.[8] Neprilysin inhibition therefore prevents the breakdown of the NPs, thereby promoting a favorable hemodynamic response of vasodilatation and maintenance of fluid homeostasis. Entresto, a combination drug composed of the neprilysin inhibitor, sacubitril, and angiotensin receptor blocker, valsartan, were

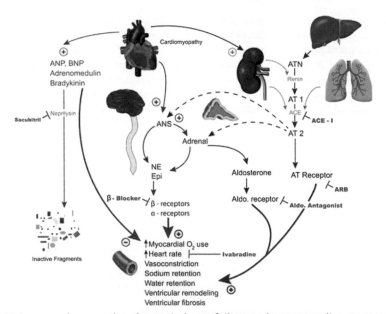

**Fig. 1.** Major neurohormonal pathways in heart failure and corresponding treatment targets. ANS, autonomic nervous system; AT, angiotensin 1; ATN, angiotensinogen; Epi, epinephrine; NE, norepinephrine. (*From* Gordin J, Fonarow G. New medications for heart failure. Trends Cardiovasc Med 2016;26:489; with permission.)

approved by the Food and Drug Administration in 2015 for use in patients with chronic systolic heart failure to reduce the risk of heart failure hospitalization and cardiovascular mortality based on the results of the PARADIGM-HF study.[9] The indication for this medication has recently been added to the 2016 ACC/AHA/Heart Failure Society of America (HFSA) Focused Update on New Pharmacotherapy for Heart Failure as part of guideline-directed medical therapy for patients with systolic heart failure.[10]

## RISK FACTORS

Understanding risk factors that predispose to developing structural heart disease and heart failure is critical for preventive strategies and early identification of disease and initiation of treatment. Based on epidemiologic studies investigating the risk of developing heart failure in populations, major risk factors associated with the development of heart failure are increasing age, particularly older than 65 years, male sex, hypertension, African American race, coronary artery disease, obesity, and diabetes mellitus.[11] Other risk factors known to cause heart failure include thyroid disease, alcohol abuse, many chemotherapeutic drugs, infectious agents, and diseases that infiltrate the heart, such as sarcoidosis, amyloidosis, and iron.[12]

## SYMPTOMS AND SIGNS

A complete history and physical examination remain the cornerstone in the evaluation of a patient suspected of having heart failure and is critical for identification of underlying structural heart disease. The primary symptoms and signs of acute heart failure are directly related to congestion and elevated filling pressures. Less commonly, the patient will present with low cardiac output. Symptoms compatible with congestion include shortness of breath at rest or with activity, orthopnea, paroxysmal nocturnal dyspnea, edema, decreased exercise tolerance, and fatigue. Less specific symptoms include early satiety, nausea, abdominal bloating, and wheezing. Important clinical signs of acute heart failure indicating high right-sided and left-sided filling pressures are elevated jugular venous pressure, edema, ascites, hepatojugular reflux, third heart sound (S3 gallop), rales, pulmonary edema, or pleural effusion on chest radiograph.[13] Rales may not be found in patients with chronic heart failure in the acute setting secondary to enhanced lymphatics.[14] Signs of reduced cardiac output include cool extremities, narrow pulse pressure, confusion, and pulsus alternans.[13] An increased jugular venous pressure and orthopnea ≥2 pillows has been demonstrated to correlate well with high pulmonary capillary wedge pressure.[15] The presence of a third heart sound or elevated jugular venous pressure is associated with increased risk of death or hospitalization for heart failure.[16] Characterization of the patient into 1 of 4 "hemodynamic profiles" based on the physical examination assessment of filling pressures and perfusion is helpful to guide therapy and has been shown to predict outcomes of death and need for urgent heart transplantation[17,18] (Fig. 2).

## EVALUATION AND DIAGNOSTIC TESTING

The role of diagnostic studies in the evaluation of a patient with heart failure is to confirm the diagnosis of heart failure, establish the etiology of heart failure, and identify comorbidities that will impact therapy. Both the 2013 American College of Cardiology Foundation (ACCF)/AHA Guideline for the Management of Heart Failure and the 2010 HFSA Comprehensive Heart Failure Practice Guideline offer similar recommendations on appropriate laboratory tests and diagnostic modalities for patients under evaluation for heart failure.[4,13] Key laboratory tests that should be performed include complete

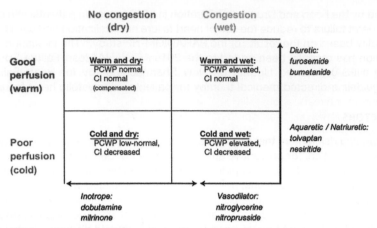

**Fig. 2.** Four hemodynamic presentations of patients with heart failure. CI, cardiac index; PCWP, pulmonary capillary wedge pressure. (*From* Pauly D. Managing acute decompensated heart failure. Cardiol Clin 2014;32:148; with permission.)

blood count, urinalysis, serum electrolytes (including calcium and magnesium), blood urea nitrogen, serum creatinine, glucose, fasting lipid profile, liver function tests, and thyroid-stimulating hormone. A 12-lead electrocardiogram (ECG) is a good preliminary test in a patient with suspected heart failure and is usually abnormal. The ECG will document the patient's baseline rhythm or underlying arrhythmia. Findings suggestive of heart failure include dyssynchrony with left bundle-branch block (LBBB), left ventricular hypertrophy (LVH), and evidence of ischemia or myocardial infarction.

A chest radiograph is useful to characterize cardiac chamber size, evaluate for pulmonary edema, and detect other causes of shortness of breath, such as pneumonia or chronic obstructive pulmonary disease. However, approximately 1 in 5 patients presenting with heart failure will lack evidence of congestion on chest radiograph, and a normal chest radiograph does not exclude heart failure.[14]

A comprehensive 2-dimensional echocardiography with Doppler is the most useful test for a patient with suspected heart failure and risk factors such as prior myocardial infarction, valvular disease, atrial arrhythmias, abnormal ECG findings such as LVH or LBBB or cardiomegaly on chest radiograph, or in the setting of newly diagnosed heart failure. Echocardiography with Doppler is recommended to characterize ventricular function, chamber size and wall thickness, wall motion, and interrogate valve function.

Current heart failure management guidelines indicate the main role for measuring BNP or N terminal pro b-type NP (NT-proBNP) is to support the diagnosis of heart failure when clinical uncertainty exists.[4,13] ProBNP is released from cardiomyocytes in response to increased left ventricular (LV) wall stretch, which is then subsequently cleaved into active BNP and inactive NT-proBNP fragment. BNP and NT-proBNP values appear to correlate reasonably well. Lower values of these peptides exclude the presence of heart failure; whereas, elevated values carry a high positive predictive value for the diagnosis of heart failure. Using a cutoff value for BNP of 100 pg/mL in patients presenting with acute dyspnea to the emergency department enrolled in the Breathing-Not-Properly Study, the sensitivity was 90%, specificity 76%, and diagnostic accuracy was 83% for heart failure.[19] With BNP levels less than 50 pg/mL, the negative predictive value was 96%. NT-proBNP has similar diagnostic accuracy for heart failure. In the PRIDE (ProBNP Investigation of Dyspnea in the

Emergency Department) study, NT-proBNP levels greater than 450 pg/mL in patients older than 50 years, greater than 900 pg/mL for patients 50 to 74 years, and greater than 1800 pg/mL in patients older than 75 years were sensitive and specific for diagnosing heart failure. NT-proBNP level less than 300 pg/mL has a very high negative predictive valve (99%) for ruling out heart failure.[20] BNP and NT-proBNP values are useful diagnostically for patients with heart failure and preserved EF. Important caveats about BNP testing to be aware of are BNP values increase with age, are lower in obese patients, and can be elevated in other cardiac and noncardiac conditions.[21]

Coronary artery disease (CAD) resulting in myocardial ischemia and infarction is a common cause of heart failure in patients with reduced as well as preserved cardiac function and should be excluded whenever possible. Based on current ACC/AHA guidelines for patients presenting with heart failure who have a history of CAD but no angina, noninvasive imaging with stress testing should be considered to rule out ischemia.[4] Coronary angiography is indicated to evaluate for occlusive CAD and potential revascularization in patients with heart failure presenting with angina or evidence of ischemia.[4]

## DIFFERENTIAL DIAGNOSIS

Patients with acute decompensated heart failure most commonly present with symptoms of worsening dyspnea and fatigue indicative of congestion. Given that shortness of breath and fatigue are not specific to heart failure, it is important to consider a broad differential diagnosis during the evaluation phase (**Box 1**). Acute respiratory distress syndrome and noncardiogenic pulmonary edema may have similar radiographic findings on chest radiograph. Elderly patients with multiple comorbidities, including diabetes, hypertension, and kidney disease, may be symptomatic due to lung disease such as chronic obstructive pulmonary disease, pneumonia, or anemia. Acute pulmonary embolism must be considered in the differential, as immobility and venous stasis seen in the patient with decompensated heart failure can predispose to thromboembolic events.

---

**Box 1**
**Differential diagnosis of symptoms and signs of heart failure**

- Coronary artery disease
- Pneumonia
- Chronic obstructive pulmonary disease
- Asthma exacerbation
- Acute respiratory distress syndrome
- Pulmonary hypertension
- Pulmonary embolus
- Anemia
- Cirrhosis
- Renal failure and nephrotic syndrome
- Thyroid disease
- Deconditioning

## MANAGEMENT

The overall management of acute heart failure focuses on addressing precipitating factors, relieving congestion, and optimizing forward cardiac output. Common precipitating factors include dietary indiscretion, nonadherence to medication, pneumonia, acute coronary syndromes, arrhythmias, uncontrolled hypertension, and worsening renal function. Physicians and patients must be aware of commonly used medications that can precipitate acute heart failure and these should be avoided (**Box 2**).[22] Nonsteroidal anti-inflammatory drugs increase sodium and water retention, decrease diuretic responsiveness, and are associated with increased cardiovascular event rates. Nondihydropyridine calcium channel blockers, diltiazem, and verapamil, due to their negative inotropic effects, can worsen heart failure and should not be used in the patients with reduced EF. If needed for blood pressure control, amlodipine is a safe alternative in patients with reduced EF.[23]

The evaluation of a patient with acute heart failure should focus on determining end-organ perfusion and degree of volume overload based on symptoms and physical examination findings. These are used to guide management decisions and provide important prognostic information (see **Fig. 2**). Patients may present with acute decompensated heart failure to the outpatient clinic. The treating physician must decide if further treatment can be safely continued on an outpatient basis or whether the patient should be referred to the emergency room for admission. Key clinical factors that would suggest outpatient management is safe include patients with a known history of heart failure presenting with mild congestion, adequate perfusion, stable vital signs, and lack of significant symptoms. Such patients can usually be treated by augmentation of their outpatient oral diuretic regimen and optimization of their vasodilator medications, with close outpatient follow-up. However, previously undiagnosed patients with decompensated heart failure, unstable vital signs, significant symptoms, acute coronary syndrome, unstable arrhythmias, nonadherence to outpatient medical regimen, and lack of response to outpatient oral diuretics should be considered for hospital admission[13] (**Box 3**). Furthermore, treating patients with acute heart failure in heart failure observation units may be an option for uncomplicated patients presenting with volume overload.[24]

---

**Box 2**
**Medications to avoid in patients with heart failure**

- Steroids
- Nonsteroidal anti-inflammatory drugs
- Nondihydropyridine calcium channel blockers (verapamil and diltiazem)
- Metformin
- Thiazolidinediones
- Amphetamines
- Tricyclic antidepressants
- Carbamazepine
- Itraconazole
- Ephedrine and pseudoephedrine
- Herbals: Ma huang, Yohimbe bark, licorice

---

**Box 3**
**Clinical factors that guide decision for hospitalization in acute heart failure**

- Newly diagnosed, symptomatic heart failure
- Significant dyspnea, pulmonary edema due to volume-overload state
- Unstable vital signs
- Worsening end-organ function (kidney, liver)
- Lack of response to outpatient diuretic regimen
- Acute coronary syndrome
- Recurrent defibrillator shocks
- New or unstable arrhythmias

---

## DIURETIC THERAPY

Diuretics are the cornerstone of therapy in acute heart failure for relief of congestion. In the outpatient setting, oral diuretics are either initiated or the maintenance dose increased with a goal to increase urine output and improve symptoms. If hospitalized for heart failure, first-line diuretic therapy is the intravenous loop diuretics, furosemide or bumetanide. Oral torsemide, another loop diuretic, may be considered in cases of poor diuretic absorption or resistance to other high-dose loop diuretics in the setting of right-sided heart failure. Ethacrynic acid, a sulfa-free loop diuretic, can be used for patients with severe sulfa allergies in whom cross-reactivity is a concern. Combining a loop diuretic with a thiazide diuretic, such as oral metolazone or intravenous (IV) chlorthalidone, should be considered in patients with an inadequate diuretic response to loop diuretics. Careful monitoring of serum electrolytes is required due to the risk of significant electrolytes losses in patients on diuretic therapy especially when thiazide and loop diuretics are used concomitantly.[25] In addition to diuretic therapy, fluid restriction (<2 L per day) and low-salt diet (<1.5 g/d) are important to assist diuresis and maintain diuretic responsiveness.

## ULTRAFILTRATION

Ultrafiltration (UF) is an extracorporeal, portable fluid removal device that can remove an adjustable amount of isotonic fluid via hydrostatic pressure forced across a semipermeable filter membrane. This device requires central IV access, trained personnel, and inpatient hospitalization and is expensive. Fluid removal rate is generally in the range of 100 to 500 mL/h with little effect on serum electrolytes.[26] Ultrafiltration may be considered for patients refractory to high-dose loop diuretic therapy who remain significantly volume overloaded.[27]

## NEUROHORMONAL INHIBITION

Upregulation of the sympathetic nervous system and renin-angiotensin-aldosterone system initially are compensatory mechanisms by which cardiac output and blood pressure are maintained at the onset of heart failure. Over time, continued activation of these systems leads to abnormal cardiac remodeling, cardiac fibrosis, and progressive heart failure.

Patients presenting with acute heart failure should be continued on their guideline-directed medical therapy when hospitalized, unless contraindicated. Published data have shown that patients who are continued on their outpatient beta-blocker therapy have superior outcomes in terms of clinical improvement of heart failure and lower mortality compared with patients whose beta-blocker dose was reduced or discontinued.[28,29] Beta-blockers should be discontinued in the setting of cardiogenic shock, hypotension, or advanced heart block. Patients with newly diagnosed systolic heart failure should be started on a low-dose, evidence-based beta-blocker (metoprolol succinate, carvedilol, or bisoprolol) after stabilization, once euvolemia is achieved, and ideally before discharge.[30]

ACE inhibitors that inhibit the renin-angiotensin hormonal axis are first-line therapy for patients with symptomatic heart failure and reduced EF. Clinical trials have demonstrated that ACE inhibitors improve symptoms, decrease risk of hospitalization, and reduce mortality in this cohort of patients.[31] Results from the CONSENSUS trial demonstrated that initiation of the ACE inhibitor, enalapril, during acute heart failure was safe and effective in improving heart failure symptoms and reducing mortality in hospitalized patients.[32] Angiotensin receptor blocker (ARB) medications should be used if patients develop a cough or angioedema with ACE inhibitors. These medications also should be initiated at low dosage and up-titrated carefully depending on renal function, serum potassium, and blood pressure response. The aldosterone antagonists, spironolactone and eplerenone, are also an important component of the guideline-directed medical regimen for patients with symptomatic heart failure and reduced EF. When added to beta-blocker therapy and renin-angiotensin inhibitors, aldosterone receptor antagonists improve heart failure functional status, risk of hospitalization, and reduce mortality.[33,34] Patients presenting with worsening renal function or hyperkalemia may require temporary cessation of ACE inhibitors, ARBs, and aldosterone receptor antagonists until kidney function improves and electrolyte abnormalities normalize.

## TRANSITION TO THE INPATIENT SETTING

As previously discussed, patients should be considered for hospitalization if they remain highly symptomatic due to volume overload and have failed a trial of oral diuretics, have unstable vital signs or acute coronary syndrome, or possess complex comorbidities that would make outpatient acute heart failure management challenging. The following sections highlight important advanced medical therapy options and rationale for invasive hemodynamic monitoring and noninvasive ventilation that may be considered in patients presenting with severe acute decompensated heart failure.

## INTRAVENOUS VASODILATORS AND INOTROPIC THERAPY

Intravenous vasodilators (nitroglycerine, nitroprusside, and nesiritide) have beneficial hemodynamic effects in acutely decompensated heart failure, such as lowering blood pressure in hypertensive patients reducing systemic vascular resistance, and improving cardiac output. Frequent monitoring of blood pressure is required when using these agents. These agents may be considered for rapid relief of dyspnea and congestion in hospitalized patients, particularly if hypertensive. Nitroglycerin activates guanylyl cyclase, increasing intracellular cyclic guanosine monophosphate levels, reducing LV filling pressures and dyspnea. Headache is a common side effect, and patients may develop tachyphylaxis within 24 hours of administration. Sodium nitroprusside breaks down to nitric oxide and acts as a potent vasodilator decreasing preload and afterload. Caution is advised when using nitroprusside in patients with renal dysfunction because of the elevated risk of thiocyanate toxicity. Nesiritide, a recombinant form of human BNP that reduces LV filling pressures through vasodilatory properties, did not have a significant impact on heart failure symptoms, hospitalization, or survival in patients with acute heart failure in the Acute Study of Clinical Effectiveness of Nesiritide and Decompensated Heart Failure (ASCEND-HF) and Renal Optimization Strategies Evaluation in Acute Heart Failure (ROSE-AHF) studies.[35–37] Because of the lack of benefit seen in these trials, nesiritide should not be routinely used in the management of acute heart failure but considered only when alternative strategies fail.

Patients with reduced EF and low cardiac output state manifested by poor perfusion and end-organ dysfunction should be considered for inotrope therapy (milrinone or dobutamine). Inotropes augment LV contractility and increase cardiac output resulting in the reduction of filling pressures and improving end-organ perfusion. Dobutamine, a beta-1 receptor agonist, acts directly on the cardiomyocyte, stimulating LV contraction and increasing myocardial work that can predispose to arrhythmias and precipitate coronary ischemia. Milrinone, a phosphodiesterase inhibitor, increases intracellular levels of cyclic adenosine monophosphate (cAMP) leading to vasodilation and increased cardiac output. If the patient is already on a beta-blocker, milrinone is the preferred inotrope to use because it would not interfere with beta-blocker therapy. Despite the short-term hemodynamic benefits of inotropic therapy, data from the Outcomes of a Prospective Trial of Intravenous. Milrinone for Exacerbations of Chronic Heart Failure (OPTIME-CHF) study demonstrated that the routine use of milrinone in decompensated heart failure did not reduce days in hospital or mortality rate. Atrial arrhythmias and hypotension occurred more often in the milrinone-treated patients.[38] These agents are not recommended for the routine management of decompensated heart failure and are generally only for short-term use when other treatments are ineffective.[39]

## INVASIVE HEMODYNAMIC MONITORING WITH PULMONARY ARTERY CATHETER

In select cases of acute heart failure when volume status is difficult to assess, with worsening symptoms or end-organ function, hypotension, or inadequate response to diuretic therapy, invasive hemodynamic monitoring can be considered to guide management. A pulmonary artery catheter is inserted usually through the internal jugular vein and direct measurements of intracardiac pressures, cardiac output, pulmonary vascular resistance, and peripheral vascular resistance are performed. Of note, based on the results from the Evaluation Study of Congestive Heart Failure and Pulmonary Artery Catheterization Effectiveness (ESCAPE) trial, the routine use of invasive hemodynamic monitoring in decompensated heart failure is not advised because it did not improve mortality or length of hospital stay compared with clinical assessment.[40]

## NONINVASIVE MECHANICAL VENTILATION

The cause of dyspnea in acutely decompensated heart failure is increased left-sided filling pressures leading to pulmonary congestion. Supplemental oxygen and noninvasive positive pressure ventilation (NIPPV) should be used in patients to help relieve symptoms and hypoxemia and in the case of NIPPV, reduce pulmonary edema and increased work of breathing. NIPPV has been shown to improve dyspnea, heart rate, and hypercapnea in acute cardiogenic pulmonary edema.[41] Patients with significant pulmonary edema and hypoxia may require mechanical ventilation until pulmonary congestion has resolved.

## REFERRAL TO HEART FAILURE SPECIALIST

Management of acute decompensated heart failure provides an opportunity to establish appropriate follow-up care, connect the patient with resources to ensure

---

**Box 4**
**Clinical characteristics that define advanced heart failure**

- Severely reduced left ventricular ejection fraction less than 30%
- Heart failure hospitalization in the past 6 months
- Significant shortness of breath or fatigue with minimal activity or at rest
- Intolerance to angiotensin-converting enzyme inhibitor/angiotensin receptor blocker/beta-blocker therapy due to hypotension and fatigue
- Dependence on high-dose loop diuretic (ie, Lasix >160 mg daily)
- Persistent symptoms despite cardiac resynchronization therapy and optimal medical therapy
- Worsening renal function
- Chronic hyponatremia
- Severely limited functional capacity based on 6-minute walk test (<300 m) or cardiopulmonary exercise test (peak $Vo_2$ <12 mL/kg/min)
- Frequent defibrillator shocks

*Adapted from* Russell S, Miller L, Pagani F. Advanced heart failure: a call to action. Congest Heart Fail 2008;14(6):319; with permission.

---

compliance, and encourage lifestyle changes that will optimize the chance for stabilization and improvement over time. Patients with "advanced heart failure," defined by severely reduced EF (EF <30%), hypotension, inability to tolerate evidence-based medical therapy, limited functional capacity, persistent symptoms during routine daily activity, poor nutritional status, and recurrent hospitalizations for heart failure portend a poor prognosis. These patients should be referred to a heart failure specialist for further evaluation and consideration for heart transplantation and/or mechanical circulatory assist device therapy (**Box 4**).[42]

## SUMMARY

Acute heart failure is a clinical syndrome marked by the development of shortness of breath secondary to increased left heart filling pressures from either reduced EF or impaired diastolic filling abnormalities. Hospitalization for acute heart failure is an indicator for increased morbidity and mortality. A thorough patient history and clinical examination are essential for the identification of risk factors, etiology of heart failure, and to define the degree of fluid overload and end-organ perfusion that will guide management decisions. Key diagnostic tests in a patient presenting with acute heart failure include a baseline assessment of cardiac structure and function with echocardiography and either stress testing or coronary angiography to define the degree of CAD. Treatment is focused on volume removal with diuretics and additional agents may be required for low cardiac output state. The long-term management goals include optimization of oral medical therapy and patient education on disease management that include compliance, proper dieting, and weight monitoring with the overall objectives to reduce heart failure symptoms, the risk of hospitalization, and improve survival.

## REFERENCES

1. Djousse L, Driver JA, Gaziano JM. Relation between modifiable lifestyle factors and lifetime risk of heart failure. JAMA 2009;302:394–400.

2. Roger VL. Epidemiology of heart failure. Circ Res 2013;113:646–59.
3. Lloyd-Jones D, Adams RJ, Brown TM, et al. Heart disease and stroke statistics—2010 update: a report from the American Heart Association. Circulation 2010;121:e46–215.
4. Yancy CW, Jessup M, Bozkurt B, et al. 2013 ACCF/AHA guideline for the management of heart failure: a report of the American College of Cardiology Foundation/American Heart Association Task Force on Practice Guidelines. J Am Coll Cardiol 2013;62:147–239.
5. Jessup M, Brozena S. Heart failure. N Engl J Med 2003;348:2007–18.
6. Daniels LB, Maisel AS. Natriuretic peptides. J Am Coll Cardiol 2007;50:2357–68.
7. Potter LR, Abbey-Hosch S, Dickey DM. Natriuretic peptides, their receptors, and cyclic guanosine monophosphate-dependent signaling functions. Endocr Rev 2006;27:47–72.
8. Potter LR. Natriuretic peptide metabolism, clearance and degradation. FEBS J 2011;278:1808–17.
9. McMurray J, Packer M, Desai A, et al. Angiotensin–neprilysin inhibition versus enalapril in heart failure. N Engl J Med 2014;371:993–1004.
10. Yancy CW, Jessup M, Bozkurt B, et al. 2016 ACC/AHA/HFSA focused update on new pharmacological therapy for heart failure: an update of the 2013 ACCF/AHA guideline for the management of heart failure: a report of the American College of Cardiology Foundation/American Heart Association Task Force on Clinical Practice Guidelines and the Heart Failure Society of America. J Am Coll Cardiol 2016;68:1476–88.
11. Rich MW. Heart failure in the 21st century: a cardiogeriatric syndrome. J Gerontol A Biol Sci Med Sci 2001;56:M88–96.
12. Bui A, Horwich T, Fonarow G. Epidemiology and risk profile of heart failure. Nat Rev Cardiol 2011;8:30–41.
13. Lindenfeld J, Albert NM, Boehmer JP, et al. Executive summary: HFSA 2010 comprehensive heart failure practice guideline. J Card Fail 2010;16:475–539.
14. Stevenson LW, Perloff JK. The limited reliability of physical signs for estimating hemodynamics in chronic heart failure. JAMA 1989;261:884–8.
15. Drazner MH, Hellkamp AS, Leier CV, et al. Value of clinician assessment of hemodynamics in advanced heart failure: the ESCAPE trial. Circ Heart Fail 2008;1(3):170–7.
16. Drazner MH, Rame JE, Stevenson LW, et al. Prognostic importance of elevated jugular venous pressure and a third heart sound in patients with heart failure. N Engl J Med 2001;345:574–81.
17. Forrester JS, Diamond G, Chatterjee K, et al. Medical therapy of acute myocardial infarction by application of hemodynamic subsets (second of two parts). N Engl J Med 1976;295:1404–13.
18. Nohria A, Tsang SW, Fang JC, et al. Clinical assessment identifies hemodynamic profiles that predict outcomes in patients admitted with heart failure. J Am Coll Cardiol 2003;41:1797–804.
19. Maisel AS, Krishnaswamy P, Nowak RM, et al. Rapid measurement of B-type natriuretic peptide in the emergency diagnosis of heart failure. N Engl J Med 2002;347:161–7.
20. Januzzi JL Jr, Camargo CA, Anwaruddin S, et al. The N-terminal Pro-BNP investigation of dyspnea in the emergency department (PRIDE) study. Am J Cardiol 2005;95:948–54.

21. Tang WH, Francis GS, Morrow DA, et al. National Academy of Clinical Biochemistry Laboratory Medicine practice guidelines: clinical utilization of cardiac biomarker testing in heart failure. Circulation 2007;116:99–109.
22. Amabile C, Spencer A. Keeping your patient with heart failure safe: a review of potentially dangerous medications. Arch Intern Med 2004;164:709–20.
23. Packer M, O'Connor C, Ghali J, et al. Effect of amlodipine on morbidity and mortality in severe chronic heart failure. N Engl J Med 1996;335:1107–14.
24. Fermann G, Collins S. Observation units in the management of acute heart failure syndromes. Curr Heart Fail Rep 2010;7:125–33.
25. Jentzer J, DeWald T, Hernandez A. Combination of loop diuretics with thiazide-type diuretics in heart failure. J Am Coll Cardiol 2010;56:1527–34.
26. Bourge R, Tallaj J. Ultrafiltration: a new approach toward mechanical diuresis in heart failure. J Am Coll Cardiol 2005;46:2052–3.
27. Fonarow G, Abraham W, Albert N, et al. Influence of beta-blocker continuation or withdrawal on outcomes in patients hospitalized with heart failure findings from the OPTIMIZE-HF program. J Am Coll Cardiol 2008;52:190–9.
28. Metra M, Torp-Pedersen C, Cleland J, et al. Should beta-blocker therapy be reduced or withdrawn after an episode of decompensated heart failure? Results from COMET. Eur J Heart Fail 2007;9:901–9.
29. Yilmaz M, Laribi S, Mebazaa A. Managing beta-blockers in acute heart failure: when to start and when to stop? Curr Heart Fail Rep 2010;7:110–5.
30. Effect of enalapril on survival in patients with reduced left ventricular ejection fractions and congestive heart failure. The SOLVD Investigators. N Engl J Med 1991; 325:293–302.
31. Effects of enalapril on mortality in severe congestive heart failure. Results of the Cooperative North Scandinavian Enalapril Survival Study (CONSENSUS). The CONSENSUS Trial Study Group. N Engl J Med 1987;316:1429–35.
32. Pitt B, Zannad F, Remme W, et al. The effect of spironolactone on morbidity and mortality in patients with severe heart failure: randomized Aldactone Evaluation Study Investigators. N Engl J Med 1999;34:709–17.
33. Zannad F, McMurray JJ, Krum H, et al. Eplerenone in patients with systolic heart failure and mild symptoms. N Engl J Med 2011;364:11–21.
34. Bart B, Goldsmith S, Lee K, et al. Ultrafiltration in decompensated heart failure with cardiorenal syndrome. N Engl J Med 2012;367:2296–304.
35. O'Connor C, Starling R, Hernandez A, et al. Effect of nesiritide in patients with acute decompensated heart failure. N Engl J Med 2011;365:32–43.
36. Gottlieb SS, Stebbins A, Voors AA, et al. Effects of nesiritide and predictors of urine output in acute decompensated heart failure: results from ASCEND-HF (Acute Study of Clinical Effectiveness of Nesiritide and Decompensated Heart Failure). J Am Coll Cardiol 2013;62:1177–83.
37. Chen HH, Anstrom KJ, Givertz MM, et al. Low-dose dopamine or low-dose nesiritide in acute heart failure with renal dysfunction: the ROSE acute heart failure randomized trial. JAMA 2013;310:2533–43.
38. Cuffe MS, Califf RM, Adams KF Jr, et al. Short-term intravenous milrinone for acute exacerbation of chronic heart failure: a randomized controlled trial. JAMA 2002;287:1541–7.
39. Mebazaa A, Parissis J, Porcher R, et al. Short-term survival by treatment among patients hospitalized with acute heart failure: the global ALARM-HF registry using propensity scoring methods. Intensive Care Med 2010;37:290–301.
40. Binanay C, Califf RM, Hasselblad V, ESCAPE Investigators and ESCAPE Study Coordinators. Evaluation study of congestive heart failure and

pulmonary artery catheterization effectiveness: The ESCAPE trial. JAMA 2005; 294:1625–33.

41. Gray A, Goodacre S, Newby D, et al. Noninvasive ventilation in acute cardiogenic pulmonary edema. N Engl J Med 2008;359:142–51.

42. Russell S, Miller L, Pagani F. Advanced heart failure: a call to action. Congest Heart Fail 2008;14:316–21.

# Outpatient Emergencies
## Anaphylaxis

Scott P. Commins, MD, PhD[a,b],*

## KEYWORDS

- IgE • Mast cell • Allergy • Tryptase • Anaphylaxis

## KEY POINTS

- Anaphylaxis is a severe allergic reaction that can be rapidly progressive and fatal. If the triggering allergen is unknown, establishing the etiology is pivotal to long-term risk management.
- There is no current diagnostic test that adequately predicts the severity of the next episode of anaphylaxis: mild events can be followed by life-threatening reactions.
- Medications and insect stings are the most common causes of anaphylaxis in adults, whereas foods are more common in children.
- Administer epinephrine intramuscularly in the mid-outer thigh and remove the inciting allergen, if possible.
- Quickly assess airway, breathing, circulation, and mentation, and summon appropriate assistance; if needed, cardiopulmonary resuscitation and summon emergency medical services.

## INTRODUCTION

Anaphylaxis is a life-threatening reaction with respiratory, cardiovascular, cutaneous, or gastrointestinal manifestations resulting from exposure to an offending agent, usually a food, insect sting, medication, or physical factor. It causes approximately 1500 deaths in the United States annually.[1,2] Occasionally, anaphylaxis can be confused with septic or other forms of shock, asthma, airway foreign body, panic attack, or other entities.[3–5] Urinary and serum histamine levels and plasma tryptase levels drawn after the onset of symptoms may assist in diagnosis as well as assessment of platelet

[a] Division of Rheumatology, Allergy and Immunology, Department of Medicine, Thurston Research Center, University of North Carolina, 3300 Thurston Building, CB 7280, Chapel Hill, NC 27599-7280, USA; [b] Division of Rheumatology, Allergy and Immunology, Department of Pediatrics, Thurston Research Center, University of North Carolina, 3300 Thurston Building, CB 7280, Chapel Hill, NC 27599-7280, USA
* Division of Rheumatology, Allergy and Immunology, Department of Medicine, Thurston Research Center, University of North Carolina, 3300 Thurston Building, CB 7280, Chapel Hill, NC 27599-7280.
E-mail address: scommins@email.unc.edu

Med Clin N Am 101 (2017) 521–536
http://dx.doi.org/10.1016/j.mcna.2016.12.003
0025-7125/17/© 2017 Elsevier Inc. All rights reserved.

activating factor.[3,6,7] Prompt treatment of anaphylaxis is critical, with intramuscular epinephrine, recumbent positioning, and intravenous fluids remaining the mainstays of acute management.[4,8] Adjunctive measures include airway protection, antihistamines, glucocorticoids, and beta-agonists.[4] Patients should be observed for delayed or protracted anaphylaxis and instructed on how to initiate urgent treatment for future episodes.[9,10]

A significant portion of the US population is at risk for anaphylaxis and these reactions are underrecognized and frequently undertreated.[2,11] Anaphylaxis is mediated by immunoglobulin E (IgE), whereas anaphylactoid reactions are not.[4] Because of their clinical similarities, the term anaphylaxis is used to refer to both conditions herein. In keeping with the theme of this collection, we focus on aspects of anaphylaxis primarily related to outpatient emergencies: symptoms, treatment, and management with less discussion devoted to diagnostic testing and consideration of differential diagnosis.

## SYMPTOMS

Anaphylaxis may include any combination of common signs and symptoms (**Table 1**).[4] Cutaneous manifestations of anaphylaxis, including urticaria and angioedema, are by far the most common, occurring in 62% to 90% of reported cases.[12] Nonetheless, the absence of cutaneous symptoms speaks against a diagnosis of anaphylaxis but does not rule it out. Severe episodes characterized by rapid cardiovascular collapse and shock can occur without cutaneous manifestations.[13] The respiratory system is also involved commonly, producing symptoms such as dyspnea, wheezing, and upper airway obstruction from edema.[12] Gastrointestinal manifestations (eg, nausea, vomiting, diarrhea, abdominal pain) and cardiovascular manifestations (eg, dizziness, syncope, hypotension) affect about one-third of patients.[14] Headache, rhinitis, substernal pain, pruritus, and seizure occur less frequently.[12] In addition, anaphylaxis can present with unusual manifestations, such as syncope, without any further sign or symptom.[15] The essentials of the history are listed in **Box 1**.

Symptom onset varies widely, but generally occurs within seconds or minutes of exposure.[2,5] A novel IgE antibody to a mammalian oligosaccharide has been

| Table 1 Signs and symptoms of anaphylaxis | |
|---|---|
| **Signs and Symptoms** | **Frequency (%)** |
| Urticaria, angioedema | 60–90 |
| Upper airway edema | 50–60 |
| Flush | 45–55 |
| Dyspnea, wheeze | 45–50 |
| Dizziness, syncope, hypotension | 30–35 |
| Nausea, vomiting, diarrhea, cramping abdominal pain | 25–35 |
| Rhinitis | 15–20 |
| Headache | 10–15 |
| Chest pain | 3–7 |
| Pruritus without rash | 2–5 |
| Palmar erythema and pruritus[a] | 35–45 |

[a] Specifically related to patients with IgE to galactose-alpha-1,3-galactose mammalian meat allergy.
Data from Refs.[2,4,12,14,51]

---

**Box 1**
**Pertinent history taking in evaluation of a patient presenting with anaphylaxis**

- Detailed history of ingestants (foods, drinks/medications) taken within 8 h before the event
- Activity in which the patient was engaged at the time of the event
- Location of the event (home, school, work, indoors/outdoors)
- Exposure to heat or cold
- Any related sting or bite (significant tick or chigger bites within prior 4 weeks)
- Time of day or night
- Duration of event
- Recurrence of symptoms after initial resolution
- Exact nature of symptoms (eg, if cutaneous, determine whether flush, pruritus, urticaria, or angioedema)
- In a woman, the relation between the event and her menstrual cycle
- Was medical care given and what treatments were administered
- How long before recovery occurred and was there a recurrence of symptoms after a symptom-free period
- The perceived level of stress by the patient before the episode
- Any recent illness or infection
- Pertinent travel history
- Description of any prior similar episodes
- Return of mild symptoms with exposure to heat, exercise or alcohol ingestion

*Adapted from* Lieberman P, Nicklas RA, Randolph C, et al. Anaphylaxis—a practice parameter update 2015. Ann Allergy Asthma Immunol 2015;115(5):353; with permission.

---

discovered that is associated with 2 distinct forms of anaphylaxis, an immediate onset of an event to cetuximab and a delayed onset of anaphylaxis, usually occurring 3 to 6 hours after the ingestion of mammalian food products (eg, beef and pork).[16,17] This red meat allergy has been associated with tick bites and seems to have significant and expanding regional prevalence in the southern and eastern United States.[18] Anaphylaxis can be protracted, lasting for more than 24 hours, or recur after initial resolution.[10]

## OUTPATIENT-BASED TREATMENT

Plan for appropriate office response to anaphylaxis by (1) educating staff and patients, (2) preparing an anaphylaxis emergency cart (**Box 2**), and (3) developing an office action plan for anaphylaxis management to maintain proficiency in anaphylaxis management.[4] At the onset of anaphylaxis, (1) administer epinephrine intramuscularly in the mid outer thigh, (2) remove the inciting allergen, if possible (eg, stop an infusion), (3) quickly assess airway, breathing, circulation, and mentation and summon appropriate assistance from staff members, and (4) start, if needed, cardiopulmonary resuscitation and summon emergency medical services (EMS).[4] After administering epinephrine, notify EMS for patients having severe anaphylaxis and/or patients not responding to epinephrine.

---

**Box 2**
**Essential elements in an outpatient office-based emergency cart to treat anaphylaxis**

Stethoscope and sphygmomanometer

Tourniquets

Syringes

IV catheters (eg, 14–18 gauge)

Aqueous epinephrine HCL (1:1000 w/v) or equivalent autoinjectable epinephrine device

Airway support devices (eg, endotracheal tubes, resuscitator bag)

Portable oxygen supply

Oral and injectable antihistamines (both $H_1$ and $H_2$)

Corticosteroids for intramuscular or intravenous injection

Ammonia inhalant pad or breakable capsule

Intravenous fluids (eg, saline)

Glucagon kit for patients on beta-blockers

Also suggested: infusion pump, external defibrillator

---

Apart from the administration of medications, it is important to remember to place and maintain patients in a supine position, unless the respiratory compromise contraindicates it, to prevent or to counteract potential circulatory collapse.[4] Place pregnant patients on their left side. As soon as possible after administering epinephrine and appropriate positioning, establishing intravenous access is essential for maintaining hemodynamic stability. Consider initiating supplemental oxygen to select patients in anaphylaxis. Rapid and ongoing assessment of the patient's airway status should be made a priority, and maintaining airway patency using the least invasive but effective method (eg, bag-valve-mask).[4,19] Intravenous fluid replacement should be initiated with normal saline for patients with circulatory collapse and for patients who do not respond to intramuscular epinephrine.[8,20] In addition to epinephrine administered for anaphylaxis, consider administering a nebulized beta$_2$-agonist (eg, albuterol) for signs and symptoms of bronchospasm.[4] In patients receiving beta-adrenergic blocking agents, administer glucagon if they have not responded to epinephrine.[21]

Administration of $H_1$ and $H_2$ antihistamines or corticosteroids should not replace epinephrine as initial therapy for anaphylaxis.[8] In fact, these agents are considered optional or adjunctive therapy. Individualize the duration of direct observation and monitoring after anaphylaxis but provide longer periods of observation for those patients with a history of risk factors for severe anaphylaxis (eg, asthma, previous biphasic reactions, or protracted anaphylaxis) for at least 4 to 8 hours or initiate transfer of such patients via EMS as soon as possible.[9,10]

Staff and patients must recognize that any significant change in clinical status or the onset or increase of symptoms, however subtle, which occurs immediately after in-office immunotherapy or diagnostic or therapeutic procedures, or possible ingestion of a known food or medication allergen, should be considered anaphylaxis.[11] Anaphylaxis must be viewed as a serious allergic reaction that is rapid in onset and may cause death for which the only treatment is epinephrine.[8,9] The anaphylaxis cart (see **Box 2**) must be inventoried on a regular basis (eg, every 3 months) and kept up to date by using the detailed listing of medications, supplies, and equipment as a checklist.

All practice settings where there is a risk for anaphylaxis should collaborate with their nursing staff to develop a customized written protocol for the management of anaphylaxis in the office. Several action plans for anaphylaxis management in the office setting have been published and a revised office-based anaphylaxis treatment protocol is presented in **Table 2**.[4] The anaphylaxis action plan should follow evidence-based guidelines and should provide a detailed stepwise approach based on symptoms and the patient's response to treatment. It can take the form of an algorithm, a table, a graph, or even a combination of these, but it must be easy to read and follow during an emergency.[19] Ideally, it would include assigned roles for each staff member, by position or name, to be followed during anaphylaxis management. Once developed, it should be posted in all patient care areas of the office and with the emergency supplies for ready access. The successful management of anaphylaxis requires that office staff must immediately activate the response team and expeditiously deliver appropriate treatment. This can be accomplished with frequent (eg, periodic), organized, mock anaphylaxis drills in which all staff members, clerical and medical, are required to participate.[19] Maintaining clinical proficiency with anaphylaxis management involves certification in basic cardiopulmonary resuscitation and, ideally, advanced life support to ensure the proper skillset for treatment of refractory anaphylaxis, including airway management, cardiac compressions, venous and intraosseous access, and parental medication calculation and delivery.[19,22]

The initial assessment and treatment of the patient in anaphylaxis involves several critical steps that should be started concomitantly (see **Table 2**).[4,19,22] Urgent treatment is based on the finding that there is often a very short time (eg, 5 minutes for an iatrogenic intravenously administered allergen such as an antibiotic and 30 minutes for food-induced anaphylaxis) from the onset of mild symptoms to respiratory or cardiac arrest.[23–27] Although removal of the inciting allergen is ideal, this will rarely apply in the office setting because parental administration or ingestion will usually have been completed before the onset of symptoms. However, with medication infusions or oral challenges with food or medications, the procedure should be stopped as soon as signs and symptoms of even mild anaphylaxis are noted.[28,29]

The first member of the office staff to recognize that the patient is experiencing anaphylaxis must be prepared to evaluate the airway, breathing, circulation, and mentation.[19] If the patient has moderate to severe anaphylaxis or is showing signs and symptoms of impending cardiopulmonary arrest, EMS must be summoned immediately in addition to all available office medical staff.[4,12] Cardiopulmonary resuscitation should be started immediately in the event of cardiopulmonary arrest, with emphasis on adequate chest compressions without interruption (**Table 3**).[19,22] Ventilations can be given once there are 2 medical staff members at the patient's side.[22]

For imminent or established cardiopulmonary arrest, rapidly establish venous access and administer an intravenous bolus dose of epinephrine because ventricular arrhythmias have been reported after epinephrine administration.[19,22,30] For adults, the dose is 1 mg intravenously (as a 1:10,000 dilution).[31,32] This can be repeated every 3 to 5 minutes as cardiopulmonary resuscitation is continued.[22,31–33] If the intravenous route is not available, epinephrine can be given by endotracheal administration if the advanced airway is in place (adult dose is 2–2.5 mg of 1:1000 diluted in 5–10 mL of sterile water).[19,22] The treatment of anaphylaxis is, at best, based on indirect and observational studies and primarily on consensus.[12] Observational studies and analysis of near-fatal and fatal reactions have shown that prompt and decisive treatment of any systemic reaction, even a mild one, with epinephrine prevents progression to more severe symptoms.[5,34] In contrast, delayed administration of epinephrine is often believed to be the major contributing factor to fatalities.[5,34]

**Table 2**
**Treatment of anaphylaxis in the physician's office**

| Immediate measures | | |
|---|---|---|
| 1 | Allergen | Remove the inciting allergen, if possible |
| 2 | Airway | Assess airway, breathing, circulation, and orientation; if needed, support the airway using the least invasive but effective method (eg, bag-valve-mask) |
| 3 | Cardiopulmonary resuscitation | Start chest compressions (100/min) if cardiovascular arrest occurs at any time |
| 4 | Epinephrine | Inject epinephrine 0.3–0.5 mg intramuscularly in the vastus lateralis (lateral thigh) |
| 5 | Get help | Summon appropriate assistance in office |
| 6 | Position | Place adults and adolescents in recumbent position; place pregnant patient on left side |
| 7a | Oxygen | Give 8–10 L/min through facemask or up to 100% oxygen as needed; monitor by pulse oximetry if available |
| 7b | Epinephrine | Repeat intramuscular epinephrine every 5–15 min for up to 3 injections if the patient is not responding |
| 7c | EMS | Activate EMS (call 911 or local rescue squad) if no immediate response to first dose of IM epinephrine or if anaphylaxis is moderate to severe |
| 7d | IV fluids | Establish intravenous line for venous access and fluid replacement; keep open with 0.9 NL saline, push fluids for hypotension or failure to respond to epinephrine using 5–10 mg/kg as quickly as possible and up to 1–2 L in the first hour |
| Additional measures | | |
| 8 | Albuterol | Consider administration of 2.5–5.0 mg of nebulized albuterol in 3 mL of saline for lower airway obstruction; repeat as necessary every 15 min |
| 9 | Glucagon | Patients on beta-blockers who are not responding to epinephrine should be given 1–5 mg of glucagon IV slowly over 5 min because rapid administration of glucagon can induce vomiting |

| | | |
|---|---|---|
| 10 | Epinephrine (infusion) | For patients with inadequate response to IM epinephrine and IV saline, give epinephrine by continuous infusion by micro-drip in office setting (infusion pump in hospital setting): add 1 mg (1 mL of 1:1000) of epinephrine to 1000 mL of 0.9 NL saline; start infusion at 2 mg/min (2 mL/min = 120 mL/h) and increase up to 10 mg/min (10 mL/min = 600 mL/h); titrate dose continuously according to blood pressure, cardiac rate and function, and oxygenation |
| 11 | Intraosseous access | If IV access is not readily available in patients experiencing refractory anaphylaxis, obtain intraosseous access for administration of IV fluids and epinephrine infusion |

**Refractory anaphylaxis**

| | | |
|---|---|---|
| 12 | Advanced airway management | Use supraglottic airway, endotracheal intubation, or cricothyroidotomy for marked stridor, severe laryngeal edema, or when ventilation using the bag-valve-mask is inadequate and EMS has not arrived |
| 13 | Vasopressors | Consider administration of dopamine (in addition to epinephrine infusion) if patient is unresponsive to above treatment; this will likely be in the hospital setting where cardiac monitoring is available |

**Optional treatment (efficacy not established)**

| | | |
|---|---|---|
| 14 | H₁ antihistamine | Consider giving 25–50 mg of diphenhydramine intravenously; use 10 mg of cetirizine if an oral antihistamine is administered; once there is full recovery, there is no evidence that this medication needs to be continued |
| 15 | Corticosteroids | Administer 1–2 mg/kg up to 125 mg per dose, IV or PO, of methylprednisolone or an equivalent formulation; once there is full recovery, there is no evidence that this medication needs to be continued |

**Observation and monitoring**

| | | |
|---|---|---|
| 16 | Observation in hospital | Transport to emergency department by EMS for further treatment and observation for ~8 h |
| 17 | Observation in office | Observe in office until full recovery + additional 30–60 min for all patients who are not candidates for EMS transport to emergency department |

*(continued on next page)*

**Table 2**
*(continued)*

Discharge management

| | | |
|---|---|---|
| 18 | Education | Educate patient and family on how to recognize and how to treat anaphylaxis |
| 19 | Autoinjectable epinephrine | Prescribe 2 doses of autoinjectable epinephrine for patients who have experienced an anaphylactic reaction and for those at risk for severe anaphylaxis; train patient, patient provider, and family on how to use the autoinjector |
| 20 | Anaphylaxis action plan | Provide patients with an action plan instructing them on how and when to administer epinephrine |

*Abbreviations:* EMS, emergency medical services; IM, intramuscular; IV, intravenous; NL, normal; PO, oral.

*Adapted from* Lieberman P, Nicklas RA, Randolph C, et al. Anaphylaxis—a practice parameter update 2015. Ann Allergy Asthma Immunol 2015;115(5):363; with permission.

**Table 3**
**Summary of adult cardiac life support recommendations**

| | Basic Cardiopulmonary Resuscitation is C-A-B (Compressions-Airway-Breathing) |
|---|---|
| Check for pulse | Take for a maximum of 10 s |
| Chest compressions | Push hard and push fast on the center of the chest<br>• Maintain rate of 100/min<br>• Compress chest 5 cm with each downstroke<br>• Allow complete chest recoil between compressions<br>• Minimize frequency and duration of any interruptions |
| Ventilations | Perform only if ≥2 rescuers are present<br>• Avoid excessive ventilation, just enough to confirm chest rise<br>• Deliver ventilation over 1 s<br>• If 3 rescuers available: 1 for compressions, 2 for bag-valve-mask and rotate positions every 2 min |
| Compression/ventilation ratio | 30/2 |
| Defibrillation | Single defibrillation using highest available energy in adults       Adult: 200 J |
| Phases of resuscitation in cardiac arrest | Electrical phase 0–4 min       Defibrillate, compressions<br>Hemodynamic phase 4–10 min after arrest       Defibrillate, compressions<br>Metabolic phase >10 min after arrest       Few patients survive |

*Data from* Refs.[4,12,19,22]

Anaphylaxis guidelines are in agreement that epinephrine should be administered intramuscularly into the lateral thigh.[4,5,14] Published studies on epinephrine pharmacokinetics in patients not in anaphylaxis have shown that intramuscular administration in the vastus lateralis muscle produces a more rapid rate of increase in blood epinephrine levels than subcutaneous or intramuscular administration in the deltoid muscle.[35,36] Unfortunately, there are no studies evaluating the pharmacokinetics of a subcutaneous injection in the lateral thigh. The adult dose of 1:1000 epinephrine is 0.2 to 0.5 mL, and the pediatric dose is 0.01 mg/kg, with a maximum of 0.3 mg.[19] A higher dose (eg, 0.5 mL) within the recommended dose range should be considered in patients with severe anaphylaxis.[4,12,19] If there has not been significant improvement in symptoms, then the dose can be repeated approximately every 5 to 15 minutes, as the physician deems to be necessary. It has been shown that a repeat dose is required up to 35% of the time.[37,38] Monitor and record the patient's blood pressure, cardiac rate and function, respiratory status, and oxygenation at frequent and regular intervals.[19] Start frequent oxygen saturation measurement, start continuous noninvasive monitoring, and obtain an electrocardiogram, if available.

There is universal agreement that most patients should be placed in a supine position during anaphylaxis.[4,5,12,14,19,39,40] However, whether to elevate the legs is controversial.[4,41,42] Although some guidelines continue to recommend the Trendelenburg position (feet are elevated 15°–30° higher than the head) for the management of shock, the American Heart Association and the American Red Cross in a 2010 consensus document concluded that there is insufficient evidence to support routine use of the Trendelenburg position in patients with shock.[30,43] If the patient is having respiratory difficulty, consider having the patient sit up.[30] In a retrospective study of 10 anaphylactic fatalities, there seemed to be an association with fatality when there was a change in position from a supine to an upright or standing position during anaphylaxis.[44] Although the investigators recommended maintaining a supine position during anaphylaxis, they did not recommend the Trendelenburg position.[44]

Administration of oxygen is the second most important therapeutic intervention, second only to epinephrine administration, for the treatment of anaphylaxis and should be considered for all patients experiencing anaphylaxis regardless of their respiratory status.[4,5,12,14,20,40] It is imperative to administer oxygen for any patient with respiratory or cardiovascular compromise and to patients who do not respond to the initial treatment with epinephrine.[19] Oxygen up to 100% should be administered at a flow rate of 6 to 10 L/min through a facemask. Ideally, oxygen saturation should be monitored and kept at 94% to 96% by oximetry.[19] In most office settings, bag-valve-mask ventilation will be the method of choice to support ventilation in the event of respiratory failure or arrest.[4,12] It is most effective when 2 individuals can support the airway.[22] One person opens the airway with the head-tilt and chin-lift maneuver and seals the mask to the face, covering the nose and mouth.[22] The second person squeezes the bag and the 2 rescuers look for adequate chest rise.[22] It is recommended that approximately 600 mL of tidal volume for 1 second using an adult (1–2 L) bag be delivered.[22,30] Supplementary oxygen at a flow rate of 10 to 12 L/min should be used.[30] Two breaths are delivered during a 3- to 4-s pause after every 30 chest compressions.[22] An oropharyngeal airway can aid in the delivery of adequate ventilation in an unconscious patient with no cough or gag reflex.[30] The training, skill, and experience of the physician should guide the selection of the most appropriate airway for the patient.[22] When the provider can ventilate the patient adequately using the bag-valve-mask, there is no evidence that the use of advanced airway measures improves survival rates of out-of-hospital cardiac arrest.[22,30,43] The incidence of complications is unacceptably high when endotracheal intubation is performed by an inexperienced provider or monitoring of the tube is inadequate.[19] Use of a supraglottic airway (eg, laryngeal mask airway), esophageal tracheal tube (Combitube), or laryngeal tube is believed to be a reasonable alternative to the endotracheal intubation and its use can be accomplished without interruption of chest compressions.[30] Upper airway obstruction (eg, severe laryngeal edema) is an absolute contraindication for endotracheal intubation.[30] It has been suggested that inhaled epinephrine or intratracheally administered epinephrine might decrease oropharyngeal edema, making airway management less difficult.[19] The use of cricothyrotomy should be reserved for life-and-death situations when obstruction (eg, angioedema) above the larynx prevents adequate ventilation, even with the endotracheal tube.[19,41]

Hypotension should be treated with rapid fluid replacement using 1 to 2 L of 0.9% normal saline, infused rapidly (eg, 5–10 mL/kg within the first 5 minutes for an adult and up to 30 mL/kg in the first hour for children).[22,30,45] Large-bore (14- to 16-gauge for adults) intravenous catheters should be used. For the normotensive patient in anaphylaxis, starting normal saline at an appropriate maintenance rate for weight (eg, 125 mL/h for adults) to maintain venous access for medications and/or rapid fluid replacement is often unnecessary.[19] Intravenous administration of epinephrine will rarely be necessary in the office setting and should be administered in a monitored setting with a programmable infusion pump to titrate appropriately.[4,12,19,40] However, if there is no response to multiple injections of intramuscular epinephrine and intravenous fluid replacement in combination with a delay in EMS response, prolonged transport, or cardiopulmonary arrest and resuscitation, then intravenous epinephrine might be needed.[19,30] There is no established dosage or regimen for intravenous epinephrine in anaphylaxis.[4,8,12,20,40] However, a prospective study demonstrated the efficacy of a 1:100,000 solution of epinephrine intravenously by infusion pump at the initial rate of 2 to 10 mg/min titrated up or down depending on the clinical response or epinephrine side effects.[46] If an infusion of epinephrine is started in the office setting, then monitor by available means (eg, every-minute blood pressure and pulse and electrocardiographic monitoring, if available) and be prepared to treat ventricular arrhythmias.[4,12,19,22,30] Other vasopressors (eg, dopamine and vasopressin) have been suggested as alternative agents to epinephrine for treatment of refractory hypotension. However, there are no controlled studies that have evaluated the efficacy of these drugs in the treatment of anaphylaxis.[30,43]

Cases of unusually severe or refractory anaphylaxis (paradoxic bradycardia, profound hypotension, and severe bronchospasm) have been reported in patients receiving beta-adrenergic blockers.[21,47] These systemic effects also have been documented with use of ophthalmic beta-blockers.[48] Greater severity of anaphylaxis observed in patients receiving beta-blockers might relate in part to a blunted response to epinephrine administered to treat anaphylaxis.[4,12] Epinephrine administered to a patient taking a beta-blocker can produce unopposed alpha-adrenergic and reflex vagotonic effects, possibly leading to hypertension and the risk of cerebral hemorrhage.[41] In patients receiving beta-blockers, increased propensity not only for bronchospasm but also for decreased cardiac contractility with perpetuation of hypotension and bradycardia is possible. There are no epidemiologic studies that have indicated that anaphylaxis occurs more frequently in patients receiving beta-blockers.[49,50] Use of selective beta$_1$-antagonists does not lower the risk of anaphylaxis because beta$_1$- and beta$_2$-antagonists can inhibit the beta-adrenergic receptor.[12] If epinephrine is ineffective in treating anaphylaxis in patients taking beta-blockers, then glucagon administration might be necessary. Glucagon can reverse refractory bronchospasm and hypotension during anaphylaxis in patients on beta-blockers by activating adenyl cyclase directly and bypassing the beta-adrenergic receptor. The recommended dosage for glucagon is 1 to 5 mg administered intravenously over 5 minutes and followed by an infusion at 5 to 15 mg/min titrated to clinical response.[4,12,30] Protection of the airway is important because glucagon can cause emesis and risk aspiration in severely drowsy or obtunded patients. Placement in the lateral recumbent position provides sufficient airway protection for most of these patients.[4,12,19]

Antihistamines, $H_1$ and $H_2$, should be considered second-line drugs in the management of anaphylaxis because there is no direct evidence to support their use in the treatment of anaphylaxis.[3–5,12,14,40] The use of the $H_1$ antihistamines is extrapolated mainly from their use in other allergic diseases (eg, urticaria or allergic rhinitis) in which they relieve itching, urticaria, flushing, sneezing, and rhinorrhea.[12] However, they do not prevent or treat upper airway obstruction or hypotension. The frequent and at times fatal error that is made by professionals and patients is to delay the administration of epinephrine while waiting for the antihistamines to relieve symptoms.[8,20,22,39,51–54] When administered as adjunctive treatment for severe anaphylaxis, only sedating antihistamines (eg, diphenhydramine) are available for intravenous administration. The dose for diphenhydramine is 25 to 50 mg in adults administered intravenously over 10 to 15 minutes.[19] When given orally, a low or nonsedating antihistamine (eg, fexofenadine) is preferred over a sedating antihistamine (eg, diphenhydramine or chlorpheniramine) to avoid somnolence, impairment of cognitive function, and a decreased ability to describe symptoms.[19] If administered parentally, then the dose of the $H_2$ antihistamine ranitidine is 1 mg/kg for adults and can be administered intramuscularly or intravenously (with slow infusion) because these administration methods have the same onset of action.[12,19]

The use of corticosteroids has no role in the acute management of anaphylaxis.[22,30] The purported evidence that they produce a decrease of biphasic or prolonged reactions is not supported by strong evidence.[8–10] Their use and dosage are extrapolated from those used for acute asthma. When administered, the intravenous or oral dosage often recommended is 1 to 2 mg/kg per dose up to 125 mg of methylprednisolone or an equivalent formulation.[19] Patients who have complete resolution of symptoms after treatment with epinephrine do not need to be prescribed antihistamines or corticosteroids thereafter.[4]

The duration of direct observation and monitoring after an episode of anaphylaxis must be individualized and based on the severity and duration of the anaphylactic event, response to treatment, pattern of previous anaphylactic reactions (eg, history of protracted or biphasic reactions), medical comorbidities, patient reliability, and access to medical care.[2,4,12,19,20,40] Patients with moderate to severe anaphylaxis should be observed for a minimum of 4 to 8 hours.[4,12,19] Mild anaphylactic symptoms that occur in a medical setting (eg, office-based allergy injection) and that rapidly resolve with treatment usually will require a relatively shorter period of observation. A longer observation, including possible hospital admission, should be considered when (1) risk factors for more severe anaphylaxis (eg, history of severe asthma) are present, (2) the allergens have been ingested, (3) more than 1 dose of epinephrine is required, (4) pharyngeal edema is present, and (5) severe or prolonged symptoms (eg, prolonged wheezing or hypotension) are noted.[4,12,14,19,40,55,56]

## FOLLOW-UP EDUCATION

As in many diseases, patient education is vital; however, owing to the potential for rapidly progressing, life-threatening reactions, proper and through patient education is a critical component in the management of anaphylaxis. Autoinjectable epinephrine should be prescribed for patients who have experienced an anaphylactic reaction and for those at increased risk for anaphylaxis. The patient must be instructed in the administration of epinephrine. Patients should be encouraged to fill this prescription immediately because up to 23% can experience a return of symptoms as a biphasic reaction, usually within 10 hours after the resolution of the presenting symptoms of anaphylaxis.[10] Two autoinjectors should be provided because up to 30% of patients who develop anaphylaxis will require more than 1 dose of epinephrine.[2,8,9,34] In the United States, autoinjectors are available in only 2 doses, 0.15 and 0.30 mg. The preferred adult dose is 0.30 mg. Although the initial anaphylaxis action plan can be provided at the point of care (eg, emergency department or primary care office), the permanent anaphylaxis action plan should be developed by the allergist working with the patient, the primary care physician, other members of the interdisciplinary clinical team, and the school, when appropriate. Education on the triggers and early signs and symptoms of anaphylaxis must be a structured, reoccurring, and scheduled process for all office staff, medical and clerical, and patients. The patient's education on anaphylaxis should start at the time of the new patient visit for all patients who present with signs and symptoms of anaphylaxis and for all patients who will be undergoing a diagnostic or treatment procedure that could result in anaphylaxis (eg, chemotherapy infusion).

### Future Considerations and Summary

Patients with anaphylaxis should be assessed and treated as rapidly as possible, because respiratory or cardiac arrest and death can occur within minutes. Anaphylaxis seems to be most responsive to treatment in its early phases, before shock has developed, based on the observation that delayed epinephrine injection is associated with fatalities. Epinephrine is life-saving in anaphylaxis. It should be injected as early as possible in the episode to prevent progression of symptoms and signs. There are no absolute contraindications to epinephrine use, and it is the treatment of choice for anaphylaxis of any severity. Patients successfully treated for anaphylaxis should be discharged with a personalized written anaphylaxis emergency action plan, an autoinjectable epinephrine, written information about anaphylaxis and its treatment, and a plan for further evaluation. Consultation with an allergist can help to (1) confirm the diagnosis of anaphylaxis, (2) identify the anaphylactic trigger through history, skin testing, and radioallergosorbent test, (3) educate the patient in the prevention and initial treatment of future episodes, and (4) aid in desensitization and pretreatment when indicated as well as, for some allergens, immunomodulation is also available to reduce the risk.[4,12]

## REFERENCES

1. Neugut AI, Ghatak AT, Miller RL. Anaphylaxis in the United States: an investigation into its epidemiology. Arch Intern Med 2001;161(1):15–21.
2. Wood RA, Camargo CA Jr, Lieberman P, et al. Anaphylaxis in America: the prevalence and characteristics of anaphylaxis in the United States. J Allergy Clin Immunol 2014;133(2):461–7.
3. Brown SG, Stone SF, Fatovich DM, et al. Anaphylaxis: clinical patterns, mediator release, and severity. J Allergy Clin Immunol 2013;132(5):1141–9.e5.
4. Lieberman P, Nicklas RA, Randolph C, et al. Anaphylaxis–a practice parameter update 2015. Ann Allergy Asthma Immunol 2015;115(5):341–84.
5. Sampson HA, Munoz-Furlong A, Campbell RL, et al. Second symposium on the definition and management of anaphylaxis: summary report–second National

Institute of Allergy and Infectious Disease/Food Allergy and Anaphylaxis Network symposium. Ann Emerg Med 2006;47(4):373–80.

6. Schwartz LB, Metcalfe DD, Miller JS, et al. Tryptase levels as an indicator of mast-cell activation in systemic anaphylaxis and mastocytosis. N Engl J Med 1987; 316(26):1622–6.

7. Vadas P, Gold M, Perelman B, et al. Platelet-activating factor, PAF acetylhydrolase, and severe anaphylaxis. N Engl J Med 2008;358(1):28–35.

8. Ellis AK, Day JH. The role of epinephrine in the treatment of anaphylaxis. Curr Allergy Asthma Rep 2003;3(1):11–4.

9. Ellis AK. Priority role of epinephrine in anaphylaxis further underscored–the impact on biphasic anaphylaxis. Ann Allergy Asthma Immunol 2015;115(3):165.

10. Ellis AK, Day JH. Incidence and characteristics of biphasic anaphylaxis: a prospective evaluation of 103 patients. Ann Allergy Asthma Immunol 2007;98(1): 64–9.

11. Altman AM, Camargo CA, Simons FE, et al. Anaphylaxis in America: a national physician survey. J Allergy Clin Immunol 2015;135(3):830–3.

12. Lieberman P, Nicklas RA, Oppenheimer J, et al. The diagnosis and management of anaphylaxis practice parameter: 2010 update. J Allergy Clin Immunol 2010; 126(3):477–80.e1-42.

13. Viner NA, Rhamy RK. Anaphylaxis manifested by hypotension alone. J Urol 1975; 113(1):108–10.

14. Sampson HA, Munoz-Furlong A, Bock SA, et al. Symposium on the definition and management of anaphylaxis: summary report. J Allergy Clin Immunol 2005; 115(3):584–91.

15. Valabhji J, Robinson S, Johnston D, et al. Unexplained loss of consciousness: systemic mastocytosis. J R Soc Med 2000;93(3):141–2.

16. Commins SP, Satinover SM, Hosen J, et al. Delayed anaphylaxis, angioedema, or urticaria after consumption of red meat in patients with IgE antibodies specific for galactose-alpha-1,3-galactose. J Allergy Clin Immunol 2009;123(2):426–33.

17. Chung CH, Mirakhur B, Chan E, et al. Cetuximab-induced anaphylaxis and IgE specific for galactose-alpha-1,3-galactose. N Engl J Med 2008;358(11):1109–17.

18. Commins SP, James HR, Kelly LA, et al. The relevance of tick bites to the production of IgE antibodies to the mammalian oligosaccharide galactose-α-1,3-galactose. J Allergy Clin Immunol 2011;127(5):1286–93.e6.

19. Campbell RL, Li JT, Nicklas RA, et al, Members of the Joint Task Force, Practice Parameter Workgroup. Emergency department diagnosis and treatment of anaphylaxis: a practice parameter. Ann Allergy Asthma Immunol 2014;113(6): 599–608.

20. Ellis AK, Day JH. Diagnosis and management of anaphylaxis. CMAJ 2003;169(4): 307–11.

21. Toogood JH. Risk of anaphylaxis in patients receiving beta-blocker drugs. J Allergy Clin Immunol 1988;81(1):1–5.

22. Berg RA, Hemphill R, Abella BS, et al. Part 5: adult basic life support: 2010 American Heart association guidelines for cardiopulmonary resuscitation and emergency cardiovascular care. Circulation 2010;122(18 Suppl 3):S685–705.

23. Commins SP, Platts-Mills TA. Allergenicity of carbohydrates and their role in anaphylactic events. Curr Allergy Asthma Rep 2010;10(1):29–33.

24. Kaliner M, Shelhamer JH, Ottesen EA. Effects of infused histamine: correlation of plasma histamine levels and symptoms. J Allergy Clin Immunol 1982;69(3): 283–9.

25. Maier S, Chung CH, Morse M, et al. A retrospective analysis of cross-reacting cetuximab IgE antibody and its association with severe infusion reactions. Cancer Med 2014;4(1):36–42.
26. Pointreau Y, Commins SP, Calais G, et al. Fatal infusion reactions to cetuximab: role of immunoglobulin e-mediated anaphylaxis. J Clin Oncol 2012;30(3):334 [author reply: 335].
27. Simon RA, Schatz M, Stevenson DD, et al. Radiographic contrast media infusions. Measurement of histamine, complement, and fibrin split products and correlation with clinical parameters. J Allergy Clin Immunol 1979;63(4):281–8.
28. Bock SA, Munoz-Furlong A, Sampson HA. Further fatalities caused by anaphylactic reactions to food, 2001-2006. J Allergy Clin Immunol 2007;119(4):1016–8.
29. Bock SA, Munoz-Furlong A, Sampson HA. Fatalities due to anaphylactic reactions to foods. J Allergy Clin Immunol 2001;107(1):191–3.
30. Neumar RW, Otto CW, Link MS, et al. Part 8: adult advanced cardiovascular life support: 2010 American Heart Association guidelines for cardiopulmonary resuscitation and emergency cardiovascular care. Circulation 2010;122(18 Suppl 3): S729–67.
31. Beavers CJ, Pandya KA. Pharmacotherapy considerations for the management of advanced cardiac life support. Nurs Clin North Am 2016;51(1):69–82.
32. Hannibal GB. 2015 advanced cardiac life support updates and strategies for improving survival after cardiac arrest. AACN Adv Crit Care 2016;27(2):241–7.
33. Orban JC, Giolito D, Tosi J, et al. Factors associated with initiation of medical advanced cardiac life support after out-of-hospital cardiac arrest. Ann Intensive Care 2016;6(1):12.
34. Rank MA, Oslie CL, Krogman JL, et al. Allergen immunotherapy safety: characterizing systemic reactions and identifying risk factors. Allergy Asthma Proc 2008;29(4):400–5.
35. Simons FE, Gu X, Simons KJ. Epinephrine absorption in adults: intramuscular versus subcutaneous injection. J Allergy Clin Immunol 2001;108(5):871–3.
36. Simons FE, Roberts JR, Gu X, et al. Epinephrine absorption in children with a history of anaphylaxis. J Allergy Clin Immunol 1998;101(1 Pt 1):33–7.
37. Manivannan V, Campbell RL, Bellolio MF, et al. Factors associated with repeated use of epinephrine for the treatment of anaphylaxis. Ann Allergy Asthma Immunol 2009;103(5):395–400.
38. Oren E, Banerji A, Clark S, et al. Food-induced anaphylaxis and repeated epinephrine treatments. Ann Allergy Asthma Immunol 2007;99(5):429–32.
39. Sampson HA, Mendelson L, Rosen JP. Fatal and near-fatal anaphylactic reactions to food in children and adolescents. N Engl J Med 1992;327(6):380–4.
40. Simons FE, Frew AJ, Ansotegui IJ, et al. Practical allergy (PRACTALL) report: risk assessment in anaphylaxis. Allergy 2008;63(1):35–7.
41. Ali J, Adam RU, Gana TJ, et al. Trauma patient outcome after the Prehospital Trauma Life Support program. J Trauma 1997;42(6):1018–21 [discussion: 1021–2].
42. Wolfl CG, Bouillon B, Lackner CK, et al. Prehospital Trauma Life Support (PHTLS): an interdisciplinary training in preclinical trauma care. Unfallchirurg 2008;111(9): 688–94 [in German].
43. Peberdy MA, Callaway CW, Neumar RW, et al. Part 9: post-cardiac arrest care: 2010 American Heart Association guidelines for cardiopulmonary resuscitation and emergency cardiovascular care. Circulation 2010;122(18 Suppl 3):S768–86.
44. Pumphrey RS. Fatal posture in anaphylactic shock. J Allergy Clin Immunol 2003; 112(2):451–2.

45. Berg MD, Schexnayder SM, Chameides L, et al. Part 13: pediatric basic life support: 2010 American Heart Association guidelines for cardiopulmonary resuscitation and emergency cardiovascular care. Circulation 2010;122(18 Suppl 3): S862–75.

46. Brown SG, Blackman KE, Stenlake V, et al. Insect sting anaphylaxis; prospective evaluation of treatment with intravenous adrenaline and volume resuscitation. Emerg Med J 2004;21(2):149–54.

47. Toogood JH. Beta-blocker therapy and the risk of anaphylaxis. CMAJ 1987; 137(7):587–8, 590–1.

48. Vander Zanden JA, Valuck RJ, Bunch CL, et al. Systemic adverse effects of ophthalmic beta-blockers. Ann Pharmacother 2001;35(12):1633–7.

49. Matasar MJ, Neugut AI. Epidemiology of anaphylaxis in the United States. Curr Allergy Asthma Rep 2003;3(1):30–5.

50. Mulla ZD, Lin RY, Simon MR. Perspectives on anaphylaxis epidemiology in the United States with new data and analyses. Curr Allergy Asthma Rep 2011; 11(1):37–44.

51. Commins SP, James HR, Stevens W, et al. Delayed clinical and ex vivo response to mammalian meat in patients with IgE to galactose-alpha-1,3-galactose. J Allergy Clin Immunol 2014;134(1):108–15.

52. Sicherer SH, Sampson HA. Food allergy: epidemiology, pathogenesis, diagnosis, and treatment. J Allergy Clin Immunol 2014;133(2):291–307 [quiz: 308].

53. Atkins D, Bock SA. Fatal anaphylaxis to foods: epidemiology, recognition, and prevention. Curr Allergy Asthma Rep 2009;9(3):179–85.

54. Yu JE, Lin RY. The epidemiology of anaphylaxis. Clin Rev Allergy Immunol 2015.

55. Boyce JA, Assa'ad A, Burks AW, et al. Guidelines for the diagnosis and management of food allergy in the United States: summary of the NIAID-sponsored expert panel report. Nutr Res 2011;31(1):61–75.

56. Simons FE, Frew AJ, Ansotegui IJ, et al. Risk assessment in anaphylaxis: current and future approaches. J Allergy Clin Immunol 2007;120(1 Suppl):S2–24.

# Outpatient Management for Acute Exacerbations of Obstructive Lung Diseases

Brenda Marsh, MD, PhD, Matthew G. Drake, MD*

## KEYWORDS

- Asthma • Chronic obstructive pulmonary disease • Exacerbation • Glucocorticoids

## KEY POINTS

- The management of acute asthma and chronic obstructive pulmonary disease exacerbations involves reversing airflow obstruction with inhaled bronchodilators and reducing airway inflammation with corticosteroids.
- Outpatient management must include an assessment of disease severity to facilitate patient triage to the appropriate level of care.
- Outpatient therapy for exacerbations should include short-term follow-up and patient education to ensure recovery and reduce risk of exacerbation recurrence.

## INTRODUCTION

Asthma and chronic obstructive pulmonary disease (COPD) are commonly encountered lung diseases in the outpatient setting. Outpatient providers must not only manage the chronic phases of these diseases but also promptly recognize and treat disease exacerbations. This review focuses on the diagnosis and management of acute exacerbations of asthma and COPD in the adult outpatient setting.

## ASTHMA EXACERBATIONS
### Disease Characteristics

Asthma is a chronic inflammatory disease of the airways characterized by excessive mucus production, bronchoconstriction (narrowing of the airways), and airway hyper-responsiveness (heightened contractile responses to stimuli). Symptom severity ranges from mild, intermittent wheezing, chest tightness, cough and dyspnea, to severe, persistent disease that limits daily activities. Asthma exacerbations are defined by worsening of symptoms outside the range of an individual's day-to-day variation.[1]

The authors have no financial or commercial conflicts of interest to declare.
Division of Pulmonary and Critical Care Medicine, Oregon Health and Science University, 3181 SW Sam Jackson Park Road, Portland, OR 97239, USA
* Corresponding author.
E-mail address: drakem@ohsu.edu

Prompt recognition and early treatment of exacerbations are vital for preventing further decompensation that, in severe cases, may be life threatening.

## Detecting Exacerbations and Assessing Severity

Asthma exacerbations present with breathlessness, wheezing, nonproductive cough, and/or chest tightness. Symptoms may develop acutely over hours or advance slowly over several days. Signs of an exacerbation include increased respiratory and heart rate, agitation, and expiratory wheezing on chest auscultation. Patients may have reduced lung function measured as a decrease in peak expiratory flow (PEF) or forced expiratory volume in 1 second ($FEV_1$). Importantly, some asthmatics have a blunted perception of their disease severity that may lead to underreporting of symptoms or delays in seeking care.[2] Thus, clinicians must be vigilant for evidence of a severe exacerbation. Pertinent risk factors for severe or fatal asthma exacerbations include a history of severe exacerbations requiring intensive care unit admission or intubation, 2 or more hospitalizations or 3 or more emergency room visits for asthma in the past year, or hospitalization in the past month for asthma (**Box 1**). In addition, improper use of asthma control medications (ie, incorrect inhaler technique, lack of a spacer), low socioeconomic status, use of 2 or more canisters of short-acting bronchodilators per month or comorbid psychiatric, cardiac, or other chronic lung conditions predispose to severe exacerbations.[3]

Asthma exacerbation severity is categorized by clinical symptoms and signs (**Table 1**). Mild exacerbations may include wheezing, cough, and chest tightness, but normal oxygen saturation and a PEF greater than 70% predicted. Patients should be able to speak in full sentences and have no shortness of breath at rest. Accessory respiratory muscle use (ie, sternocleidomastoid retractions) should be absent. Moderate exacerbations may involve mild shortness of breath at rest, use of accessory muscles, elevated heart and respiratory rate, and a PEF between 40% and 69% predicted. Severe exacerbations may include dyspnea at rest, speaking in 1- to 2-word sentences, accessory muscle use, and agitation. Pulsus paradoxus (>25 mm Hg), PEF less

---

**Box 1**
**Risk factors for fatal asthma: components of the personal and medical history that should alert practitioners to an increased risk for fatal asthma exacerbations**

Prior severe exacerbation requiring:
- Intensive care admission
- Intubation

2 + hospitalizations in past year

Asthma-related hospitalization or emergency room care in past month

3 + emergency room visits in past year

Current use or recent withdrawal of systemic corticosteroids

2 + refills of short-acting $beta_2$ agonist per month

Reduced perception of degree of airflow obstruction

Illicit drug use

Low socioeconomic status

Medical comorbidities:
- Psychiatric disorder
- Cardiovascular disease
- Other chronic lung disease

**Table 1**
**Categories of asthma exacerbation severity**

| Severity | Symptoms | Signs | Functional Assessment |
|---|---|---|---|
| Mild | Breathlessness with walking | Respiratory rate >20 | PEF ≥70% predicted |
| | Speaks in full sentences | No accessory muscle use | O$_2$ saturation >95% |
| | Alert or mild agitation | End expiratory wheeze | Paco$_2$ <42 mm Hg[a] |
| | | Heart rate <100 | Pao$_2$ >80 mm Hg[a] |
| Moderate | Breathlessness at rest | Respiratory rate >20 | PEF 40%–69% predicted |
| | Speaks in short phrases | Use of accessory muscles | O$_2$ saturation >90% |
| | Alert, but agitated | Diffuse expiratory wheeze | Paco$_2$ <42 mm Hg[a] |
| | | Heart rate >100 | Pao$_2$ >65 mm Hg[a] |
| | | Pulsus paradoxus (10–25 mm Hg) | |
| Severe | Marked breathlessness at rest | Respiratory rate >30 | PEF <40% predicted |
| | Speaks in 1–2 word phrases | Pronounced accessory muscle use with respiration | O$_2$ saturation <90% |
| | Agitated or altered mentation | Prominent inspiratory and expiratory wheeze | Paco$_2$ >42 mm Hg[a] |
| | | Heart rate >120 | Pao$_2$ <65 mm Hg[a] |
| | | Pulsus paradoxus (>25 mm Hg) | |

Assessment tool to help identify exacerbation severity and guide decision regarding level of care and treatment.

Blood gas measurements assume patient is breathing room air at sea level.

The presence of multiple parameters increases likelihood for that category of exacerbation. Some patients may have severe exacerbations without meeting criteria above.

*Abbreviations:* Paco$_2$, partial pressure of arterial carbon dioxide; Pao$_2$, partial pressure of arterial oxygen.

[a] Laboratory test not necessary for most evaluations.

than 40% predicted, and arterial oxygen saturation <90% may be present. Notably, up to half of asthmatics with severe exacerbations lack these abnormalities[4]; thus, an absence of symptoms should not provide reassurance if the clinician suspects a severe exacerbation.

## Evaluation

Prompt identification of an exacerbation is critical for timely triage and treatment. Clinicians should obtain a history of asthma symptoms and the time of their onset, recent exposure to exacerbation triggers, response to initial treatments, and medical comorbidities. Clinicians must apply these findings to determine exacerbation severity (**Fig. 1**).

A focused physical examination should evaluate for findings consistent with an asthma exacerbation and exclude alternative diagnoses. It is important to recognize wheezing is not specific for the diagnosis of asthma. Pneumonia, pneumothorax or upper airway obstruction due to epiglottitis, foreign body impaction, or vocal cord dysfunction should be ruled out. Evaluating volume status, capillary refill, and jugular venous distention for evidence of heart failure is necessary, as is excluding cardiac ischemia. Neck and jaw pain, diaphoresis, left-sided chest pressure, and palpitations should prompt an electrocardiogram and measurement of serum

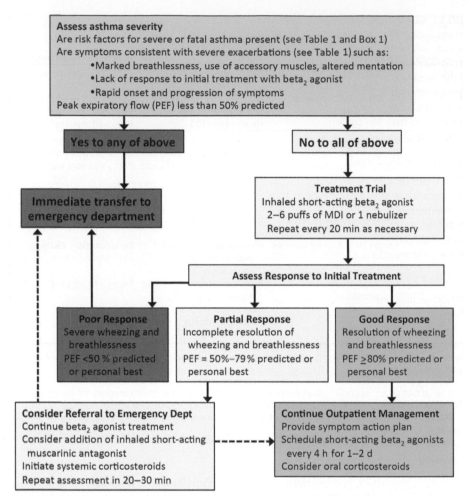

**Fig. 1.** Initial management of acute asthma exacerbation. Algorithm for outpatient assessment, triage, management, and re-evaluation of asthma exacerbations. (*Adapted from* National Heart Lung and Blood Institute. National Asthma Education and Prevention Program Expert Panel 3, Guidelines for the Diagnosis and Management of Asthma. 2007. Available at: http://www.nhlbi.nih.gov/files/docs/guidelines/asthgdln.pdf. Accessed August, 2016.)

troponins. That said, most patients presenting with asthma exacerbations do not require laboratory testing, and testing should not delay treatment. Arterial blood gas measurement is not routinely recommended, but can be considered when there is concern for carbon dioxide retention ($Paco_2$ >42 mm Hg). $Paco_2$ is typically low during an exacerbation due to an increase in respiratory drive. An elevated $Paco_2$ should raise concern for impending respiratory failure. Chest radiographs are also not routinely recommended unless the presentation suggests pneumonia, congestive heart failure, pneumothorax, pneumomediastinum, or atelectasis is present.[5]

When possible, lung function measurement using PEF or $FEV_1$ enables an objective assessment of exacerbation severity. Furthermore, repeated measurement

30 to 60 minutes following initial treatments can help determine subsequent care needs (see **Fig. 1**). For example, a PEF of 50% to 79% predicted requires prompt treatment with short-acting bronchodilators. Improvement in PEF after treatment to greater than 80% predicted suggests the patient is safe for home management. Conversely, a decrease in PEF despite treatment warrants transfer to the emergency department. When a PEF remains reduced, but stable after treatment, clinicians must weigh symptom severity, risk factors for severe asthma, and the likelihood that the patient will adhere to treatment and follow-up when determining the next step in care.

## Management Strategy

The treatment strategy for asthma exacerbations regardless of severity involves rapid reversal of airflow obstruction with short-acting bronchodilators and, in some cases, treatment with systemic corticosteroids. The dose, frequency, and location of these interventions vary depending on severity of symptoms. Initial treatment at home or in the outpatient clinic is reasonable for mild or moderate exacerbations, whereas severe exacerbations should be treated in the emergency department.

### Inhaled Short-Acting Bronchodilators

Short-acting beta$_2$ agonists are the cornerstone of therapy for all asthma exacerbations.[6] Albuterol should be given either as 2 to 6 puffs repeated every 20 minutes via metered dose inhaler (MDI) with a spacer, or 2.5 to 5 mg of nebulized albuterol (**Table 2**). Albuterol administered via MDI is equivalent to nebulized albuterol.[7] However, nebulizer therapy may be preferable for patients unable to effectively perform MDI treatments due to agitation or distress.

The patient's response to initial treatment guides further management. For example, if symptoms do not improve or if PEF does not increase to 50% to 79% predicted after 2 albuterol treatments, an emergency department evaluation is warranted.[8] If patients partially respond to initial treatments, scheduling a short-acting beta$_2$ agonist every 3 to 4 hours is reasonable until PEF returns to baseline. Adding the muscarinic antagonist ipratropium may be beneficial when used concurrently with albuterol and has been shown to reduce the need for hospitalization in children.[5,9] However, ipratropium should not replace beta$_2$ agonist therapy except in rare instances where a contraindication to albuterol exists (ie, medical allergy).[10,11] Long-acting bronchodilators are not recommended in place of short-acting bronchodilators during acute asthma exacerbations.

### Corticosteroids

When symptoms cannot be controlled with bronchodilators alone, systemic corticosteroids should be initiated. The optimal dose and duration of steroid treatments are not defined.[12] Guidelines recommend a 5- to 7-day nontapering course of oral prednisone (1 mg/kg per day or 40–60 mg/d) (see **Table 2**). Lower doses (≤80 mg/d methylprednisolone or ≤400 mg/d hydrocortisone) were equally efficacious compared with higher steroid doses.[13] Furthermore, oral steroids have similar efficacy to comparable doses of intravenous steroids. In patients who may have difficulty reliably taking medications, a single intramuscular dose of corticosteroid (160 mg methylprednisolone) can be considered as an alternative to oral therapy.[14]

There is insufficient evidence to support adding or increasing inhaled corticosteroids in place of or in combination with systemic corticosteroids during acute exacerbations.[15] In one study, quadrupling the dose of inhaled corticosteroid in mild asthma

**Table 2**
**Commonly prescribed medications for obstructive lung disease exacerbations**

| Medication | Dose | Comments |
|---|---|---|
| Inhaled short-acting beta$_2$-agonist | | |
| Albuterol | MDI (90 µg/puff) 2–6 puffs every 20 min | Use spacer |
| | Nebulizer (2.5–5 mg/3 mL) 1 vial every 20 min | Alternative: 10–15 mg/h continuous |
| Levalbuterol (R-albuterol) | MDI (45 µg/puff) 2–6 puffs every 20 min | Use spacer |
| | Nebulizer (1.25–2.5 mg/3 mL) 1 vial every 20 min | Comparable efficacy to albuterol; has not been evaluated as continuous |
| Anticholinergics | | |
| Ipratropium bromide | MDI (18 µg/puff) 2–4 puffs every 20 min | Repeat for 3 doses |
| | Nebulizer (0.25–0.5 mg/mL) 1 vial every 20 min | Repeat for 3 doses |
| Combination therapy | | |
| Ipratropium bromide with Albuterol | Respimat inhaler Ipratropium 20 µg/Albuterol 100 µg 1–2 puffs every 20 min | Repeat × 3 doses Respimat propellant-free formulation has replaced MDI formulation |
| | Nebulizer Ipratropium 0.5 mg/Albuterol 3 mg per 3 mL 1 vial every 20 min | Repeat × 3 doses |
| Systemic corticosteroids | | |
| Prednisone oral formulation | 40–60 mg/d by mouth | Can be divided into 2 doses; continue for 5–10 d |
| Methylprednisolone parenteral formulation | 40–60 mg/d intravenous | Can be divided into 2 doses; continue for 5–10 d |
| Methylprednisolone Intramuscular formulation | 160 mg intramuscular once | Similar efficacy to 160 mg oral taper over 8 d |

Short-acting bronchodilators and systemic corticosteroids are the cornerstones of therapy for both asthma and COPD exacerbations.

exacerbations reduced the need for oral corticosteroids.[16] Conversely, in another study, doubling an inhaled steroid did not impact systemic corticosteroids use.[17] That said, patients previously on inhaled corticosteroids should continue them during treatment with systemic steroids.

## Antibiotics

Antibiotics are not recommended for asthma exacerbations unless a concurrent bacterial infection is present.[8,18] Unlike viral infections that commonly trigger exacerbations, bacterial infections are rare.

## Leukotriene Receptor Antagonists

Leukotriene antagonists are not recommended for outpatient management of mild or moderate asthma exacerbations despite their role in chronic allergic asthma treatment.[19–21]

## Biologics

Monoclonal antibody therapies targeting immunoglobulin E and interleukin-5 are approved for chronic asthma treatment. However, antibody treatments are not indicated for acute asthma exacerbations and should not be initiated until an exacerbation has resolved.

## Other Treatments

Antihistamines, mucolytics, and intravenous or nebulized magnesium are not recommended for outpatient asthma exacerbation management.[8] Likewise, methylxanthines (theophylline) and racemic epinephrine have serious risk for toxicity and are not recommended.[22] Supplemental oxygen or noninvasive positive pressure ventilation may be necessary for severe asthma exacerbations, but their use should be limited to hospital-based settings with intensive monitoring.

## Treatment Goals and Follow-up

Treatment goals include relief of dyspnea and wheezing, improvement in PEF to >80% predicted and, when applicable, resolution of hypoxemia. Following initial treatments at home or in clinic, repeated assessments should be conducted every 30 to 60 minutes until it is deemed safe to continue outpatient management. Failure to respond to bronchodilators warrants transfer to the emergency department. Alternatively, patients appropriate for home management must have a clear follow-up plan. The timing for follow-up is based on symptom severity. For moderate exacerbations, follow-up by phone or in person within 24 to 48 hours is reasonable. Mild exacerbations may be re-evaluated at later intervals. Patients should understand treatment goals and warning signs (ie, worsening of symptoms) that should prompt urgent medical attention. The decision to manage an exacerbation at home must account for the patient's risk for severe exacerbations, their likely adherence to the treatment plan, and their social support system.

## Patient Education and Risk Reduction

Asthmatics are at increased risk for returning to the emergency department if they have inadequate knowledge of their disease, lack an action plan should symptoms worsen, use inhalers incorrectly, or are re-exposed to triggers like tobacco smoke.[5] Patient education should address these risk factors by providing (1) an asthma action plan that instructs the patient to modify their treatment based on symptoms and/or PEF (examples available through the National Heart Lung and Blood Institute at http://www.nhlbi.nih.gov/files/docs/public/lung/asthma_actplan.pdf); (2) instructions on proper inhaler technique including use of a spacer; and (3) individualized, written medication instructions.

# CHRONIC OBSTRUCTIVE PULMONARY DISEASE EXACERBATIONS
## Disease Characteristics

COPD is characterized by chronic bronchitis (bronchial inflammation) and emphysema (alveolar destruction) that causes airflow obstruction and difficulty breathing. COPD typically develops in older patients with a history of cigarette smoking. Exacerbations of COPD symptoms are associated with accelerated respiratory decline, decreased quality of life,[23] and increased mortality.[24] Hence, treatment and prevention of exacerbations are important parts of outpatient management. COPD exacerbations are commonly triggered by upper respiratory infections due to viruses and bacteria.[25] Environmental exposure to tobacco smoke, air pollution, or ozone, and comorbid medical conditions, such as congestive heart failure, arrhythmias, or pulmonary embolism, can also trigger exacerbations.[26] One-third of COPD exacerbations have no identifiable cause.

### Detecting Exacerbations and Assessing Severity

COPD exacerbations are defined by acute worsening of respiratory symptoms beyond typical day-to-day variations that prompt a change in medication.[27] Specific symptoms include increased dyspnea, increased sputum volume and purulence, wheezing, cough, and chest tightness (**Table 3**). Signs include increased work of breathing, decreased oxygen saturation, and increased respiratory or heart rate. No biomarkers adequately identify exacerbations[28]; thus the diagnosis is based on clinical factors. Early recognition of exacerbations is essential to enable prompt treatment, reduce the risk of hospitalization, and improve quality of life.[29]

All patients with COPD may develop an exacerbation, although severe baseline COPD and those with a history of exacerbations are at increased risk.[30] Other risk factors include current smoking, body mass index less than 18.5 kg/m$^2$, reduced baseline activity level, poor social support, underutilization of long-term oxygen therapy, and medical comorbidities, including cardiovascular and cerebrovascular disease.[30–33]

### Evaluation

The initial evaluation of a suspected COPD exacerbation includes an assessment of exacerbation severity and exclusion of alternative diagnoses (see **Table 3**; **Table 4**). Most exacerbations (~80%) can be treated safely as outpatients, but severe

**Table 3**
**Presenting features of chronic obstructive pulmonary disease exacerbation**

| Symptoms and Signs | Differential Diagnoses[a] |
|---|---|
| Pulmonary | Pneumonia |
| Breathlessness | Congestive heart failure |
| Increased sputum volume | Pleural effusion |
| Increased sputum purulence | Pneumothorax |
| Expiratory wheeze | Pulmonary embolism |
| Cough | Cardiac ischemia |
| Increased work of breathing | Arrhythmia |
| Respiratory rate >20 | |
| Cardiac | |
| Chest tightness | |
| Heart rate >110 | |
| Psychiatric | |
| Confusion | |
| Sleepiness | |
| Insomnia | |
| Systemic | |
| Fatigue | |
| Malaise | |

Pulmonary and extra-pulmonary manifestations of COPD exacerbation. Patients with COPD often have several comorbidities, hence alternative diagnoses may need to be ruled out.

[a] Differential diagnoses listed are only some of the potential diseases that can present with symptoms and signs similar to COPD exacerbations.

**Table 4**
**Characteristics of severe chronic obstructive pulmonary disease exacerbation**

| Risk Factors | Signs | Indications for Hospital Admission |
|---|---|---|
| Age >75 | Lung function tests | Marked increase in symptoms |
| Severe baseline COPD Use of long-term oxygen therapy | PEF <100 L/min, $FEV_1$ <1 L arterial blood gas | Severe baseline COPD; new physical signs |
| Medical comorbidities | $Pao_2$ <60 mmHg or $Spo_2$ <90% | Peripheral edema |
| | pH<7.3 | Cyanosis |
| | $Paco_2$ >50 mm Hg | Altered mental status |
| | Chest radiograph | Failure to respond to initial medical management |
| | Pneumonia or alternative diagnosis present | Significant medical comorbidities |
| | Electrocardiogram | New arrhythmia |
| | Arrhythmia/ischemia | Hemodynamic instability |
| | Electrolyte disturbances | Age >75 |
| | Nutritional deficiencies | Insufficient home support |

Assessment tool to help identify exacerbation severity and guide decision regarding level of care.

exacerbations require a higher level of care (**Fig. 2**). Factors that predispose to severe exacerbations include age greater than 75, severe baseline COPD ($FEV_1$ <50% predicted), use of long-term oxygen therapy, and medical comorbidities, particularly cardiovascular disease.[34] Similarly, marked increases in symptoms, new resting dyspnea, abnormal physical signs (ie, cyanosis, arrhythmia), a history of frequent exacerbations, insufficient home support, and failure to respond to initial treatment should prompt consideration for transfer to the emergency department (see **Table 4**).[27]

Physical examination findings during a COPD exacerbation include elevated respiratory rate (>20 breaths per minute), elevated heart rate (>100 beats per minute), and hypoxemia (oxygen saturation <92% measured by pulse oximetry) (see **Table 3**). Severe exacerbations may present with altered mental status, accessory respiratory muscles use, cyanosis, and hemodynamic instability.[27]

Although not routinely recommended, an arterial blood gas measurement can be obtained to evaluate for acute respiratory acidosis. If present, hospital transfer for initiation of noninvasive positive pressure ventilation should be considered. Furthermore, cardiovascular complications, such as heart failure or ischemia,[35] present concurrently with exacerbations, require careful evaluation of the patient's cardiac status. Obtaining a chest radiograph, electrocardiogram, complete blood count, complete metabolic panel, brain natriuretic peptide, and serum troponins may help clarify the diagnosis.

## Management Strategy

COPD treatment goals are similar to those in asthma exacerbation: to maximize bronchodilation while reducing airway inflammation. Unlike asthma, however, many patients with COPD will benefit from antibiotic treatment.[27]

### Inhaled Short-Acting Bronchodilators

COPD exacerbations should be treated with short-acting bronchodilators delivered via an MDI or nebulizer (see **Table 2**). Albuterol and ipratropium are most

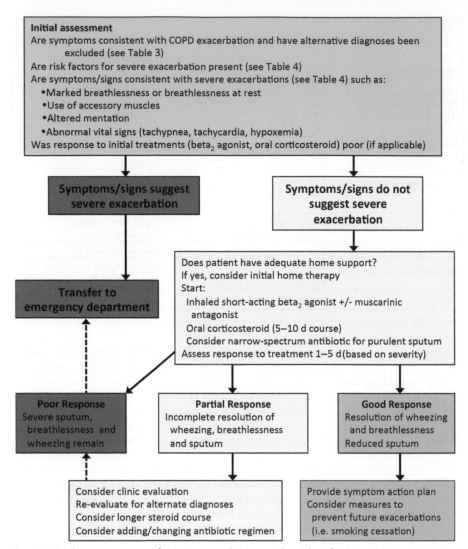

**Fig. 2.** Initial management of COPD exacerbations. Algorithm for outpatient assessment, triage, management, and re-evaluation of COPD exacerbations. Guidelines should be adapted to individual patient requirements.

commonly used and have similar treatment effects despite differing mechanisms of action. There is not a recommendation to start one over the other. Furthermore, the combination of albuterol and ipratropium is not superior to single-drug treatment.[36] Despite this, guidelines recommend combining them once the maximal dose of initial bronchodilator has been reached.[37] Levalbuterol is an alternative to albuterol and has similar efficacy, but remains considerably more expensive. Bronchodilator administration via an MDI with a spacer has similar benefit to administration via nebulizer when equivalent doses are compared,[7] but nebulizers should be considered for patients who have difficulty coordinating MDI use.

### Inhaled Long-Acting Bronchodilators

Guidelines recommend starting a long-acting bronchodilator during an exacerbation in patients not already using one. Formoterol and tiotropium, alone or in combination, may improve $FEV_1$ in this setting.[38]

### Corticosteroids

Most studies of systemic steroids in COPD exacerbations have evaluated hospitalized patients; few have assessed steroids in the outpatient setting.[39] Nonetheless, corticosteroids are recommended for outpatient COPD exacerbations to improve dyspnea and lung function while decreasing exacerbation duration and rate of treatment failure.[40] Oral steroids are equally efficacious to intravenous formulations, and short courses (5 days) are as effective as longer ones (14 days).[40,41] Guidelines vary regarding dosing, but generally 30 to 40 mg of oral prednisone is sufficient (see **Table 2**).[27,37,42] One study suggested that increasing the dose of inhaled corticosteroids may be as effective as adding systemic steroids,[43] but more data are required before recommending this option.

### Antibiotics

More than half of COPD exacerbations are attributed to bacterial infection of the lower airways,[25] typically from *Streptococcus pneumoniae*, *Haemophilus influenzae*, *Moraxella catarrhalis*, *Pseudomonas aeruginosa*, and *Chlamydophila pneumoniae*. Hence, unlike in asthma, antibiotic treatment improves time to exacerbation resolution and decreases relapse rates in hospitalized patients; the data are less clear for outpatients with mild to moderate exacerbations.[44] Purulent sputum may correlate with bacterial growth, and patients without purulent sputum improve without antibiotic treatment.[45] Indeed, guidelines use purulent sputum as the indication for initiating antibiotics for mild and moderate COPD exacerbations.[27,42]

In choosing an antibiotic, one should consider likely bacteria present in the airways, local antibiotic resistance patterns, and prior treatment failures. For example, in patients with purulent sputum, no recent treatment failure, and low community antibiotic resistance, it is reasonable to treat with doxycycline or azithromycin. Patients who fail treatment or who live in areas with high levels of bacterial resistance may require a broader spectrum agent such as a respiratory fluoroquinolone.[27,37,42] Optimal antibiotic duration is unclear, but typically involves 5 to 10 days of therapy.

### Supplemental Oxygen

Supplemental oxygen is indicated for arterial oxygen saturations less than 88% (or $Pao_2$ <60 mm Hg). Patients currently on oxygen therapy may require temporary increases in oxygen supplementation. Oxygen flow should be titrated to target oxygen saturations between 88% and 92% to reduce the potential risk of worsening respiratory acidosis.[46]

### Tobacco Cessation

Smokers should be encouraged to quit. Behavioral counseling (ie, smoking cessation groups) and pharmacotherapy (ie, varenicline, bupropion, or nortriptyline) should be offered.[47]

### Other Therapies

Theophylline is not recommended for COPD exacerbations due to a lack of benefit and high risk of adverse events.[48] Mucolytics may be offered to improve sputum clearance, but have no known benefit for improving exacerbation outcomes. Similarly, chest physiotherapy does not decrease exacerbation duration or improve lung function.

### Treatment Goals and Follow-up

Treatment goals include reversal of acute symptoms, minimizing exacerbation duration, and reducing the risk of treatment failure. Clinicians and patients must agree on a timeline for re-evaluation and discuss symptoms that warrant urgent medical attention, such as fatigue, and worsening dyspnea and mucus production. Failure to improve after 1 to 3 days should prompt additional treatment, including antibiotics (if not already started), switching to broad-spectrum antibiotics (when receiving a narrow-spectrum agent), and evaluating for alternative diagnoses. Treatment failure may require a hospital assessment.

### Patient Education and Risk Reduction

Preventing future COPD exacerbations is a primary goal for outpatient clinicians. Prevention begins with patient education. Clinic visits provide an opportunity to teach proper inhaler technique, provide nutrition counseling, and most importantly, discuss smoking cessation. Smoking cessation reduces the risk of exacerbation, and risk reduction correlates with the duration of abstinence.[49] Pharmacotherapies for treating chronic COPD are reviewed elsewhere, but long-acting beta$_2$ agonists, muscarinic receptor antagonists, and/or inhaled corticosteroids should all be considered.[50,51] Influenza vaccination decreases exacerbation rates and should be given annually.[52] Patients with 2 or more exacerbations per year despite inhaler therapy may benefit from a continuous macrolide,[53] roflumilast,[54] or mucolytics. Pulmonary rehabilitation improves quality of life, decreases hospital admissions and mortality when started within 4 weeks of an exacerbation, and thus, should also be considered.[55] Finally, patients may benefit from an outpatient action plan that prompts changes in medication at the onset of exacerbation symptoms (examples available through the American Lung Association at http://www.lung.org/assets/documents/copd/copd-action-plan.pdf). Self-management plans that include the option of starting oral corticosteroids with or without antibiotics have been shown to decrease exacerbation duration, emergency room visits, and hospitalization.[56]

### SUMMARY

Primary care providers are on the front line of asthma and COPD treatment. Effective management of obstructive lung disease exacerbations requires prompt diagnosis, appropriate triage based on exacerbation severity, and timely initiation of bronchodilators, anti-inflammatory therapies, and in some cases, antibiotics.

### REFERENCES

1. Reddel HK, Taylor DR, Bateman ED, et al. An official American Thoracic Society/European Respiratory Society statement: asthma control and exacerbations: standardizing endpoints for clinical asthma trials and clinical practice. Am J Respir Crit Care Med 2009;180(1):59–99.
2. Rubinfeld AR, Pain MC. Perception of asthma. Lancet 1976;1(7965):882–4.
3. Papiris S, Kotanidou A, Malagari K, et al. Clinical review: severe asthma. Crit Care 2002;6(1):30–44.
4. Kelsen SG, Kelsen DP, Fleeger BF, et al. Emergency room assessment and treatment of patients with acute asthma. Adequacy of the conventional approach. Am J Med 1978;64(4):622–8.

5. Camargo CA Jr, Rachelefsky G, Schatz M. Managing asthma exacerbations in the emergency department: summary of the National Asthma Education and Prevention Program Expert Panel Report 3 guidelines for the management of asthma exacerbations. Proc Am Thorac Soc 2009;6(4):357–66.

6. Newhouse MT, Dolovich MB. Control of asthma by aerosols. N Engl J Med 1986; 315(14):870–4.

7. Turner MO, Patel A, Ginsburg S, et al. Bronchodilator delivery in acute airflow obstruction. A meta-analysis. Arch Intern Med 1997;157(15):1736–44.

8. National Asthma Education and Prevention Program, Third Expert Panel on the Diagnosis and Management of Asthma. Expert Panel Report 3: Guidelines for the Diagnosis and Management of Asthma. Bethesda (MD): National Heart, Lung, and Blood Institute (US); 2007. Available from: https://www.ncbi.nlm.nih.gov/books/NBK7232/. Accessed August 26, 2016.

9. Rodrigo GJ, Castro-Rodriguez JA. Anticholinergics in the treatment of children and adults with acute asthma: a systematic review with meta-analysis. Thorax 2005;60(9):740–6.

10. Rodrigo GJ, Rodrigo C. First-line therapy for adult patients with acute asthma receiving a multiple-dose protocol of ipratropium bromide plus albuterol in the emergency department. Am J Respir Crit Care Med 2000;161(6):1862–8.

11. Stoodley RG, Aaron SD, Dales RE. The role of ipratropium bromide in the emergency management of acute asthma exacerbation: a metaanalysis of randomized clinical trials. Ann Emerg Med 1999;34(1):8–18.

12. Normansell R, Kew KM, Mansour G. Different oral corticosteroid regimens for acute asthma. Cochrane Database Syst Rev 2016;(5):CD011801.

13. Manser R, Reid D, Abramson M. Corticosteroids for acute severe asthma in hospitalised patients. Cochrane Database Syst Rev 2001;(1):CD001740.

14. Lahn M, Bijur P, Gallagher EJ. Randomized clinical trial of intramuscular vs oral methylprednisolone in the treatment of asthma exacerbations following discharge from an emergency department. Chest 2004;126(2):362–8.

15. Edmonds ML, Milan SJ, Brenner BE, et al. Inhaled steroids for acute asthma following emergency department discharge. Cochrane Database Syst Rev 2012;(12):CD002316.

16. Oborne J, Mortimer K, Hubbard RB, et al. Quadrupling the dose of inhaled corticosteroid to prevent asthma exacerbations: a randomized, double-blind, placebo-controlled, parallel-group clinical trial. Am J Respir Crit Care Med 2009; 180(7):598–602.

17. Harrison TW, Oborne J, Newton S, et al. Doubling the dose of inhaled corticosteroid to prevent asthma exacerbations: randomised controlled trial. Lancet 2004; 363(9405):271–5.

18. Graham V, Lasserson T, Rowe BH. Antibiotics for acute asthma. Cochrane Database Syst Rev 2001;(3):CD002741.

19. Schuh S, Willan AR, Stephens D, et al. Can montelukast shorten prednisolone therapy in children with mild to moderate acute asthma? A randomized controlled trial. J Pediatr 2009;155(6):795–800.

20. Watts K, Chavasse RJ. Leukotriene receptor antagonists in addition to usual care for acute asthma in adults and children. Cochrane Database Syst Rev 2012;(5):CD006100.

21. Ram FS, Cates CJ, Ducharme FM. Long-acting beta2-agonists versus antileukotrienes as add-on therapy to inhaled corticosteroids for chronic asthma. Cochrane Database Syst Rev 2005;(1):CD003137.

22. Nair P, Milan SJ, Rowe BH. Addition of intravenous aminophylline to inhaled beta(2)-agonists in adults with acute asthma. Cochrane Database Syst Rev 2012;(12):CD002742.
23. Cote CG, Dordelly LJ, Celli BR. Impact of COPD exacerbations on patient-centered outcomes. Chest 2007;131(3):696–704.
24. Gunen H, Hacievliyagil SS, Kosar F, et al. Factors affecting survival of hospitalised patients with COPD. Eur Respir J 2005;26(2):234–41.
25. Shimizu K, Yoshii Y, Morozumi M, et al. Pathogens in COPD exacerbations identified by comprehensive real-time PCR plus older methods. Int J Chron Obstruct Pulmon Dis 2015;10:2009–16.
26. Medina-Ramon M, Zanobetti A, Schwartz J. The effect of ozone and PM10 on hospital admissions for pneumonia and chronic obstructive pulmonary disease: a national multicity study. Am J Epidemiol 2006;163(6):579–88.
27. Vestbo J, Hurd SS, Agusti AG, et al. Global strategy for the diagnosis, management, and prevention of chronic obstructive pulmonary disease: GOLD executive summary. Am J Respir Crit Care Med 2013;187(4):347–65.
28. Brightling CE. Biomarkers that predict and guide therapy for exacerbations of chronic obstructive pulmonary disease. Ann Am Thorac Soc 2013;10(Suppl): S214–9.
29. Wilkinson TM, Donaldson GC, Hurst JR, et al. Early therapy improves outcomes of exacerbations of chronic obstructive pulmonary disease. Am J Respir Crit Care Med 2004;169(12):1298–303.
30. Hurst JR, Vestbo J, Anzueto A, et al. Susceptibility to exacerbation in chronic obstructive pulmonary disease. N Engl J Med 2010;363(12):1128–38.
31. Garcia-Aymerich J, Farrero E, Felez MA, et al. Risk factors of readmission to hospital for a COPD exacerbation: a prospective study. Thorax 2003;58(2):100–5.
32. Garcia-Aymerich J, Monso E, Marrades RM, et al. Risk factors for hospitalization for a chronic obstructive pulmonary disease exacerbation. EFRAM study. Am J Respir Crit Care Med 2001;164(6):1002–7.
33. Yang H, Xiang P, Zhang E, et al. Predictors of exacerbation frequency in chronic obstructive pulmonary disease. Eur J Med Res 2014;19:18.
34. Quintana JM, Esteban C, Unzurrunzaga A, et al. Predictive score for mortality in patients with COPD exacerbations attending hospital emergency departments. BMC Med 2014;12:66.
35. MacDonald MI, Shafuddin E, King PT, et al. Cardiac dysfunction during exacerbations of chronic obstructive pulmonary disease. Lancet Respir Med 2016; 4(2):138–48.
36. McCrory DC, Brown CD. Anti-cholinergic bronchodilators versus beta2-sympathomimetic agents for acute exacerbations of chronic obstructive pulmonary disease. Cochrane Database Syst Rev 2002;(4):CD003900.
37. Snow V, Lascher S, Mottur-Pilson C, Joint Expert Panel on Chronic Obstructive Pulmonary Disease of the American College of Chest Physicians and the American College of Physicians-American Society of Internal Medicine. Evidence base for management of acute exacerbations of chronic obstructive pulmonary disease. Ann Intern Med 2001;134(7):595–9.
38. Di Marco F, Verga M, Santus P, et al. Effect of formoterol, tiotropium, and their combination in patients with acute exacerbation of chronic obstructive pulmonary disease: a pilot study. Respir Med 2006;100(11):1925–32.
39. Aaron SD, Vandemheen KL, Hebert P, et al. Outpatient oral prednisone after emergency treatment of chronic obstructive pulmonary disease. N Engl J Med 2003;348(26):2618–25.

40. Walters JA, Tan DJ, White CJ, et al. Systemic corticosteroids for acute exacerbations of chronic obstructive pulmonary disease. Cochrane Database Syst Rev 2014;(9):CD001288.

41. Walters JA, Tan DJ, White CJ, et al. Different durations of corticosteroid therapy for exacerbations of chronic obstructive pulmonary disease. Cochrane Database Syst Rev 2014;(12):CD006897.

42. Standards for the diagnosis and management of patients with COPD. 2004. Available at: https://www.thoracic.org/copd-guidelines/resources/copddoc.pdf. Accessed August, 2016.

43. Maltais F, Ostinelli J, Bourbeau J, et al. Comparison of nebulized budesonide and oral prednisolone with placebo in the treatment of acute exacerbations of chronic obstructive pulmonary disease: a randomized controlled trial. Am J Respir Crit Care Med 2002;165(5):698–703.

44. Vollenweider DJ, Jarrett H, Steurer-Stey CA, et al. Antibiotics for exacerbations of chronic obstructive pulmonary disease. Cochrane Database Syst Rev 2012;(12):CD010257.

45. Stockley RA, O'Brien C, Pye A, et al. Relationship of sputum color to nature and outpatient management of acute exacerbations of COPD. Chest 2000;117(6): 1638–45.

46. Austin MA, Wills KE, Blizzard L, et al. Effect of high flow oxygen on mortality in chronic obstructive pulmonary disease patients in prehospital setting: randomised controlled trial. BMJ 2010;341:c5462.

47. Warnier MJ, van Riet EE, Rutten FH, et al. Smoking cessation strategies in patients with COPD. Eur Respir J 2013;41(3):727–34.

48. Barr RG, Rowe BH, Camargo CA. Methylxanthines for exacerbations of chronic obstructive pulmonary disease. Cochrane Database Syst Rev 2003;(2):CD002168.

49. Au DH, Bryson CL, Chien JW, et al. The effects of smoking cessation on the risk of chronic obstructive pulmonary disease exacerbations. J Gen Intern Med 2009; 24(4):457–63.

50. Appleton S, Poole P, Smith B, et al. Long-acting beta2-agonists for poorly reversible chronic obstructive pulmonary disease. Cochrane Database Syst Rev 2006;(3):CD001104.

51. Karner C, Chong J, Poole P. Tiotropium versus placebo for chronic obstructive pulmonary disease. Cochrane Database Syst Rev 2014;(7):CD009285.

52. Poole PJ, Chacko E, Wood-Baker RW, et al. Influenza vaccine for patients with chronic obstructive pulmonary disease. Cochrane Database Syst Rev 2006;(1):CD002733.

53. Herath SC, Poole P. Prophylactic antibiotic therapy for chronic obstructive pulmonary disease (COPD). Cochrane Database Syst Rev 2013;(11):CD009764.

54. Martinez FJ, Calverley PM, Goehring UM, et al. Effect of roflumilast on exacerbations in patients with severe chronic obstructive pulmonary disease uncontrolled by combination therapy (REACT): a multicentre randomised controlled trial. Lancet 2015;385(9971):857–66.

55. Kon SS, Canavan JL, Man WD. Pulmonary rehabilitation and acute exacerbations of COPD. Expert Rev Respir Med 2012;6(5):523–31 [quiz: 531].

56. Effing T, Kerstjens H, van der Valk P, et al. (Cost)-effectiveness of self-treatment of exacerbations on the severity of exacerbations in patients with COPD: the COPE II study. Thorax 2009;64(11):956–62.

# Psychiatric Emergencies
## Assessing and Managing Suicidal Ideation

Andrea N. Weber, MD, MME[a,b], Maria Michail, PhD[c],
Alex Thompson, MD, MBA, MPH[b],
Jess G. Fiedorowicz, MD, PhD[a,b,d,e],*

## KEYWORDS

- Depression • Mental health • Prevention • Primary health care • Risk assessment
- Suicide

## KEY POINTS

- Screening tools, including but not limited to the Patient Health Questionnaire 9 and the Columbia Suicide Severity Rating Scale, may identify individuals at risk and in need of further assessment.
- The suicide risk assessment involves a clinical judgment based on an individualized evaluation of various risk and protective factors for suicide.
- There exist a variety of interventions to modify suicide risk and that should be tailored to the individual's risk profile.

## INTRODUCTION

Suicide is a complex personal and sociologic phenomenon accounting for 1.6% of all deaths in the United States. According to the Centers for Disease Control and Prevention (CDC), there were 42,773 suicides reported in the United States in 2014 (a rate of 13.4 per 100,000), which represents a 24% increase since 1999. Suicide is the 10th leading cause of death in all age groups, with approximately 50% of those deaths involving firearms. Firearms account for 55% of suicides in men, whereas poisoning is the most common means of suicide in women. For people aged 10 to 34 years,

[a] Department of Internal Medicine, The University of Iowa, 200 Hawkins Drive, Iowa City, IA 52242, USA; [b] Department of Psychiatry, Carver College of Medicine, The University of Iowa, 200 Hawkins Drive, Iowa City, IA 52242, USA; [c] School of Health Sciences, University of Nottingham, D17 Institute of Mental Health, Innovation Park, Triumph Road, Nottingham, NG7 2TU, UK; [d] Department of Epidemiology, College of Public Health, The University of Iowa, 145 North Riverside Drive, 100 CPH, Iowa City, IA 52242, USA; [e] Abboud Cardiovascular Research Center, Carver College of Medicine, The University of Iowa, 2269 Carver Biomedical Research Building, Iowa City, IA 52242, USA
* Corresponding author. Department of Psychiatry, The University of Iowa, 200 Hawkins Drive, Iowa City, IA 52242.
*E-mail address:* jess-fiedorowicz@uiowa.edu

Med Clin N Am 101 (2017) 553–571
http://dx.doi.org/10.1016/j.mcna.2016.12.006
0025-7125/17/Published by Elsevier Inc.
medical.theclinics.com

suicide remains the second leading cause of death behind unintentional injury. For those aged 35 to 54 years, it is the fourth leading cause of death in the United States, killing more people than liver disease, diabetes, stroke, or infection.[1]

Although suicidal ideation remains the most common psychiatric emergency encountered by mental health providers, its management and risk factors are more commonly treated by primary care providers. More than 90% of individuals who complete suicide present to their primary care provider within weeks to months of their death.[2–5] Primary care providers with practices of approximately 2000 patients, on average, lose a patient to suicide every 3 years.[6] Growing requirements for depression screening in primary care render screening, assessing, and managing suicidal ideation and behaviors a more common element of practice. However, most providers fail to screen for suicidal ideation and consider themselves unprepared to do so. When evaluating standardized patients presenting with depressive symptoms, only 36% of providers screened for suicidal ideation, with many potential barriers identified.[7] More than 40% of patients who present to primary care are hesitant to discuss their depressive symptoms, noting stigma, belief that depression is not a primary care problem, and belief that they should be able to control their own symptoms.[8] Many providers lack the time, space, access to subspecialty care, and mental health training to appropriately assess and manage suicidal patients.[9,10] In a study of 50 primary care providers who lost a patient to suicide, 88% of these patients endorsed suicidal ideation at their last visit, but such comments were at times thought to be attention seeking or not significantly different from baseline. Providers also struggled with limited access to mental health services for their patients.[5] This challenge is also described when working with adolescent populations in which risk factors are often interpreted as attention seeking or part of normal development. In younger populations, open communication can be difficult and involving a support system can be more challenging.[11]

The aforementioned challenges make the process of assessing for suicide risk a daunting task for busy practitioners. This article summarizes the latest evidence and guidelines for suicide risk assessment and management with a focus for application in busy outpatient settings.

## CHALLENGE

Suicidal ideation and behaviors, akin to the symptoms of an acute coronary syndrome or stroke, require immediate attention. However, unlike their vascular emergency counterparts, no evidence-based algorithms exist to reliably assess, manage, and prevent suicide.[12] The low frequency of suicide is partly responsible for this difficulty. Suicides accounted for 1.6% of all deaths in the United States in 2014. Even in a high-risk demographic, such as older men, the overall prevalence of suicide is very low, particularly within a narrow time frame. Even when protocols have been applied to an inpatient psychiatric population with a high baseline risk for suicide, positive predictive values remain less than 11%.[13] Adding to the complexity, the impact of many of the variables associated with suicide at a population level may vary at the level of the individual. For instance, marriage is generally protective of suicide,[14] but for a given patient it may be a key stressor driving suicidal thoughts, the primary reason to not act on suicidal thoughts, and everything in between. This possibility necessitates a contextual model of clinical decision making in what has been called the quintessential clinical judgment.[15]

Although the ability to predict suicide may seem grim, there has been increasing evidence that education of primary care providers, population-based suicide prevention strategies (such as media desensationalization and gun reform), and collaborative care models can reduce the rate of suicide through the identification and modification of certain risk factors and limiting access to lethal means.

## MANAGEMENT GOALS

Management of suicide includes screening for suicidal ideation or behaviors, performing an assessment of the individual's current risk of imminent harm, and creating a treatment plan in collaboration with the patient and any involved supports. This process needs to be individualized; collaborative; and completed using a calm, cooperative, and curious interview style.

### Screening Goals

The goal of suicide screening is to determine whether an actionable risk is present. In a primary care setting, this screen should be efficient, easily completed by front-office staff, and have high sensitivity (or low false-negative rate).[16]

### How to Screen

The Patient Health Questionaire-9 (PHQ-9) is a quick, subjective reporting scale that can be incorporated into the medical record. Affirmative responses to item 9 regarding thoughts of death or self-harm have hazard ratios of 10 and 8.5 for attempts and deaths in a community setting, respectively.[17] It is in the public domain and available with instructions through the Substance Abuse and Mental Health Services Administration (SAMSHA) Web site (www.integration.samhsa.gov/images/res/PHQ%20-%20Questions.pdf). Although many clinics defer to the PHQ-2 for depression screening, the cutoff for further depression assessment is typically 3 and can miss 50% to 60% of patients who would otherwise endorse suicidal ideation on item 9 of the extended version.[18]

The Columbia Suicide Severity Rating Scale (C-SSRS) is a public forum questionnaire that can help screen for suicide and form a detailed account of an individual's suicidal ideations or behaviors. It is easy to administer with minimal training, available in multiple languages, and easily included in an electronic medical record. In studies, it has reported sensitivity of 67%, specifically of 76%, positive predictive values of 14%, and negative predictive values of 98%.[19,20]

**Table 1** includes types of screening questions that can help identify current suicide risk factors and depressive symptoms while enabling the general practitioner to discuss sensitive topics in an honest and comfortable environment.[21]

### Who to Screen

There is no current consensus on who should be screened for suicidal ideation or plans. The World Health Organization (WHO) currently recommends that all individuals more than 10 years of age with any mental health disorder, epilepsy, interpersonal conflict, recent severe life event, or other risk factor for suicide should be asked about thoughts or plans to self-harm or attempt suicide.[20] Similarly, the Joint Commission recommends that all individuals with a behavioral or emotional disorder be screened for suicide.[22] In an updated review, the United States Protective Task Force found insufficient evidence to recommend suicide screening for the general population, noting that routine screening does not identify individuals at risk for suicide more than screening individuals with mental health disorders, emotional distress, or a history of suicide attempts.[23] Only the CDC currently recommends that all primary physicians screen the general population for both depression and suicide.[22]

| Table 1 Examples of screening questions to identify risk factors for suicide | |
|---|---|
| Home | Where do you live and who lives with you? How do you get along with each member? Who could you go to if you needed help with a problem? |
| Education/ employment | What do you like about school (or work)? What are you good and not good at? How do you get along with teachers and other students (boss and coworkers)? |
| Activities | What sort of things do you do in your spare time? Do you belong to any clubs, groups, and so forth? What sort of things do you like to do with friends? |
| Drugs | Many young people at your age are starting to experiment with cigarettes or alcohol. Have you tried these or other drugs like marijuana, injection drugs, or other substances? How much are you taking and how often? |
| Sexuality | Some young people are getting involved in sexual relationships. Have you had a sexual experience with a guy or a girl or both? |
| Suicide/safety | What sort of things do you do if you are feeling sad, angry, or hurt? Some people who feel really down often feel like hurting themselves or even killing themselves. Have you ever felt this way? Have you ever tried to hurt yourself? Do you have access to firearms in your home or the home of a friend or family member? |

In addition to the guidelines discussed earlier, specific complaints or patient characteristics may warrant suicide screening. These include:

- Changes in mood, including any depressive symptoms, emotional distress, anger, irritability, or aggression[24,25]
- Anxiety or agitation[26,27]
- Sleep complaints[24]
- Evidence of unpredictable or impulsive behavior[25]
- Sudden change in life circumstances[28]
- Increase in alcohol or other drug use
- Increasing health care use, including hospitalizations, office visits, and emergency room visits[29]
- Therapy nonadherence, including medications, physical therapy, and psychotherapy
- Presentation because of family/friend; more than 50% of individuals who presented to primary care providers before suicide were convinced to do so by family or friends[30]

Despite concerns reported by both patients and general practitioners, a systematic review found no significant increase in suicidal ideation or behaviors when patients were asked about suicide, regardless of age, current level of depression, or history of suicidal behaviors.[31,32]

### Assessment Goals

After screening has identified an individual at risk, a formal suicide risk assessment should occur with the following goals: identify modifiable and fixed risk factors; identify protective factors; clarify the current level of suicidal intent and planning; and estimate the current risk as low, moderate, or high to guide treatment and disposition.

## Current Assessment Guidelines

In a 2014 review of 10 published guidelines on suicide assessment and management, recommendations varied in length, depth, and content covered. Guidelines ranged from 15 to 190 pages and although most discussed evidence-based treatments for suicidal ideation and behaviors, few offered recommendations on how to select treatment and less than 60% included a standardized method of determining risk.[33] The published guidelines and resources that included sections on recommended risk categorizations and/or recommended interventions are included in **Table 2**.

## How to Assess

Interviews between care providers and suicidal patients need to maintain or enhance the therapeutic alliance. All assessments should be conducted with curiosity, concern, calmness, and acceptance of the individual's current emotional and cognitive state.[34] Patients with suicidal ideation may feel hopeless, desperate, or cognitively overwhelmed, interfering with their ability to comprehend and convey these thoughts to others. Clinicians should stay attuned to their own reactions that may be nontherapeutic, such as hostility, avoidance of negative feelings, or the blurring of professional roles, possibly as a way to take on a savior role.[34]

| Table 2 | |
| --- | --- |
| Published guidelines and resources for suicide risk assessment | |
| **Name** | **Sources** |
| Practice Parameter for Assessment and Treatment of Children and Adolescents with Suicidal Behaviors | American Academy of Child and Adolescent Psychiatry |
| Practice Guideline for the Assessment and Treatment of Patients with Suicidal Behaviors | American Psychiatric Association |
| Clinical Practice Guidelines for Assessment and Management of Patients at Risk for Suicide | Department of Veterans Affairs, Department of Defense |
| Assessment and Care of Adults at Risk for Suicidal Ideation and Behavior | Registered Nurses' Association of Ontario |
| Core Competencies for Assessment and Management of Suicide | American Association of Suicidology |
| National Suicide Prevention Lifeline Suicide Risk Assessment Standards Packet | National Suicide Prevention Lifeline, SAMSHA |
| SAFE-T | SAMSHA |
| Suicide Prevention: Saving Lives One Community at a Time | AFSP |
| Suicide and the Elderly | AFSP |
| IASP Guidelines for Suicide | IASP |
| Suicide Care in Systems Framework | National Action Alliance for Suicide Prevention, Clinical Care and Intervention Task Force |

*Abbreviations:* AFSP, American Foundation for Suicide Prevention; IASP, International Association for Suicide Prevention; SAFE-T, Suicide Assessment Five-step Evaluation and Triage.

In adolescent populations, the HEADSS (home, education and employment, activities, drugs, sexuality, and suicide and safety [see **Table 1**]) assessment was developed in the Australian primary care setting to assess the psychosocial needs of younger populations and guide decision making. The primary goal of any adolescent patient interview is to understand the developmental perspective of the patient while empowering the patient to participate in their health care, discuss sensitive topics with minimal discomfort, and to ultimately take any signs or symptoms of distress seriously.[35] In collaboration with general practitioners and the Charles Walker Memorial Trust (CWMT), an interactive, case-based toolkit entitled The CWMT GP Toolkit - The Mental Health Consultation (With a Young Person) is available publicly and online (http://www.cwmt.org.uk/wp-content/uploads/2014/01/GPToolkit2013.pdf).

### Risk Factors

One challenge with suicide risk factor assessment is that many risk factors are static, not modifiable, and are limited in helping determine who needs a higher level of care. In a 1983 study, 30 suicides were documented in 803 veterans considered at high risk based on risk factors, but another 37 suicides were also completed in those not considered to be high risk by risk factors.[13]

In contrast, some risk factors may be more acute or subacute, indicating a heightened risk for suicide in the near term.[36] Some of these more acute risk factors, referred to as warning signs, were identified by a consensus panel formed by the American Association of Suicidology to help clinicians appreciate what the patient is doing or saying in the present moment that may acutely increase the risk.[37] There is concern that, even in the setting of significant protective factors, acute risk factors can significantly increase an individual's risk for suicide.[38]

**Table 3** includes validated risk factors for suicide, separated by those associated with more acute suicide risk. Risk factors with asterisks represent factors that are potentially modifiable in the immediate clinical setting.

- Prior suicide attempt remains the strongest predictor of future attempts and completions.[39] There is increasing correlation between suicidal ideation and behaviors, especially for patients presenting in an emergency room setting.[40,41]

| Table 3 Summary of suicide risk factors | |
| --- | --- |
| **Suicide Risk Factors** | |
| **Chronic** | **Acute** |
| Prior attempts | Suicidal ideation |
| Recent hospitalization | Purposelessness |
| Living alone | Insomnia* |
| Family history of suicide | Anxiety, agitation* |
| LGBTQ population | Trapped feeling |
| Adverse childhood events | Nonadherence to care |
| Stressful life events | Withdrawal |
| Mental illness* | Anger, rage, revenge seeking |
| Physical illness* | Recklessness |
| Unemployment | Mood and personality changes |
| Advancing age | Substance use* |
| | Hopelessness* |

Asterisks represent factors that are potentially modifiable in the immediate clinical setting.
*Abbreviation:* LGBTQ, lesbian, gay, bisexual, transgender, queer or questioning.

Although most individuals who self-harm do not go on to commit suicide, repeated self-harm even without intention to end life is a predictor of suicide and is typically present within the 12 months preceding suicide in young people.[42,43] However, more than 90% of suicides are completed on the first or second attempt.[44]

- Suicidal ideation, in contrast with a history of suicide attempts, may represent an increase in suicide risk, especially if this ideation has developed into the seeking of means to perform the action, increasing discussion about death, and rehearsal behaviors.[37] There is no documented difference between passive or active suicidal ideation in suicide course or outcome; as such, both should hold weight in suicide assessment.[45,46]

- Stressful life events must be considered within the circumstance and age of the patient. Common adolescent events include bullying (either as victim or perpetrator), disciplinary actions, legal issues, school difficulties, romantic break-ups, assaults, or problems relating to home life.[47,48] For adults, financial difficulties, relationship losses, unemployment, and intimate partner violence all increase the risk for suicide attempts.[23,49–51] These events may ultimately resolve with time and action, but during a visit with a primary care provider they are unlikely to be modifiable.

- All psychiatric disorders, with the exception of intellectual disability and later-course dementias, are associated with an increased risk of suicidal ideation, attempts, and completions.[39,52,53] This risk is significantly greater during active periods of illness and correlates with severity of illness.[48,54] Hopelessness in the setting of depression increases the risk for suicide and is typically modifiable with treatment of the mental health disorder.[25,40]

- Physical illnesses, such as pulmonary disease, cancer, stroke, diabetes, ischemic heart disease, and spine disorders, are all independently associated with suicide completion.[55] Suicide decedents tend to spend more time in the hospital for both medical and psychiatric reasons in the months before their deaths, endorse lower global quality of life assessment scores, and have more physical impairment.[29,53] Similar risk for depression and suicide is also found in adolescent populations with chronic physical illnesses.[56] Although some illnesses cannot be cured, the amount of disability or functioning may be modifiable with therapy.

- High-risk substance use or use disorders, including alcohol, prescription drugs, and illicit drugs, are associated with increased suicide risk, both in adult and adolescent populations.[53,57] Twenty percent of suicides occur while individuals are intoxicated.[58] Increasing substance use despite worsening mood symptoms, associated dysfunction, and increasing suicidal ideation may lead to a more acute suicide risk compared with a previous baseline level of use.[37]

- Members of the LGBTQ (lesbian, gay, bisexual, transgender, queer or questioning) community may be at increased risk for suicide, especially if they have not found acceptance within their community and main support systems. This risk factor should be considered within the environment of the patient.[59,60]

### Protective Factors

Similar to risk factors, most individuals have both modifiable and nonmodifiable protective factors that may be enhanced during periods of acute distress to help prevent against suicide. The following questions can help elicit these factors[36,61]:

1. What keeps you going during difficult times?
2. What are your reasons for living?

3. What has kept you from acting on those thoughts?
4. What or who do you rely on for support during times like these?

Established protective factors against suicide are provided in **Table 4**, separated by modifiability.

| Table 4 Protective factors for suicide | |
| --- | --- |
| **Suicide Protective Factors** | |
| **Nonmodifiable** | **Potentially Modifiable** |
| Female gender | Interpersonal support |
| Marriage | Positive coping skills |
| Children | Life satisfaction |
| Pregnancy | |
| Religion/spirituality | |

Similar to risk factors, protective factors have to be considered within the context of the patient. For example, social obligation to a spouse is protective against suicide, but the presence of high conflict or violence within the relationship significantly increases suicide risk.[34,61] Responsibility to children is thought to be protective in suicide, except in cases of postpartum mood and psychotic disorders, teen pregnancy, and extreme economic hardships.[34,62] Although pregnancy and motherhood has been studied as a protective factor, suicide remains the leading cause of maternal death in industrialized countries and vigilance in assessing for antepartum and postpartum depression and anxiety cannot be overemphasized.[61,63,64]

### Suicidal Evaluation

Part of a suicide risk assessment is gaining a clear understanding of the individual's desire to complete suicide, capability to do so, and current suicidal intent. Some questions that can help elicit this information are[36,61,65]:

1. Why do you want to die?
2. Have you done anything in preparation for your death?
3. On a scale of 1 to 10, where would you rate your seriousness or wish to die?
4. Have you tried out any particular method or taken steps in rehearsal for suicide?

### Determining Level of Risk

The overall goal at this point is that the primary care provider has been able to adequately identify key risk factors, both modifiable and acute, and protective factors in order to rate the individuals current risk of suicide. This acute, current risk may differ from the patient's chronic level of suicide risk, the latter typically being based on static demographic factors that are not modifiable.[66] There can be ambiguity around risk factors and what may define a chronic and hard-to-manage risk versus an acute risk that must be dealt with immediately, necessitating clinical judgment. As for many assessment and screening tools, the authors propose that overall risk be defined as a manageable 3 levels (low, medium, or high). Individuals at the lowest and highest risk may be easiest to identify and those at more moderate levels of risk may require greater assessment to discern the appropriate management strategy.[65]

### Managing Level of Risk

**Table 5** has been modified and adapted from Bryan and Rudd[66] 2006 and the Suicide Assessment Five-step Evaluation and Triage (SAFE-T) protocol developed through

**Table 5**
**Levels of suicide risk**

| Acute Risk Level | Characteristics of Level | | | Recommended Response |
|---|---|---|---|---|
| | Protective Factors | Acute Risk Factors | Suicidal Evaluation | |
| Mild | Easily identifiable, multiple protective factors | Few risk factors, mild mood symptoms, evidence of self-control | Ideation limited in frequency, intensity, or duration. No plan or intent | 1. Frequent outpatient follow-up, monitoring for any change in risk<br>2. Further evaluation of mood symptoms<br>3. Consider psychiatric referral |
| Moderate | Some identifiable protective factors | Baseline chronic risk factors. Minimal mood symptoms. Maintained self-control. Rare acute risk factors | Frequent suicidal ideation, still limited in intensity and duration. May have plan, but no intent | 1. Increase frequency/duration of visits. Repeated evaluation of need for hospitalization<br>2. Involve family and support system<br>3. Means restriction<br>4. Review emergency protocols, such as emergency rooms and crisis services<br>5. Control mood symptoms with medications and/or psychotherapy<br>6. Frequent follow-up with phone calls or nursing visits (if available)<br>7. Consider psychiatric referral and/or hospitalization, especially if risk increasing with reevaluation |
| Severe | Minimal protective factors endorsed | Multiple acute risk factors or high-acuity risk factor. Poor self-control, either at baseline or caused by substances | Frequent, intense, persistent suicidal ideation with plans. May discuss intent, but has no gathered means or had rehearsal behaviors | 1. Evaluation for inpatient hospitalization, either by on-site psychiatric professional or through an emergency room<br>2. Do not leave patient alone in the office during assessment<br>3. Hospitalization may be indicated even if involuntarily<br>4. Means restriction for acute period following hospitalization |

SAMSHA.[33,66] Both were chosen because of their descriptions of different risk categorizations and their concise response recommendations based on these categories. Although neither has been studied to predict or prevent suicide, they offer explicit guidance for busy general practitioners.

Although most providers may think that the primary purpose of a risk assessment is to determine disposition (home vs hospital), it should also be used to help guide other interventions, both pharmacologic and nonpharmacologic, and regardless of setting.

## NONPHARMCOLOGIC INTERVENTIONS

Brief therapeutic interventions, such as psychotherapy, case management, or supportive telephone calls and letters, are more effective for long-term suicide prevention when they are directed toward the symptoms of suicide, rather than indirectly targeting symptoms associated with suicide, such as depression or hopelessness.[20,67,68] These methods address suicide risk head-on in collaboration with patients in order to prevent suicide. The following interventions may be used as tools.

### Safety Plan

Safety plans are prioritized lists of coping strategies and sources of support used during or preceding a suicidal crisis.[69] Steps in creating a safety plan include:

1. Recognize warning signs
2. Identify and use internal coping strategies
3. Use interpersonal supports as a means of distraction from unpleasant thoughts or urges
4. Contact friends or family to help resolve the crisis
5. Contact a mental health provider/agency
6. Reduce potential use of lethal means

Ideally, these steps should be detailed, written, kept in a personal spot, and followed in a stepwise fashion until the crisis resolves.[70] Safety plans have been shown to reduce suicide attempts, completions, depressive symptoms, anxiety, and hopelessness within 3 months compared with interventions without safety plans.[71] Safety plans should not be confused with so called no-harm or contracts for safety, which have not been shown to reduce suicide or suicidal behavior, offering only false reassurance to providers.[47] An example of a template for a safety plan can be found online at http://www.sprc.org/sites/default/files/Brown_StanleySafetyPlanTemplate.pdf.

### Means Restriction

Access to lethal means of suicide remains a significant risk factor for all age groups, and interventions that minimize these means remain the most impactful form of primary prevention against suicide.[47,72] Firearms are of specific importance, because they remain the most common suicidal method and account for more than 50% of suicide-related deaths, following by suffocation, hanging, poisoning, and overdose.[73] If guns remain in the home, they should be unloaded, locked, and stored separately from ammunition.[74] Restricting access to drugs and alcohol has also been shown to reduce suicide rates, especially when substance abuse is considered a risk factor or warning sign for the individual.[75]

### Psychotherapy

In a pooled sample of 11 trials, psychotherapy regardless of methodology was shown to roduoo suicide attempts by more than 30%.[73,76] The most robust literature exists for the ability of cognitive behavior therapy, dialectical behavioral therapy, and problem-solving therapy to reduce self-harm, suicide behavior, and suicidal ideation.[77–80]

Although primary care providers are unlikely to be providing psychotherapy, successful referrals to qualified individuals may be enhanced by the provider's knowledge and confidence in its effectiveness in addition to a therapeutic alliance. The risk of suicide attempts increases the month before and after starting treatment, regardless of whether treatment is medications or psychotherapy, making close follow-up very important.[81]

### Follow-up Care

Intensive management that includes weekly follow-up and assertive outreach by clinic personal after missed appointments has been shown to significantly reduce suicide rates in the United Kingdom.[82] Other follow-up interventions, such as telephone calls, letters, and postcards, have shown some benefit for reducing repeat suicide attempts.[20,83]

National crisis lines are also effective at reducing people's sense of crisis, confusion, helplessness, and suicidality. This effect is improved when a standardized suicide risk assessment algorithm has been implemented.[84]

### Referral to Mental Health Provider

In addition to the suggested interventions for referral given in **Table 5**, referral can be considered for any patient at risk of suicide.[85] Physicians should refer patients to mental health providers when patients are past the primary physicians' comfort level, following failed response to treatment trials for a psychiatric disorder, if the patient's suicidal thoughts are persistent, if there is suspicion for current psychotic symptoms (hallucinations, delusions, disorganized thinking), or when hospitalization may be warranted.[65,85,86]

Collaborative care models, which place mental health services within the primary care setting, also reduce suicidal ideation and depression within primary care populations.[87] These models have been shown to be cost-effective and should be advocated by primary physicians when possible because they have not been disseminated as widely as the evidence warrants.

## PHARMACOLOGIC INTERVENTION

Because more than 90% of patients who complete suicide have a mental health diagnosis at their time of death, aggressive, evidence-based treatment of mental health disorders should also be discussed during treatment planning.[88] Despite concerns about increased suicide risk with antidepressant medications, which primarily reflects acute increases in suicidal ideation and attempts in trials of pediatric samples,[89] multiple studies have found them protective against suicidal thoughts, behaviors, and attempts in all age groups, and most strongly and consistently in adults, especially older adults, when used to treat mood and anxiety disorders.[90–96] Selective serotonin-reuptake inhibitors are preferred to tricyclic antidepressants (TCAs) in suicidal patients because of their lower risk in overdose. TCAs and other medications with increased risk in overdose should be prescribed in limited supplies while acute suicide risk remains increased.[20] When indicated, there is evidence supporting a reduction in risk of suicide for patients treated with clozapine or lithium.[97] As with psychotherapy, there is evidence that suicide attempts are increased in the month before treatment, the month after treatment, after discontinuation of medications, and after any dose change. Close follow-up and monitoring are warranted during treatment.[98]

Some pharmacologic interventions may be harmful. After adjusting for mental health diagnoses, a current prescription for any sedative or hypnotic was associated with a 4-fold increase in suicide risk, especially in patients more than 65 years old.[99,100]

## DOCUMENTATION

Once a suicide risk assessment and treatment plan have been completed, it is important to document this plan in detail for the protection of both the patient and the health care team. Documentation should include[34]:

- Summary of presenting complaints.
- Evaluation of current risk factors, protective factors, and warning signs.
- Listing of individuals who participated in the evaluation, including patient's family, friends, and any consultants.
- Summary of treatment options discussed with the patient, including any suggestions or recommendation for hospitalization, if applicable.
- Review of treatment plan agreed on with the patient, including why this plan provides the safest treatment in the least restrictive environment. Treatment plan may include:
  1. Starting medications and/or therapy
  2. Means restriction (ideally with verification from support system that it will be completed)
  3. Substance use reduction or formal treatment
  4. Safety plan creation (make a copy and scan into medical record)
  5. Referral to mental health provider
  6. Hospitalization
- Include plan for follow-up (next appointment, any follow-up phone calls, or other planned out-of-clinic contacts).

The goal of documentation is to clarify the clinical reasoning behind the assessment with a plan that logically follows. From a medicolegal perspective, physicians cannot be expected to predict suicide outcomes in which high-risk individuals may not act and low-risk individuals complete suicide.[13,101] Although legal standards of care vary, a documented suicide risk assessment that captures the clinical decision making should suffice.[102] Given the aforementioned need to contextualize the risk assessment within the story of a particular patient, the assessment need not list every risk and protective factor, but can highlight those key risk and protective factors deemed most relevant for the case. Examples of documented suicide risk assessment can be found in **Box 1**.

## EVALUATION AND EDUCATION

Although many primary care providers think they are unprepared for assessing and managing suicidal patients, they often start with a strong therapeutic alliance, which has been independently shown to decrease suicidal ideation in the primary care population.[103] Physician education programs, both through postgraduate training and continuing medical education, can achieve clinical outcomes similar to those of psychiatrists in the treatment of depression, reduced suicide rates, and increased subjective competency such that providers are more willing to assess and treat suicidal patients.[72,104,105]

> **Box 1**
> **Example of documented suicide risk assessments**
>
> This 30-year-old married woman presents with a major depressive disorder and seems to be a low suicide risk. She denies suicidal ideation, has no history of attempts, and is responsible for 2 children. She has recently started on sertraline and is hopeful about her future. She can be managed safely as an outpatient.
>
> The patient is a 67-year-old married, retired male construction worker who has ischemic cardiomyopathy and recent increased use of alcohol, placing him at a moderate to high risk of suicide. He has no history of suicide attempts and a strong support system. He had a recent hospitalization for a myocardial infarction, during which he developed a depressive syndrome and he seems increasingly hopeless about the future, particularly surrounding his medical bills and debt. While intoxicated last week, he reported having vague and fleeting suicidal thoughts but denies any past or current intent of acting on these thoughts. His wife is not aware of any acute evidence of dangerousness and was willing to secure the patient's firearms and excess medications. He was offered hospitalization, but declined. There is insufficient evidence of acute dangerousness to warrant involuntary hospitalization. Patient agrees to quit drinking and engage in close follow-up for his depression with referral to a psychiatrist. He verbalizes intent to seek emergent assistance if feeling unsafe.

## FUTURE CONSIDERATIONS/SUMMARY

Suicide risk assessment is distinct from assessing risk for other conditions, such as cardiovascular risk. There are a multitude of factors that must be considered without a clear algorithm that exists or can be developed. This challenge can prove daunting for many clinicians without some template for stratification of risk from which to tailor the appropriate management, but this process is like the many decisions that clinicians must make on a daily basis for which clinical judgment is paramount. Suicide risk assessment similarly requires clinicians to exercise their clinical judgment and to weigh the relevance of evidence-based risk and protective factors for the assessment of a particular patient's risk. Interventions can have a positive impact[97] and this article is dedicated to the cadres of clinicians willing to make the effort to save the lives of patients suffering so profoundly as to take their own, at times not even knowing which lives were spared.

## REFERENCES

1. Center for Disease Control and Prevention, National Center for Injury Prevention and Control. "Ten Leading Causes of Death by Age Group, United States - 2014." National Vital Statistics, National Center for Health Statistics. 2016. Available at: https://www.cdc.gov/injury/wisqars/pdf/leading_causes_of_death_by_age_group_2014-a.pdf.
2. Ahmedani BK, Simon GE, Stewart C, et al. Health care contacts in the year before suicide death. J Gen Intern Med 2014;29(6):870–7.
3. Luoma JB, Martin CE, Pearson JL. Contact with mental health and primary care providers before suicide: a review of the evidence. Am J Psychiatry 2002; 159(6):909–16.
4. Pearson A, Saini P, Da Cruz D, et al. Primary care contact prior to suicide in individuals with mental illness. Br J Gen Pract 2009;59(568):825–32.
5. Saini P, Chantler K, Kapur N. General practitioners' perspectives on primary care consultations for suicidal patients. Health Soc Care Community 2016; 24(3):260–9.

6. Diekstra RF. Epidemiology of suicide. Encephale 1996;22(Spec No 4):15–8 [in French].

7. Feldman MD, Franks P, Duberstein PR, et al. Let's not talk about it: suicide inquiry in primary care. Ann Fam Med 2007;5(5):412–8.

8. Bell RA, Franks P, Duberstein PR, et al. Suffering in silence: reasons for not disclosing depression in primary care. Ann Fam Med 2011;9(5):439–46.

9. Leahy D, Schaffalitzky E, Saunders J, et al. Role of the general practitioner in providing early intervention for youth mental health: a mixed methods investigation. Early Interv Psychiatry 2015. [Epub ahead of print].

10. Saini P, Windfuhr K, Pearson A, et al. Suicide prevention in primary care: general practitioners' views on service availability. BMC Res Notes 2010;3:246.

11. Michail M, Tait L. Exploring general practitioners' views and experiences on suicide risk assessment and management of young people in primary care: a qualitative study in the UK. BMJ Open 2016;6(1):e009654.

12. Cornette MM, Schlotthauer AE, Berlin JS, et al. The public health approach to reducing suicide: opportunities for curriculum development in psychiatry residency training programs. Acad Psychiatry 2014;38(5):575–84.

13. Pokorny AD. Prediction of suicide in psychiatric patients. Report of a prospective study. Arch Gen Psychiatry 1983;40(3):249–57.

14. Smith JC, Mercy JA, Conn JM. Marital status and the risk of suicide. Am J Public Health 1988;78(1):78–80.

15. Practice guideline for the assessment and treatment of patients with suicidal behaviors. Am J Psychiatry 2003;160(Suppl 11):1–60.

16. Crawford MJ, Thana L, Methuen C, et al. Impact of screening for risk of suicide: randomised controlled trial. Br J Psychiatry 2011;198(5):379–84.

17. Simon GE, Coleman KJ, Rossom RC, et al. Risk of suicide attempt and suicide death following completion of the Patient Health Questionnaire depression module in community practice. J Clin Psychiatry 2016;77(2):221–7.

18. Inagaki M, Ohtsuki T, Yonemoto N, et al. Validity of the Patient Health Questionnaire (PHQ)-9 and PHQ-2 in general internal medicine primary care at a Japanese rural hospital: a cross-sectional study. Gen Hosp Psychiatry 2013;35(6):592–7.

19. Mundt JC, Greist JH, Jefferson JW, et al. Prediction of suicidal behavior in clinical research by lifetime suicidal ideation and behavior ascertained by the electronic Columbia-Suicide Severity Rating Scale. J Clin Psychiatry 2013;74(9):887–93.

20. Bolton JM, Gunnell D, Turecki G. Suicide risk assessment and intervention in people with mental illness. BMJ 2015;351:h4978.

21. Carr-Gregg MR, Enderby KC, Grover SR. Risk-taking behaviour of young women in Australia: screening for health-risk behaviours. Med J Aust 2003;178(12):601–4.

22. Bono V, Amendola CL. Primary care assessment of patients at risk for suicide. J Am Acad Physician Assist 2015;28(12):35–9.

23. O'Connor E, Gaynes BN, Burda BU, et al. Screening for and treatment of suicide risk relevant to primary care: a systematic review for the U.S. Preventive Services Task Force. Ann Intern Med 2013;158(10):741–54.

24. Denneson LM, Kovas AE, Britton PC, et al. Suicide risk documented during veterans' last Veterans Affairs health care contacts prior to suicide. Suicide Life Threat Behav 2016;46(3):363–74.

25. Morriss R, Kapur N, Byng R. Assessing risk of suicide or self harm in adults. BMJ 2013;347:f4572.

26. McDowell AK, Lineberry TW, Bostwick JM. Practical suicide-risk management for the busy primary care physician. Mayo Clin Proc 2011;86(8):792–800.
27. Dobscha SK, Denneson LM, Kovas AE, et al. Correlates of suicide among veterans treated in primary care: case-control study of a nationally representative sample. J Gen Intern Med 2014;29(Suppl 4):853–60.
28. Lemieux AM, Saman DM, Lutfiyya MN. Men and suicide in primary care. Dis Mon 2014;60(4):155–61.
29. Chock MM, Bommersbach TJ, Geske JL, et al. Patterns of health care usage in the year before suicide: a population-based case-control study. Mayo Clin Proc 2015;90(11):1475–81.
30. Owens C, Lambert H, Donovan J, et al. A qualitative study of help seeking and primary care consultation prior to suicide. Br J Gen Pract 2005;55(516):503–9.
31. Bajaj P, Borreani E, Ghosh P, et al. Screening for suicidal thoughts in primary care: the views of patients and general practitioners. Ment Health Fam Med 2008;5(4):229–35.
32. Dazzi T, Gribble R, Wessely S, et al. Does asking about suicide and related behaviours induce suicidal ideation? What is the evidence? Psychol Med 2014; 44(16):3361–3.
33. Bernert RA, Hom MA, Roberts LW. A review of multidisciplinary clinical practice guidelines in suicide prevention: toward an emerging standard in suicide risk assessment and management, training and practice. Acad Psychiatry 2014; 38(5):585–92.
34. Fowler JC. Suicide risk assessment in clinical practice: pragmatic guidelines for imperfect assessments. Psychotherapy (Chic) 2012;49(1):81–90.
35. Sanci L, Young D. Engaging the adolescent patient. Aust Fam Physician 1995; 24(11):2027–31.
36. Rudd MD, Berman AL, Joiner TE Jr, et al. Warning signs for suicide: theory, research, and clinical applications. Suicide Life Threat Behav 2006;36(3): 255–62.
37. Rudd MD. Suicide warning signs in clinical practice. Curr Psychiatry Rep 2008; 10(1):87–90.
38. Berman AL, Silverman MM. Suicide risk assessment and risk formulation part II: suicide risk formulation and the determination of levels of risk. Suicide Life Threat Behav 2014;44(4):432–43.
39. Harris EC, Barraclough B. Suicide as an outcome for mental disorders. A meta-analysis. Br J Psychiatry 1997;170:205–28.
40. Wang Y, Bhaskaran J, Sareen J, et al. Predictors of future suicide attempts among individuals referred to psychiatric services in the emergency department: a longitudinal study. J Nerv Ment Dis 2015;203(7):507–13.
41. Younes N, Melchior M, Turbelin C, et al. Attempted and completed suicide in primary care: not what we expected? J Affect Disord 2015;170:150–4.
42. Gunnell D, Ho D, Murray V. Medical management of deliberate drug overdose: a neglected area for suicide prevention? Emerg Med J 2004;21(1):35–8.
43. Hawton K, Houston K, Shepperd R. Suicide in young people. Study of 174 cases, aged under 25 years, based on coroners' and medical records. Br J Psychiatry 1999;175:271–6.
44. Parra Uribe I, Blasco-Fontecilla H, García-Parés G, et al. Attempted and completed suicide: not what we expected? J Affect Disord 2013;150(3):840–6.
45. Schulberg HC, Lee PW, Bruce ML, et al. Suicidal ideation and risk levels among primary care patients with uncomplicated depression. Ann Fam Med 2005;3(6): 523–8.

46. Baca-Garcia E, Perez-Rodriguez MM, Oquendo MA, et al. Estimating risk for suicide attempt: are we asking the right questions? Passive suicidal ideation as a marker for suicidal behavior. J Affect Disord 2011;134(1–3):327–32.

47. Gray BP, Dihigo SK. Suicide risk assessment in high-risk adolescents. Nurse Pract 2015;40(9):30–7 [quiz: 37–8].

48. Fordwood SR, Asarnow JR, Huizar DP, et al. Suicide attempts among depressed adolescents in primary care. J Clin Child Adolesc Psychol 2007;36(3):392–404.

49. Cohen A, Chapman BP, Gilman SE, et al. Social inequalities in the occurrence of suicidal ideation among older primary care patients. Am J Geriatr Psychiatry 2010;18(12):1146–54.

50. Devries KM, Mak JY, Bacchus LJ, et al. Intimate partner violence and incident depressive symptoms and suicide attempts: a systematic review of longitudinal studies. PLoS Med 2013;10(5):e1001439.

51. Gallego JA, Rachamallu V, Yuen EY, et al. Predictors of suicide attempts in 3.322 patients with affective disorders and schizophrenia spectrum disorders. Psychiatry Res 2015;228(3):791–6.

52. Corson K, Denneson LM, Bair MJ, et al. Prevalence and correlates of suicidal ideation among Operation Enduring Freedom and Operation Iraqi Freedom veterans. J Affect Disord 2013;149(1–3):291–8.

53. Ashrafioun L, Pigeon WR, Conner KR, et al. Prevalence and correlates of suicidal ideation and suicide attempts among veterans in primary care referred for a mental health evaluation. J Affect Disord 2016;189:344–50.

54. Holma KM, Melartin TK, Haukka J, et al. Incidence and predictors of suicide attempts in DSM-IV major depressive disorder: a five-year prospective study. Am J Psychiatry 2010;167(7):801–8.

55. Crump C, Sundquist K, Sundquist J, et al. Sociodemographic, psychiatric and somatic risk factors for suicide: a Swedish national cohort study. Psychol Med 2014;44(2):279–89.

56. Greydanus D, Patel D, Pratt H. Suicide risk in adolescents with chronic illness: implications for primary care and specialty pediatric practice: a review. Dev Med Child Neurol 2010;52(12):1083–7.

57. Jenkins AL, Singer J, Conner BT, et al. Risk for suicidal ideation and attempt among a primary care sample of adolescents engaging in nonsuicidal self-injury. Suicide Life Threat Behav 2014;44(6):616–28.

58. Perlis RH, Miyahara S, Marangell LB, et al. Long-term implications of early onset in bipolar disorder: data from the first 1000 participants in the Systematic Treatment Enhancement Program for Bipolar Disorder (STEP-BD). Biol Psychiatry 2004;55(9):875–81.

59. Bjorkenstam C, Andersson G, Dalman C, et al. Suicide in married couples in Sweden: is the risk greater in same-sex couples? Eur J Epidemiol 2016;31(7):685–90.

60. Haas AP, Eliason M, Mays VM, et al. Suicide and suicide risk in lesbian, gay, bisexual, and transgender populations: review and recommendations. J Homosex 2011;58(1):10–51.

61. Menon V. Suicide risk assessment and formulation: an update. Asian J Psychiatr 2013;6(5):430–5.

62. Malone KM, Oquendo MA, Haas GL, et al. Protective factors against suicidal acts in major depression: reasons for living. Am J Psychiatry 2000;157(7):1084–8.

63. Howard LM, Flach C, Mehay A, et al. The prevalence of suicidal ideation identified by the Edinburgh Postnatal Depression Scale in postpartum women in

primary care: findings from the RESPOND trial. BMC Pregnancy Childbirth 2011;11:57.

64. Castro E, Couto T, Brancaglion MY, et al. Suicidality among pregnant women in Brazil: prevalence and risk factors. Arch Womens Ment Health 2016;19(2): 343–8.

65. Fiedorowicz JG, Weldon K, Bergus G. Determining suicide risk (hint: a screen is not enough). J Fam Pract 2010;59(5):256–60.

66. Bryan CJ, Rudd MD. Advances in the assessment of suicide risk. J Clin Psychol 2006;62(2):185–200.

67. Meerwijk EL, Parekh A, Oquendo MA, et al. Direct versus indirect psychosocial and behavioural interventions to prevent suicide and suicide attempts: a systematic review and meta-analysis. Lancet Psychiatry 2016;3(6):544–54.

68. Cuijpers P, de Beurs DP, van Spijker BA, et al. The effects of psychotherapy for adult depression on suicidality and hopelessness: a systematic review and meta-analysis. J Affect Disord 2013;144(3):183–90.

69. Wilcox HC, Wyman PA. Suicide prevention strategies for improving population health. Child Adolesc Psychiatr Clin N Am 2016;25(2):219–33.

70. Stanley EY. Safety in action: a practical application. Occup Health Saf 2012; 81(10):52–4.

71. Wang YC, Hsieh LY, Wang MY, et al. Coping card usage can further reduce suicide reattempt in suicide attempter case management within 3-month intervention. Suicide Life Threat Behav 2016;46(1):106–20.

72. Mann JJ, Apter A, Bertolote J, et al. Suicide prevention strategies: a systematic review. JAMA 2005;294(16):2064–74.

73. LeFevre ML, U.S. Preventive Services Task Force. Screening for suicide risk in adolescents, adults, and older adults in primary care: U.S. Preventive Services Task Force recommendation statement. Ann Intern Med 2014;160(10):719–26.

74. Jena AB, Prasad V. Primary care physicians' role in counseling about gun safety. Am Fam Physician 2014;90(9):619–20.

75. Wasserman D, Varnik A. Suicide-preventive effects of perestroika in the former USSR: the role of alcohol restriction. Acta Psychiatr Scand Suppl 1998;394:1–4.

76. Almeida OP, Pirkis J, Kerse N, et al. A randomized trial to reduce the prevalence of depression and self-harm behavior in older primary care patients. Ann Fam Med 2012;10(4):347–56.

77. Lai MH, Maniam T, Chan LF, et al. Caught in the web: a review of web-based suicide prevention. J Med Internet Res 2014;16(1):e30.

78. Watts S, Newby JM, Mewton L, et al. A clinical audit of changes in suicide ideas with internet treatment for depression. BMJ Open 2012;2(5) [pii: e001558].

79. Tarrier N, Taylor K, Gooding P. Cognitive-behavioral interventions to reduce suicide behavior: a systematic review and meta-analysis. Behav Modif 2008;32(1): 77–108.

80. Linehan MM, Comtois KA, Murray AM, et al. Two-year randomized controlled trial and follow-up of dialectical behavior therapy vs therapy by experts for suicidal behaviors and borderline personality disorder. Arch Gen Psychiatry 2006; 63(7):757–66.

81. Simon GE, Savarino J. Suicide attempts among patients starting depression treatment with medications or psychotherapy. Am J Psychiatry 2007;164(7): 1029–34.

82. While D, Bickley H, Roscoe A, et al. Implementation of mental health service recommendations in England and Wales and suicide rates, 1997-2006: a cross-sectional and before-and-after observational study. Lancet 2012;379(9820):1005–12.

83. Carter G, Reith DM, Whyte IM, et al. Repeated self-poisoning: increasing severity of self-harm as a predictor of subsequent suicide. Br J Psychiatry 2005;186:253–7.

84. Joiner T, Kalafat J, Draper J, et al. Establishing standards for the assessment of suicide risk among callers to the national suicide prevention lifeline. Suicide Life Threat Behav 2007;37(3):353–65.

85. NICE. Depression in adults: recognition and management. In: National Institute for Health and Care Excellence, editor. 2009. Available at: https://www.nice.org.uk/guidance/cg90.

86. Bronheim HE, Fulop G, Kunkel EJ, et al. The Academy of Psychosomatic Medicine practice guidelines for psychiatric consultation in the general medical setting. The Academy of Psychosomatic Medicine. Psychosomatics 1998; 39(4):S8–30.

87. Unützer J, Tang L, Oishi S, et al. Reducing suicidal ideation in depressed older primary care patients. J Am Geriatr Soc 2006;54(10):1550–6.

88. Griffiths JJ, Zarate CA Jr, Rasimas JJ. Existing and novel biological therapeutics in suicide prevention. Am J Prev Med 2014;47(3 Suppl 2):S195–203.

89. Bridge JA, Iyengar S, Salary CB, et al. Clinical response and risk for reported suicidal ideation and suicide attempts in pediatric antidepressant treatment: a meta-analysis of randomized controlled trials. JAMA 2007;297(15):1683–96.

90. Bennett K, Rhodes AE, Duda S, et al. A youth suicide prevention plan for Canada: a systematic review of reviews. Can J Psychiatry 2015;60(6):245–57.

91. Gibbons RD, Hur K, Bhaumik DK, et al. The relationship between antidepressant prescription rates and rate of early adolescent suicide. Am J Psychiatry 2006; 163(11):1898–904.

92. Gibbons RD, Brown CH, Hur K. Is the rate of suicide among veterans elevated? Am J Public Health 2012;102(Suppl 1):S17–9.

93. Khan A, Khan S, Kolts R, et al. Suicide rates in clinical trials of SSRIs, other antidepressants, and placebo: analysis of FDA reports. Am J Psychiatry 2003; 160(4):790–2.

94. Leon AC, Solomon DA, Li C, et al. Antidepressants and risks of suicide and suicide attempts: a 27-year observational study. J Clin Psychiatry 2011;72(5):580–6.

95. Leon AC, Fiedorowicz JG, Solomon DA, et al. Risk of suicidal behavior with antidepressants in bipolar and unipolar disorders. J Clin Psychiatry 2014;75(7): 720–7.

96. Gibbons RD, Brown CH, Hur K, et al. Suicidal thoughts and behavior with antidepressant treatment: reanalysis of the randomized placebo-controlled studies of fluoxetine and venlafaxine. Arch Gen Psychiatry 2012;69(6):580–7.

97. Zalsman G, Hawton K, Wasserman D, et al. Suicide prevention strategies revisited: 10-year systematic review. Lancet Psychiatry 2016;3(7):646–59.

98. Valuck RJ, Libby AM, Orton HD, et al. Spillover effects on treatment of adult depression in primary care after FDA advisory on risk of pediatric suicidality with SSRIs. Am J Psychiatry 2007;164(8):1198–205.

99. Carlsten A, Waern M. Are sedatives and hypnotics associated with increased suicide risk of suicide in the elderly? BMC Geriatr 2009;9:20.

100. Didham R, Dovey S, Reith D. Characteristics of general practitioner consultations prior to suicide: a nested case-control study in New Zealand. N Z Med J 2006;119(1247):U2358.

101. Hughes DH. Can the clinician predict suicide? Psychiatr Serv 1995;46(5): 449–51.

102. Simon R, Shuman DW. The standard of care in suicide risk assessment: an elusive concept. CNS Spectr 2006;11(6):442–5.
103. Bryan CJ, Corso KA, Corso ML, et al. Therapeutic alliance and change in suicidal ideation during treatment in integrated primary care settings. Arch Suicide Res 2012;16(4):316–23.
104. Schulberg HC, Block MR, Madonia MJ, et al. Treating major depression in primary care practice. Eight-month clinical outcomes. Arch Gen Psychiatry 1996;53(10):913–9.
105. Graham RD, Rudd MD, Bryan CJ. Primary care providers' views regarding assessing and treating suicidal patients. Suicide Life Threat Behav 2011;41(6): 614–23.

# Recognizing and Caring for the Intoxicated Patient in an Outpatient Clinic

Joseph H. Donroe, MD, MPH[a],*, Jeanette M. Tetrault, MD[b]

## KEYWORDS

- Intoxication • Withdrawal • Substance use disorder • Outpatient • Opioid • Alcohol
- Marijuana • Sedative

## KEY POINTS

- Intoxication or withdrawal from addictive substances is included in the differential diagnosis of patients presenting with altered mental status.
- In the treatment of intoxicated patients, outpatient practitioners should address the original reason for the clinic visit, triage appropriately to home or a higher level of care, and consider treatment of substance withdrawal.
- One of the most important aspects of management of the intoxicated patient is the follow-up assessment for substance use disorders, with initiation of treatment when indicated.
- Physicians should be familiar with the medico-legal aspects of caring for an intoxicated patient, including issues related to privacy, informed consent, and patient/public safety.

## INTRODUCTION

The diagnosis of substance-related intoxication or withdrawal should be considered in patients presenting to an outpatient practice with altered mental status (AMS). Despite the potentially time-consuming and disruptive nature of these visits, outpatient practitioners (OP) have important advantages when caring for intoxicated patients. First, OPs may have a preexisting relationship with the patient and therefore may be more apt to note mild or moderate intoxication. Second, OPs can ensure appropriate follow-up care with the intoxicated patient and perform the critically important assessment for unhealthy substance use and facilitate treatment.

This article reviews the presenting features and management of intoxicated patients, discusses physician responsibilities toward providing care to these patients

The authors have nothing to disclose.
[a] Department of Internal Medicine, Yale New Haven Hospital, St. Raphael Campus, Yale University School of Medicine, Office M330, 1450 Chapel Street, New Haven, CT 06511, USA;
[b] Department of Internal Medicine, Yale University School of Medicine, 367 Cedar Street, Suite 305, New Haven, CT 06510, USA
* Corresponding author.
*E-mail address:* joseph.donroe@yale.edu

Med Clin N Am 101 (2017) 573–586
http://dx.doi.org/10.1016/j.mcna.2016.12.012
0025-7125/17/© 2017 Elsevier Inc. All rights reserved.

medical.theclinics.com

including medico-legal aspects, and highlights the importance of ensuring a follow-up assessment for underlying substance use disorders (SUD).

## SYMPTOMS
### Recognizing the Intoxicated Patient

Alcohol, opioid, marijuana, and prescription sedative use is common and the most likely intoxicating substances to present to a primary care clinic.[1] The diagnosis of substance intoxication, according to the fifth edition of the Diagnostic and Statistical Manual of Mental Disorders (DSM V), has 4 criteria[2]:

1. Recent ingestion of the substance
2. Clinically significant problematic behaviors or psychological changes that develop during or shortly after use of the substance
3. Evident substance-specific intoxication syndromes (see below)
4. Symptoms that are not attributable to another medical condition and are not better explained by another mental disorder, including intoxication with another substance

### Intoxication Syndromes

Intoxication syndromes (**Table 1**) can range in symptom severity from mild alterations in behavior and mental status to life-threatening overdose. Additionally, polysubstance use is common, and patients may present under the influence of 2 or more substances. Other acute medical conditions can also present similarly to intoxication from drugs and alcohol; thus, a broad differential diagnosis must be entertained for anyone presenting to clinic with AMS.

### Alcohol

Ethyl alcohol, or ethanol, primarily acts as a central nervous system depressant. Early symptoms and signs of intoxication include disinhibition and behavioral arousal followed by the sedative effects as the blood alcohol level increases.[3] The literature suggests that observers are inaccurate when attempting to assess degree of alcohol

| Table 1 | | | |
|---|---|---|---|
| **Intoxication syndromes** | | | |
| | **Alcohol/Sedatives** | **Opioids** | **Marijuana** |
| Symptoms | Disinhibition | Euphoria | Impaired concentration |
| | Behavioral arousal | Dysphoria | Impaired attention |
| | Impaired concentration | Apathy | Decreased reaction time |
| | Impaired memory | Psychomotor agitation | Euphoria |
| | Mood lability | Psychomotor retardation | Relaxation |
| | | Drowsiness | Paranoia |
| | | Impaired attention | Anxiety |
| | | Impaired memory | Increased appetite |
| | | | Nausea |
| Signs | Sedation | Sedation | Odor of marijuana |
| | Conjunctival injection | Miotic pupils | Tachycardia |
| | Odor alcoholic beverage | Decreased respiratory rate | Orthostatic hypotension |
| | Slurred speech | Track marks | Dry mouth |
| | Impaired gait/balance | | Conjunctival injection |
| | Nystagmus | | |

*Adapted from* American Psychiatric Association. Diagnostic and statistical manual of mental disorder. 5th edition. Arlington (VA): American Psychiatric Association; 2013.

intoxication, including a poor correlation between behavior and BAL.[4-6] Nonetheless, cited signs and symptoms include impaired memory and attention, personality and behavior change, mood lability, impaired judgment, conjunctival injection, the odor of an alcoholic beverage, speech abnormalities such as slurring, impaired gait and balance, and nystagmus.[2,4,7,8]

### Marijuana

Marijuana exerts its intoxicating effects primarily through the interaction between delta 9-tetrahydrocannabinol (THC) and central nervous system cannabinoid receptors. THC dose dependently impairs psychomotor functioning, with a particular impact on executive functioning, including attention and concentration, decision making, impulsivity and inhibition, risk taking, object distance and shape discrimination, reaction time, and perceptual-motor coordination.[3,9] Clinical intoxication can include euphoria, relaxation, and increased appetite but also occasionally paranoia, anxiety, and nausea. Physical findings may include the distinct odor of recent marijuana inhalation, tachycardia, orthostatic hypotension, dry mouth, and conjunctival injection.[2]

### Opioids

Opioid intoxication can result from illicit (eg, heroin) and licit (eg, prescription opioids) use and misuse. Importantly with prescribed opioids, not all intoxication represents intentional opioid misuse. For example, intoxication in patients on stable doses of opioids prescribed for chronic pain can result if new medications are prescribed that influence opioid metabolism or have an additive sedating effect (eg, benzodiazepines), a new medical condition develops, or the patient is intoxicated with an additional substance. Behavior or psychological changes associated with opioid intoxication include slurred speech, euphoria, apathy, dysphoria, psychomotor agitation or retardation, drowsiness, and impaired attention and memory.[2,10] On examination, the OP may identify miotic pupils, decreased respiratory rate, and track marks from injection drug use.[2,10] The clinical hallmark of opioid overdose is pinpoint pupils, bradypnea, and depressed mental status.

### Prescription Sedatives

Prescription sedatives include benzodiazepines, benzodiazepine–like drugs (eg, sleep aides such as zolpidem), and barbiturates among others.[2] Signs and symptoms of intoxication are similar to those of alcohol intoxication and include slurred speech, incoordination, unsteady gait, nystagmus, impaired memory and attention, and sedation.[2] OPs should be particularly aware of the potential for intoxication and overdose resulting from co-administered opioids and prescription sedatives. This condition may result from intentional drug misuse or from the treatment of co-occurring disorders by multiple providers. A common scenario is for an OP to prescribe opioids unaware that a psychiatrist is also prescribing sedatives, highlighting the importance of reviewing prescription monitoring programs when available. When taken together, the respiratory depressant effects of opioids and sedatives are augmented.[11]

## DIAGNOSTIC TESTING/EVALUATION

The common clinical thread for intoxicated states is the presence of alterations in behavior and mental state; thus the initial evaluation is similar to any patient presenting with AMS. Evaluation begins with behavioral observation, vital signs, and history taking. If recent substance use is suspected, patients should be asked about it directly, including which substances, amount, time of most recent use, and method of administration.

Because intoxicated patients may have impaired memory, concentration, and attention, other sources of information, such as family or friends, are often necessary to provide a more complete history. Privacy considerations for the intoxicated patient are further discussed below. A directed physical examination should be performed looking for potential sources of AMS (eg, infection, head injury, and track marks) and sequelae of AMS (eg, injury). The original reason for the patient visit may have some bearing on diagnostic considerations and should be elucidated.

Pulse oximeters and glucometers are usually readily available in the outpatient setting. Oxygenation and blood sugar should be checked so as not to miss hypoxemia and hypoglycemia as etiologies of AMS. If rapid urine toxicology testing is available, it can be a useful evaluation tool and should be used. A review of the prescription monitoring programs when available can be a helpful adjunct if opioid, benzodiazepine, or medical marijuana intoxication is suspected.

## DIFFERENTIAL DIAGNOSIS

The differential diagnosis of patients presenting with apparent intoxication is broad and includes other etiologies that cause AMS. Diagnoses that can mimic acute intoxication are listed in **Table 2** and fit broadly into categories of neurologic, endocrine, infectious, metabolic, trauma, cardiopulmonary, and psychiatric disorders.[8,12]

| Table 2 Differential diagnosis for patient presenting with altered mental status | |
| --- | --- |
| **System** | **Disease** |
| Toxic/metabolic | Intentional intoxication<br>Unintentional intoxication (eg, carbon monoxide)<br>Withdrawal syndrome<br>Medication side effect<br>Electrolyte disturbance<br>Hypoglycemia<br>Dehydration<br>Hepatic encephalopathy<br>Uremia |
| Endocrine | Hypo or hyperthyroid<br>Diabetic ketoacidosis<br>Hyperglycemic, hyperosmolar state |
| Infectious | Meningitis<br>Encephalitis<br>Pneumonia<br>Urinary tract infection<br>Sepsis |
| Cardiopulmonary | Congestive heart failure<br>Myocardial infarction<br>Hypercarbia |
| Mental health | Cognitive impairment<br>Depression<br>Mania<br>Schizophrenia |
| Neurologic | Stroke<br>Seizure |
| Trauma | Head injury |

## MANAGEMENT

For patients suspected of intoxication in the outpatient settings, OPs should consider how best to manage the presenting concern, manage the suspected intoxication and withdrawal, and provide follow-up assessment for the underlying SUD.

### Management of the Presenting Concern

An attempt should be made to elucidate the primary reason for the office visit and then decide what aspects of care can and should be delivered given the patient's degree of intoxication. Given the effects of acute intoxication on memory, attention, and decision making, counseling is best deferred to a follow-up visit. Patients presenting to the OP for urgent care with apparent mild intoxication and an acute minor illness, such as streptococcal pharyngitis, can be reasonably treated provided the physician can take an accurate history and perform the necessary physical examination. If medications are prescribed, every effort should be made to contact a close relation who can ensure that treatment instruction are understood and can be followed. Follow-up with the patient is essential to ensure that care plans were followed.

### Management of Suspected Intoxication

Intoxicated patients with abnormal vital signs, patients for whom an accurate history cannot be obtained, or those who have any red flag signs (**Box 1**) should be referred immediately to a higher level of care. Beyond this, there is scant literature describing a suggested approach to treating intoxicated patients in the outpatient setting. One study conducted in Norway describes the management of suspected poisonings in an outpatient urgent care center.[13] Although the investigators conclude that outpatient treatment of acutely poisoned patients can be done safely, nonhospitalized patients in the study were observed for an average of 3 hours and 55 minutes, and the clinic had the capacity to administer emergency medications such as naloxone and intravenous

---

**Box 1**
**Red flag signs in the intoxicated patient indicating need for triage to hospital**

Respiratory depression (respiratory rate <12)

Hypoxemia

Oversedation

Pyrexia

Hypotension

Tachycardia

Symptomatic hypoglycemia

Evidence of head injury

Suicidal ideation

Physician uncertainty as to cause of AMS

Certain patient with withdrawal from alcohol, opioids, or prescription sedatives[a]

[a] Refer to text for general guidelines on which patient in acute withdrawal should be referred to inpatient management.

fluids, making it perhaps only generalizable to certain acute care clinics.[13] Factors in the study associated with hospitalization were gamma hydroxybutyrate poisoning (odds ratio [OR], 19.0; confidence interval [CI], 11.3–32.0), hallucinations (OR, 9.6; CI, 5.0–18.5), suicide attempt (OR, 6.9; CI, 4.2–11.4), hypoglycemia (OR, 6.5; CI, 1.8–23.7), and Glasgow Coma Scale score less than or equal to 7 (OR, 6.5; CI, 3.7–11.6). Nineteen percent of patients discharged home re–presented within 1 week, primarily because of a new poisoning event.[13]

## Management of Suspected Withdrawal

Withdrawal from addictive substances should be considered in patients suspected of intoxication. Certain patients with alcohol or opioid withdrawal can be effectively treated in the outpatient setting.[14,15] Signs and symptoms of specific acute withdrawal syndromes are presented in **Table 3**. Because polysubstance use is common, OPs should consider the potential of withdrawal from multiple drugs. Although a comprehensive review of the outpatient management of substance withdrawal is beyond the scope of this article, we highlight some general principles.

The goals of withdrawal management are to stabilize the patient, provide therapies to make the withdrawal process more comfortable and prevent withdrawal-related complications (eg, seizures), and engage the patient in longitudinal treatment of underlying SUDs when present.[15,16] The presence of withdrawal alone does not necessarily indicate an SUD, however, because patients taking opioids or benzodiazepines as prescribed may develop dependence and undergo subsequent withdrawal if the medication is stopped. The treatment of withdrawal in the ambulatory setting should generally be planned rather than impromptu. Additionally, management of potentially life-threatening withdrawal syndromes, such as alcohol withdrawal syndrome, should only be attempted in the ambulatory setting if a helpful support network is available to the patient, and the patient is willing to follow treatment recommendations, including daily clinic visits.[15]

| Table 3 Withdrawal syndromes | | | |
|---|---|---|---|
| | **Alcohol/Sedatives** | **Opioids** | **Marijuana** |
| Symptoms | Nausea | Nausea | Nausea |
| | Vomiting | Vomiting | Decreased appetite |
| | Palpitations | Diarrhea | Diarrhea |
| | Insomnia | Insomnia | Insomnia |
| | Anxiety | Muscle aches | Anxiety |
| | Confusion | Abdominal pain | Irritability |
| | | Dysphoria | Restlessness |
| | | | Depressed mood |
| Signs | Diaphoresis | Diaphoresis | Diaphoresis |
| | Fever | Fever | Fever |
| | Tremor | Lacrimation | Tremor |
| | Tachycardia | Rhinorrhea | |
| | Hypertension | Mydriasis | |
| | Seizure | Piloerection | |
| | Delirium | Yawning | |
| | Hallucinations | | |
| | Death | | |

*Adapted from* American Psychiatric Association. Diagnostic and statistical manual of mental disorder. 5th edition Arlington (VA): American Psychiatric Association; 2013; with permission.

Certain patients with acute withdrawal may not be good candidates for treatment in the ambulatory setting. Patients already in severe withdrawal or those at risk for complicated withdrawal (**Box 2**), including those with certain medical or psychiatric conditions, and polysubstance use, should be referred for inpatient withdrawal management.[15–17] Clinical assessment tools can be useful for judging the severity of withdrawal, and the Clinical Institute Withdrawal Assessment for Alcohol, Revised and the Clinical Opioid Withdrawal Scale are both validated for use in the outpatient setting.[16]

## Follow-up Assessment for Substance Use Disorder

Although intoxication does not necessarily imply SUD, the rate of current and future problematic substance use is higher in patients who present intoxicated to a health care facility.[18,19] The OP is well positioned to perform the necessary follow-up assessment, treatment, or referral to specialist services and begin to intervene on this chronic medical condition.

### Assessing severity of substance use in the clinic

Several evidence-based instruments screen for severity of substance use; however, patients who have presented intoxicated to a health care facility can be assumed to have already screened positive. The next step is to assess the extent of the problem. In a nonjudgmental tone, begin by asking permission to speak with the patient about his or her alcohol or other substance use. A comprehensive assessment is multidimensional and should include the frequency and types of substances used, the extent to which substance use has negatively affected the patient's life, evidence of physiologic dependence, motivation to change, the patient's personal strengths and resources, and triggering or reinforcing factors for ongoing substance use.[20–22]

SUDs are defined as a problematic pattern of substance use leading to significant impairment or harm. The fifth edition of the Diagnostic and Statistical Manual of Mental Disorders lists 11 diagnostic criteria that fit into 4 categories:

- Impaired control over substance use
  Craving
  Using the substance in larger amount or for a longer period than intended
  A persistent desire or unsuccessful attempts to cut down

---

**Box 2**
**Risk factors for complicated alcohol withdrawal**[a]

Multiple previous episodes of alcohol withdrawal

Prior episodes of complicated alcohol withdrawal

Concomitant use of other intoxicating substances, including other sedatives

History of black outs

Chronic, large-quantity alcohol ingestion

Certain medical conditions: acute illness, poorly controlled diabetes, coronary artery disease, congestive heart failure, chronic obstructive pulmonary disease, cirrhosis, pregnancy

Certain psychiatric conditions: suicidal or homicidal ideation, psychosis

[a] Complicated withdrawal is defined as alcohol withdrawal–induced hallucinosis, seizure, or delirium tremens.

A great deal of time spent activities to obtain, use, or recover from the substance
- Substance use despite impaired social functioning
  Use resulting in failure to fulfill major obligations
  Continued use despite persistent or recurrent social or interpersonal problems
  Social, recreational or occupational activities given up or reduced due to substance use
- Substance use despite actual or potential significant harm
  Recurrent use in physically hazardous situations
  Continued use despite knowledge of physical or psychological problems resulting from the substance
- Development of physiologic dependence
  Development of tolerance
  Development of withdrawal

2-3 positive responses represent mild, 4-5 moderate, and 6 or more severe SUD.[23] Patient not meeting at least 2 diagnostic criteria may still have unhealthy substance use, however.

SUDs are diagnosed according to the fifth edition of the Diagnostic and Statistical Manual of Mental Disorders diagnostic criteria, with 2 to 3 positive responses representing mild, 4 to 5 moderate, and 6 or more severe SUD.[2] Patients not meeting at least 2 diagnostic criteria may still have unhealthy substance use, however. For instance, according to guidelines from the National Institute on Alcohol Abuse and Alcoholism, low-risk alcohol consumption is defined as drinking less than 5 standard drinks per day and 14 standard drinks per week (men), and less than 4 standard drinks per day and 7 standard drinks per week (women, elderly). Exceeding these limits is termed *at risk* or *hazardous* drinking. The term *unhealthy alcohol use* refers to both at-risk drinking and alcohol use disorder. Any patient with opioid, marijuana, or prescription sedative intoxication should be considered at risk for an SUD.

### Treatment of underlying unhealthy substance use

Determining the degree of substance use will ultimately help the OP decide on the next steps in treatment.[20] Available evidence supports the use of brief behavioral counseling interventions for patients with at-risk alcohol use, although evidence that it influences subsequent illicit drug use is less robust.[24–27] Behavioral intervention uses motivational interviewing techniques to enhance patients' motivations for change and contain the following core elements[22]:

1. An empathic approach
2. An emphasis on self-efficacy and personal responsibility in making a behavior change
3. Direct feedback on substance use relative to healthy norms and the impact of substance use on the patient's health
4. Specific advice recommending reduction or cessation or substance use
5. Providing a menu of different means toward behavior change if the patient so desires

Patients with SUD are unlikely to respond to behavioral intervention alone, and evidence-based treatment options within the toolkit of the nonaddiction specialist OP include pharmacotherapy such as naltrexone and buprenorphine (**Box 3**), encouragement of 12-step facilitation programs such as Alcoholics Anonymous, cognitive behavioral therapy, and referral to specialized addiction treatment practices.[20,22] A review of these modalities is beyond the scope of this article.

---

**Box 3**
**Pharmacologic options for the treatment of Alcohol and Opioid Use Disorder**

US Food and Drug Administration approved treatment options for patients with AUD include naltrexone (which can be prescribed as a daily pill or monthly intramuscular injection), acamprosate, and disulfiram. Additionally, there is mounting evidence for gabapentin, topiramate, baclofen, ondansetron, and varenicline in the management of AUD.[20] Offering pharmacotherapy for patients with AUD does not require any special training on the part of the OP.

US Food and Drug Administration–approved treatment of OUDs includes methadone and buprenorphine. Although methadone for OUD can only be prescribed from a registered methadone treatment program, buprenorphine can be prescribed by OPs in ambulatory practice after obtaining a Drug Enforcement Agency waiver following a brief certification process, which can be completed online. As of 2016, prescribing privileges have been expanded to include nurse practitioners and physician assistants.

---

*Naloxone*

OPs should consider prescribing naloxone to any patient suspected of opioid intoxication, whether from illicit opioid use or prescription opioid misuse. In 2015, the United States Department of Health and Human Services announced targeted initiatives aimed at reducing opioid overdose related deaths, and 1 of 3 priorities is to increase the use of naloxone.[28] Available evidence supports the use of naloxone rescue kits to reduce opioid overdose death.[29] Currently, naloxone rescue kits can be prescribed as an intramuscular injection that the patient draws up into a syringe from a medication vial, an intramuscular auto-injector, and intranasal formulations. Formulations vary with regard to pricing, insurance coverage, and complexity of administration.[29]

## MEDICO-LEGAL ASPECTS

In addition to the clinical responsibilities to patients, several legal issues are pertinent to the care of intoxicated patients of which OPs should be aware. Many scenarios will not fit neatly into existing medico-legal precedent, and there are state-to-state variations on legal interpretation of laws pertaining to physician responsibility. It is abundantly clear, however, that careful documentation of the OPs concerns, evaluation of decision-making capacity, and rationale for management decisions are essential to protect the OP from a medico-legal standpoint.

### Informed Consent

The ability to consent to or refuse care depends on the patient's competency, defined as the patient's ability to reasonably understand the nature of his or her condition, the nature of any proposed treatment, and the consequences of refusing or agreeing to any proposed treatment.[30,31] The evaluation of competency is a clinical one and requires careful physician assessment. The presence of an intoxicating substance alone is not sufficient to deem someone incompetent nor is a specific blood or urine toxin level.[32]

In the landmark case of *Craig L. Miller v. Rhode Island Hospital*, an invasive procedure was performed in the emergency department on an intoxicated patient despite patient refusal. The treating physician deemed the patient not competent to refuse care based on his degree of intoxication. In the resulting legal case, the court held that, "A patient's intoxication may have the propensity to impair the patient's ability to give informed consent" and decided in favor of the defendant physician and hospital.[30,31,33] Because this case involved management of a potentially life-threatening illness, nonemergent procedures that would occur in the outpatient setting should be deferred to a time when the patient is not acutely intoxicated.

### Health Insurance Portability and Accountability Act

In light of the intoxicated patient's impaired capacity to provide an accurate history or understand discharge instructions, it may be necessary to request information from or give information to relations of the patient. Verbal permission from the patient is adequate and should be documented; however, if permission cannot be obtained (eg, refusal or too cognitively impaired), according to section 164.510(b) (3) of the Health Insurance Portability and Accountability Act (HIPAA) Privacy Rule, the OP is permitted to disclose information to relatives if determined that such disclosure is in the best interest of the patient.[34] This provision specifically applies to when the patient's decision-making capacity is impaired by the influence of alcohol or drugs and only applies to protected health information directly relevant to the current circumstances.[34]

If the intoxicated patient is assessed by the OP to be a threat to self or others, HIPAA also allows for disclosure of protected health information to law enforcement officials "to prevent or lessen a serious and imminent threat to self or others" (C.F.R. 164.512(j) (1) (i)).[35] This may be applicable in the case of the intoxicated patient who insists on driving home (see later discussion).

### Leaving the Clinic

Alcohol use is a well-establish risk factor for motor vehicle–related injuries, for an intoxicated driver and an intoxicated pedestrian.[36,37] Available evidence also supports driving under the influence of other drugs, including marijuana and opioids, as an important risk factor for road traffic injuries.[38–42] When discharging the patient from clinic, the OP must consider whether the patient's degree of intoxication poses a threat to self or to others. For example, the patient may be sufficiently intoxicated to be at risk of personal injury while walking home or causing harm to self and others if insisting on driving from clinic.

After appropriately discussing concerns and advising the intoxicated patient against walking or driving, there are 3 safe discharge options from the perspective of risk of injury to others or self. The first is to observe the patient in clinic until the risk has resolved. This generally will take several hours, and the outpatient practice may not have the capacity to do this. The second is to transfer the patient to a higher level of care for further observation. The third is to insist that the patient be driven home by a friend or family member or take public transportation.

Two cases highlight potential physician legal risk in this scenario. The first is *Coombes v. Florio* in which a Massachusetts physician failed to warn a patient not to drive while taking prescribed medications that have sedating side effects, and the patient subsequently hit and killed a pedestrian.[43] In this case, the court referred to a similar judgment in which "the general requirement [is] that when a doctor knows, or reasonably should know that his patient's ability to drive has been affected, he has a duty to the driving public as well as to the patient to warn his patient of that fact".[44] The second case is *Kowalski v. St. Francis Hospital and Health Centers* in which an intoxicated patient left from a New York emergency department against medical advice and was subsequently struck by a car and paralyzed. In this case, the court ruled in favor of the hospital, stating that the physician had no duty to involuntarily hold an intoxicated patient against his will after the person had voluntarily brought himself in.[45] A key distinction in this case is that patient originally brought himself to the emergency department, and the ruling may not apply to a patient who was brought to a medical facility by a third party.

State-to-state variation exists as to the OP's legal responsibility to ensure the safety of both the patient and bystanders if the intoxicated patient was to injure self or others immediately after leaving the office. OPs managing office practices should be aware of these laws and develop office policies for the safe discharge of intoxicated patients. If the patient declines the OP's advice to not drive home and if the OP can reasonably foresee "serious and imminent danger," then HIPAA allows for security or police to be alerted.

## FUTURE CONSIDERATIONS/SUMMARY

Recognizing an acute intoxication syndrome when patients present to an outpatient clinical practice with behavior or mental status changes requires initial consideration of a broad differential diagnosis. After a thorough evaluation, early management may include triage to a higher level of care, provision of treatment of the presenting concern, and consideration of treatment of potential substance withdrawal. Additionally, there are medico-legal aspects of caring for intoxicated patients related to privacy, informed consent, and risk of harm to self and others after leaving clinic with which OPs should become familiar. Clear documentation of decision making is essential in these cases. Finally, one of the most important aspects of caring for an intoxicated patient is the subsequent assessment for unhealthy substance use or SUD followed by initiation of treatment when indicated.

Given the prevalence of an SUD and the potential for OPs to have a critical role in managing these chronic medical conditions, the authors urge OPs to become familiar with their pharmacologic and nonpharmacologic management. Evidence-based medications are available for the treatment of both alcohol use disorders (AUD) and opioid use disorders (OUDs), and OPs should consider offering these treatments when indicated. Additionally, OPs should seek opportunities to become certified buprenorphine prescribers to expand treatment options for patients with OUDs.

## REFERENCES

1. Substance Abuse and Mental Health Services Administration. Results from the 2014 National Survey on Drug Use and Health: Detailed Tables. 2014. Available at: http://www.samhsa.gov/data/sites/default/files/NSDUH-DetTabs2014/NSDUH-DetTabs2014.htm#tab1-1a. Accessed August 1, 2016.
2. American Psychiatric Association. Diagnostic and statistical manual of mental disorders. 5th edition. Arlington (VA): American Psychiatric Association; 2013.
3. Herron AJ, Brennan T, American Society of Addiction Medicine. The ASAM essentials of addiction medicine. 2nd edition. Philadelphia: Wolters Kluwer; 2015.
4. Rubenzer S. Judging intoxication. Behav Sci Law 2011;29(1):116–37.
5. Okruhlica L, Slezakova S. Clinical signs of alcohol intoxication and importance of blood alcohol concentration testing in alcohol dependence. Bratisl Lek Listy 2013;114(3):136–9.
6. Pechansky F, Von Diemen L, Soibelman M, et al. Clinical signs of alcohol intoxication as markers of refusal to provide blood alcohol readings in emergency rooms: an exploratory study. Clinics (Sao Paulo) 2010;65(12):1391–2.
7. Pitzele HZ, Tolia VM. Twenty per hour: altered mental state due to ethanol abuse and withdrawal. Emerg Med Clin North Am 2010;28(3):683–705.
8. Vonghia L, Leggio L, Ferrulli A, et al. Acute alcohol intoxication. Eur J Intern Med 2008;19(8):561–7.

9.  Crean RD, Crane NA, Mason BJ. An evidence based review of acute and long-term effects of cannabis use on executive cognitive functions. J Addict Med 2011;5(1):1–8.

10. Ries R, Miller SC, Saitz R, et al, American Society of Addiction Medicine. The ASAM principles of addiction medicine. 5th edition. Philadelphia: Wolters Kluwer Health/Lippincott Williams & Wilkins; 2014.

11. Jones JD, Mogali S, Comer SD. Polydrug abuse: a review of opioid and benzo-diazepine combination use. Drug Alcohol Depend 2012;125(1–2):8–18.

12. Nordstrom K, Zun LS, Wilson MP, et al. Medical evaluation and triage of the agitated patient: consensus statement of the american association for emergency psychiatry project Beta medical evaluation workgroup. West J Emerg Med 2012; 13(1):3–10.

13. Vallersnes OM, Jacobsen D, Ekeberg O, et al. Outpatient treatment of acute poisoning by substances of abuse: a prospective observational cohort study. Scand J Trauma Resusc Emerg Med 2016;24(1):76.

14. Hayashida M, Alterman AI, McLellan AT, et al. Comparative effectiveness and costs of inpatient and outpatient detoxification of patients with mild-to-moderate alcohol withdrawal syndrome. N Engl J Med 1989;320(6):358–65.

15. Substance Abuse and Mental Health Services Administration. Detoxification and substance abuse treatment. Treatment improvement protocol (TIP) series, No. 45. HHS Publication No. (SMA) 13-4131. Rockville (MD): Substance Abuse and Mental Health Services Administration; 2006.

16. Muncie HL Jr, Yasinian Y, Oge L. Outpatient management of alcohol withdrawal syndrome. Am Fam Physician 2013;88(9):589–95.

17. Maldonado JR, Sher Y, Ashouri JF, et al. The "Prediction of Alcohol Withdrawal Severity Scale" (PAWSS): systematic literature review and pilot study of a new scale for the prediction of complicated alcohol withdrawal syndrome. Alcohol 2014;48(4):375–90.

18. Adam A, Faouzi M, Yersin B, et al. Women and men admitted for alcohol intoxication at an emergency department: alcohol use disorders, substance use and health and social status 7 years later. Alcohol Alcohol 2016;51(5):567–75.

19. D'Onofrio G, Bernstein E, Bernstein J, et al. Patients with alcohol problems in the emergency department, part 1: improving detection. SAEM Substance Abuse Task Force. Society for Academic Emergency Medicine. Acad Emerg Med 1998;5(12):1200–9.

20. Edelman EJ, Fiellin DA. In the clinic. Alcohol use. Ann Intern Med 2016;164(1): ITC1–16.

21. Willenbring ML, Massey SH, Gardner MB. Helping patients who drink too much: an evidence-based guide for primary care clinicians. Am Fam Physician 2009; 80(1):44–50.

22. Miller WR, Forcehimes A, Zweben A. Treating addiction: a guide for professionals. New York: Guilford Press; 2011.

23. Hasin DS, O'Brien CP, Auriacombe M, et al. DSM-5 criteria for substance use disorders: recommendations and rationale. The American journal of psychiatry 2013;170(8):834–51.

24. Jonas DE, Garbutt JC, Amick HR, et al. Behavioral counseling after screening for alcohol misuse in primary care: a systematic review and meta-analysis for the u.s. preventive services task force. Ann Intern Med 2012;157(9):645–54.

25. Bogenschutz MP, Donovan DM, Mandler RN, et al. Brief intervention for patients with problematic drug use presenting in emergency departments: a randomized clinical trial. JAMA Intern Med 2014;174(11):1736–45.

26. Roy-Byrne P, Bumgardner K, Krupski A, et al. Brief intervention for problem drug use in safety-net primary care settings: a randomized clinical trial. JAMA 2014; 312(5):492–501.

27. Saitz R, Palfai TP, Cheng DM, et al. Screening and brief intervention for drug use in primary care: the ASPIRE randomized clinical trial. JAMA 2014;312(5): 502–13.

28. United States Department of Health and Human Services. HHS takes strong steps to address opioid-drug related overdose, death and dependence. 2015. Available at: http://www.hhs.gov/about/news/2015/03/26/hhs-takes-strong-steps-to-address-opioid-drug-related-overdose-death-and-dependence.html. Accessed August 4, 2016.

29. Lim JK, Bratberg JP, Davis CS, et al. Prescribe to prevent: overdose prevention and naloxone rescue kits for prescribers and pharmacists. J Addict Med 2016; 10(5):300–8.

30. Hartman KM, Liang BA. Exceptions to Informed Consent in Emergency Medicine. Hosp Physician 1999;35(3):53–9.

31. Thomas J, Moore G. Medical-legal issues in the agitated patient: cases and caveats. West J Emerg Med 2013;14(5):559–65.

32. Aldridge J, Charles V. Researching the intoxicated: Informed consent implications for alcohol and drug research. Drug Alcohol Depend 2008;93(3):191–6.

33. Miller v. Rhode Island Hospital, 625 A.2d 778 (R.I. 1993).

34. United States Department of Health and Human Services. HIPAA Privacy Rule and Sharing Information Related to Mental Health. 2014. Available at: http://www.hhs.gov/hipaa/for-professionals/special-topics/mental-health/. Accessed August 2, 2016.

35. United States Department of Health and Human Services. Where the HIPAA Privacy Rule applies, does it permit a health care provider to disclose protected health information (PHI) about a patient to law enforcement, family members, or others if the provider believes the patient presents a serious danger to self or others? 2008. Available at: http://www.hhs.gov/hipaa/for-professionals/faq/520/does-hipaa-permit-a-health-care-provider-to-disclose-information-if-the-patient-is-a-danger/. Accessed August 2, 2016.

36. Ostrom M, Eriksson A. Pedestrian fatalities and alcohol. Accid Anal Prev 2001; 33(2):173–80.

37. Živković V, Lukić V, Nikolić S. The influence of alcohol on pedestrians: a different approach to the effectiveness of the new traffic safety law. Traffic Inj Prev 2016; 17(3):233–7.

38. Li G, Brady JE, Chen Q. Drug use and fatal motor vehicle crashes: a case-control study. Accid Anal Prev 2013;60:205–10.

39. Asbridge M, Hayden JA, Cartwright JL. Acute cannabis consumption and motor vehicle collision risk: systematic review of observational studies and meta-analysis. BMJ 2012;344:e536.

40. Romano E, Torres-Saavedra P, Voas RB, et al. Drugs and alcohol: their relative crash risk. J Stud Alcohol Drugs 2014;75(1):56–64.

41. Elvik R. Risk of road accident associated with the use of drugs: a systematic review and meta-analysis of evidence from epidemiological studies. Accid Anal Prev 2013;60:254–67.

42. Hels T, Lyckegaard A, Simonsen KW, et al. Risk of severe driver injury by driving with psychoactive substances. Accid Anal Prev 2013;59:346–56.

43. Coombes v. Florio, 877 N.E.2d 567 (Mass. 2007).

44. Lockey CJ, Resnick PR. Physicians' Duty to Prevent Harm to Nonpatients. J Am Acad Psychiatry Law 2008;36(4):580–3.
45. West JC. Case law update. Kowalski v St. Francis Hospital & Health Centers, 2013 NY Slip Op 04756 (NY June 26, 2013). J Healthc Risk Manag 2014;33(4): 47–8.

# Management of Hyperglycemic Crises
## Diabetic Ketoacidosis and Hyperglycemic Hyperosmolar State

Maya Fayfman, MD, Francisco J. Pasquel, MD, MPH,
Guillermo E. Umpierrez, MD, CDE*

## KEYWORDS

- Hyperglycemic emergencies • Diabetic ketoacidosis
- Hyperglycemic hyperosmolar state • Management of hyperglycemic emergencies
- Diabetes

## KEY POINTS

- Hyperglycemic emergencies are life-threatening complications of diabetes.
- This article reviews diabetic ketoacidosis and hyperglycemic hyperosmolar state addressing historical context, epidemiology, clinical features, and guidelines for management.

## INTRODUCTION

Diabetic ketoacidosis (DKA) and hyperglycemic hyperosmolar state (HHS) are the most serious and life-threatening hyperglycemic emergencies in patients with diabetes. Although DKA and HHS are often discussed as separate entities, they represent points along a spectrum of hyperglycemic emergencies owing to poorly controlled diabetes. Both DKA and HHS can occur in patients with type 1 diabetes (T1D) and type 2 diabetes (T2D); however, DKA is more common in young people with T1D and HHS is more frequently reported in adult and elderly patients with T2D. In many patients, features of the 2 disorders with ketoacidosis and hyperosmolality may also coexist. The frequency of DKA has increased by 30% during the past decade, with more than 140,000 hospital admissions per year in the United States.[1,2] The rate of hospital admissions for HHS is lower than for DKA, accounting for less than 1% of all diabetes-related admissions.[3,4] Both disorders are characterized by insulinopenia

Division of Endocrinology and Metabolism, Department of Medicine, Emory University School of Medicine, 69 Jesse Hill Jr. Drive Southeast, 2nd Floor, Atlanta, GA 30303, USA
* Corresponding author. Emory University School of Medicine, 49 Jesse Hill Jr. Drive Southeast, 2nd Floor, Atlanta, GA 30303.
E-mail address: Geumpie@emory.edu

Med Clin N Am 101 (2017) 587–606
http://dx.doi.org/10.1016/j.mcna.2016.12.011
0025-7125/17/© 2016 Elsevier Inc. All rights reserved.

and severe hyperglycemia. Early diagnosis and management are paramount to improve patient outcomes. The mainstays of treatment in both DKA and HHS are aggressive rehydration, insulin therapy, electrolyte replacement, and discovery and treatment of underlying precipitating events. Herein we review the epidemiology, pathogenesis, diagnosis, and provide practical recommendations for the management of patients with hyperglycemic emergencies.

## HISTORICAL REVIEW OF DIABETIC COMAS

The first detailed clinical description of diabetic coma in an adult patient with severe polydipsia, polyuria, and a large amount of glucose in the urine followed by progressive decline in mental status and death was reported by August W. von Stosch in 1828.[5] This publication was followed by several case reports describing young and adult patients with newly diagnosed or with established diabetes who presented with an abrupt clinical course of excessive polyuria, glycosuria, coma, and death.[6–8] In 1874, The German physician Adolf Kussmaul reported that many cases of diabetic coma were preceded by deep and frequent respiration and severe dyspnea.[9,10] Kussmaul breathing rapidly became one of the hallmarks of diabetic coma. Shortly after that, it was reported that in many of these patients, the urine contained large amounts of acetoacetic acid and β-hydroxybutyric acid.[11,12] Dr Julius Dreshfeld in 1886 was the first to provide a comprehensive description of the 2 different categories of diabetic coma,[13] one with Kussmaul breathing and positive ketones and the other, an unusual type of diabetic coma in older, well-nourished individuals, characterized by severe hyperglycemia and glycosuria but without Kussmaul breathing, fruity breath odor, or a positive urine acetone test.

Before the discovery of insulin in 1921, the mortality rate of patients with DKA was greater than 90%. The first successful case of DKA treated with insulin was reported by Banting and associates[14] in a 14-year-old boy who presented with a blood glucose of 580 mg/dL and strongly positive urinary ketones at the Toronto General Hospital in 1923. These authors reported a dramatic improvement in glycosuria along with disappearance of acetone bodies in the urine after a few doses of pancreatic extract injections.[14] After the discovery of insulin, the mortality rate associated with diabetic comas decreased dramatically to 60% in 1923 and 25% by the 1930s,[15] 7% to 10% in the 1970s[16,17] and is currently less than 2% in patients for DKA[1,18,19] and between 5% and 16% in patients with HHS.[20,21]

## EPIDEMIOLOGY

Although DKA occurs more commonly in patients with autoimmune T1D, the cumulative number of cases of DKA reported in patients with T2D represents at least one-third of all cases.[22] Global epidemiologic studies have reported on the incidence of DKA among patients with T1D. An analysis from the Prospective Diabetes Registry in Germany including 31,330 patients reported a DKA admission rate of 4.81 per 100 patient-years (95% confidence interval [CI], 4.51–5.14).[23] Individuals with the highest risk included those with high hemoglobin A1c (HbA1c), longer diabetes duration, adolescents, and girls.[23] Multinational data from 49,859 children (<18 years) with T1D across 3 registries and 5 nations similarly found higher odds of DKA among females (odds ratio [OR], 1.23; 99% CI, 1.10–1.37), ethnic minorities (OR, 1.27; 99% CI, 1.11–1.44), and among those with an HbA1c of 7.5% or greater (OR, 2.54 [99% CI, 2.09–3.09] for an HbA1c from 7.5 to <9% and OR 8.74 [99% CI, 7.18–10.63] for an HbA1c of ≥9.0%).[24] Data from the T1D Exchange Clinic Network including 2561 patients, shows that young adults (18–25 years) have the highest occurrence of

DKA (approximately 5%) defined as 1 or more events in the prior 3 months.[25] HHS typically occurs in older patients with T2D[20]; however, it is being recognized as an emerging problem in children and young adults.[26]

Similar mortality rates have been reported in European countries, but the reported mortality continues to be higher than 10% in Indonesia and sub-Saharan African countries.[27,28] HHS occurs most commonly in older patients with T2D with an intercurrent illness such as an infection, surgery, or ischemic events, and is associated with a higher mortality rate than DKA. Mortality in patients with HHS is reported between 5% and 16%, which is about 10 times higher than the mortality in patients with DKA.[20,21,29] The cause of death in patients with DKA and HHS rarely results from the metabolic complications of hyperglycemia or metabolic acidosis, but relates to the underlying precipitating cause, severity of dehydration, and advanced age.[1,4,30]

Treatment of patients with DKA and HHS is associated with substantial mortality and health care costs. DKA is the leading cause of mortality among children and young adults with T1D, accounting for approximately 50% of all deaths in diabetic patients younger than 24 years of age.[1] In the United States, the overall inpatient DKA mortality is less than 1%,[1,2] but a higher rate is reported among elderly patients with life-threatening illnesses.[1,2,31,32] Similar mortality rates have been reported in European countries, but the reported mortality continues to be higher than 10% in countries with limited acute care resources.[28] A history of recurrent DKA episodes increases substantially the long-term mortality after discharge, particularly among young, socially disadvantaged adults with very high HbA1c.[33] In a retrospective review from the United Kingdom, the long-term mortality after a single episode of DKA was 5.2% (4.1 years of follow-up [range, 2.8–6.0]) compared with 23.4% in those with recurrent DKA admissions (2.4 years of follow-up [range, 2.0–3.8]; hazard ratio, 6.18).[33]

Inpatient mortality has been reported in 5% to 16% of patients with HHS, a rate that is approximately 10-fold higher than that reported for DKA.[20,21,29] The prognosis and outcome of patients with HHS is determined by the severity of dehydration, presence of comorbidities and advanced age. In addition, patients with a history of HHS are at significant risk of mortality after hospitalization, in particular those with multiple episodes. Compared with patients with diabetes without HHS, a recent study reported that, after adjustment for age, sex, selected comorbidities, and monthly income, the mortality hazard ratio was 2.8 and 4.5 times higher in subjects with one episode and 2 or more episodes of hyperglycemic crisis, respectively.[34] National data shows a decrease in deaths related to both hyperglycemic crises with an absolute decline of 529 deaths in the period of 1990 to 2010 (2.7 fewer cases per 10,000; 95% CI, 2.4–3.0).[35]

Treatment of hyperglycemic crises represents a substantial economic burden, with an estimated total annual hospital cost of $2.4 billion.[1] In the United States, it is estimated that DKA episodes represent more than $1 of every $4 spent on direct medical care for adult patients with T1D and $1 of every $2 in those patients with multiple DKA episodes.[36]

## PRECIPITATING CAUSE

The most common precipitating causes of DKA reported in different epidemiologic studies worldwide are shown in **Table 1**. DKA is the initial presentation of diabetes in approximately 15% to 20% of adults and in approximately 30% to 40% of children with T1D.[4,37,38] Infection is the most common cause of DKA around the world; however, poor adherence to insulin treatment is the most common precipitating cause

**Table 1**
**Precipitating causes of diabetic ketoacidosis by country**

| Precipitating Causes, % | Australia | Brazil | China | Indonesia | Korea | Nigeria | Spain | Syria | Taiwan | USA |
|---|---|---|---|---|---|---|---|---|---|---|
| Newly diagnosed diabetes mellitus | 5.7 | 12.2 | NR | 3.3 | NR | NR | 12.8 | NR | 18.2 | 17.2–23.8 |
| Infection | 28.6 | 25.0 | 39.2 | 58.3 | 25.3 | 32.5 | 33.2 | 47.8 | 31.7 | 14.0–16.0 |
| Poor adherence to treatment | 40.0 | 39.0 | 24.0 | 13.3 | 32.7 | 27.5 | 30.7 | 23.5 | 27.7 | 41.0–59.6 |
| Other | 25.7 | 15.0 | 10.9 | 17.1 | 11.2 | 4.8 | 23.3 | 7.8 | 6.2 | 9.7–18.0 |
| Unknown | NA | 8.8 | 25.9 | 8.0 | 30.8 | 34.6 | NA | 20.9 | 16.2 | 3.0–4.2 |

*Abbreviations:* NA, not applicable; NR, not reported.
*Adapted from* Umpierrez G, Korytkowski M. Diabetic emergencies-ketoacidosis, hyperglycaemic hyperosmolar state and hypoglycaemia. Nat Rev Endocrinol 2016;12(4):223; with permission.

of DKA in young patients with T1D and in inner city populations in the United States.[39–41] According to a recent report from a safety net hospital in Atlanta, insulin discontinuation accounted for 56% of patients with their first and 78% of patients with multiple DKA episodes.[39] Other potential precipitants of DKA included infections (14%) and noninfectious illnesses (4%)[39] such as acute myocardial infarction, neurovascular accidents, alcohol use, and pancreatitis.[42] Psychological risk factors including depression and eating disorders have been reported in up to 20% of recurrent episodes of ketoacidosis in young patients.[39,43,44] Insulin pump malfunction has long been recognized as a cause of DKA[45,46] owing to the short-acting insulin formulation used in pumps; however, this is not a common event with newer, improved pump technology.[47,48]

Urinary tract infection and pneumonia are common precipitating causes of HHS,[46,49] as well as acute cardiovascular events and other concomitant medical illnesses.[20,50] Poor adherence to medical therapy and new diabetes onset are less common precipitating cause of HHS than DKA.[49]

Several medications that altered carbohydrate metabolism may precipitate the development of DKA and HHS, including glucocorticoids, beta-blockers, thiazide diuretics, certain chemotherapeutic agents,[50,51] and atypical antipsychotics.[52–55] One large retrospective review from the UK reported that hyperglycemic emergencies occurred at a rate of 1 to 2 per 1000 person-years after initiation of antipsychotics.[56] Of the antipsychotics, olanzapine and risperidone were associated with the greatest risk.[56]

Recently, the sodium glucose cotransporter 2 (SGLT-2) inhibitors, a new class of oral antidiabetic agents that lower plasma glucose by inhibiting proximal tubular reabsorption of glucose in the kidney, have been associated with DKA in patients with T1D and T2D.[57,58] An atypical presentation of DKA, which can lead to delayed recognition and treatment, has been referred to as "euglycemic DKA" owing to only mild to moderate elevations in blood glucose reported in many cases.[57] Compiled data from randomized studies with the use of SGLT-2 inhibitors reported a very low incidence of DKA in patients with T2D (approximately 0.07%[59,60]); however, the risk of ketosis and DKA is higher in patients with T1D. About 10% of patients with T1D treated with SGLT-2 inhibitors develop ketosis and 5% require hospital admission for DKA.[57] Potential mechanisms have been proposed, including higher glucagon levels, reduction of daily insulin requirement leading to a decrease in the suppression of lipolysis and ketogenesis, and decreased urinary excretion of ketones.[58,61]

## PATHOPHYSIOLOGY

The 2 most important pathophysiologic mechanisms for DKA and HHS are significant insulin deficiency and increased concentration of counterregulatory hormones such as glucagon, catecholamines, cortisol, and growth hormone (**Fig. 1**).[62–64] The insulin deficiency of DKA can be absolute in patients with T1D or relative as observed in patients with T2D in the presence of stress or intercurrent illness.[65] Insulin deficiency coupled with increased counterregulatory hormones lead to increased hepatic glucose production owing to increased hepatic gluconeogenesis and glycogenolysis,[66] as well as reduced glucose use in peripheral tissues, in particular muscle.[67] Insulinopenia also leads to activation of hormone-sensitive lipase and accelerated breakdown of triglycerides to free fatty acids (FFAs).[68] In the liver, FFAs are oxidized to ketone bodies, a process predominantly stimulated by glucagon[69,70] and increased glucagon/insulin ratio.[71] The increased glucagon/insulin ratio lowers the activity of malonyl coenzyme A, the enzyme that modulates movement of FFA into the hepatic mitochondria where

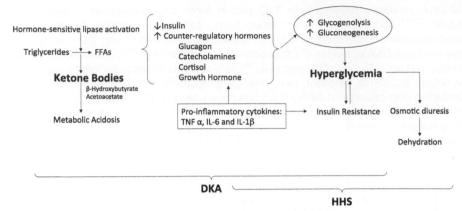

**Fig. 1.** Pathogenesis of hyperglycemic emergencies. Hyperglycemia and accumulation of ketones bodies result from a relative or absolute insulin deficiency and excess counterregulatory hormones (glucagon, cortisol, catecholamines, and growth hormone). Increased ketone bodies and diabetic ketoacidosis (DKA). Decrease in insulin levels combined with increase in counterregulatory hormones, particularly epinephrine causes the activation of hormone sensitive lipase in adipose tissue and breakdown of triglyceride into glycerol and FFAs. In the liver, FFAs are oxidized to ketone bodies, a process predominantly stimulated by glucagon. The 2 major ketone bodies are β-hydroxybutyrate and acetoacetic acid. Accumulation of ketone bodies leads to a decrease in serum bicarbonate concentration and metabolic acidosis. Higher insulin levels present in hyperglycemic hyperosmolar state (HHS) inhibit ketogenesis and limit metabolic acidosis. When insulin is deficient, hyperglycemia develops as a result of 3 processes: increased gluconeogenesis, accelerated glycogenolysis, and impaired glucose use by peripheral tissues. Hyperglycemia causes osmotic diuresis that leads to hypovolemia, decreased glomerular filtration rate and worsening hyperglycemia. TNF, tumor necrosis factor.

fatty acid oxidation takes place. The increased production of ketone bodies (acetoacetate and β-hydroxybutyrate), 2 strong acids, leads to reduction of bicarbonate and metabolic acidosis.

Several mechanisms have been proposed to explain the absence or minimal presence of ketone bodies in patients with HHS including higher levels of circulating insulin, lower levels of counterregulatory hormones and FFAs, and inhibition of lipolysis by the hyperosmolar state (see **Fig. 1**). Of them, higher insulin secretion seems to be the most important mechanism to prevent ketosis in HHS compared to patients with DKA.[64] This is owing to the fact that the antilipolytic effect of insulin is about one-tenth that of glucose use.

## Oxidative Stress and Inflammation

Several experimental and clinical studies have shown that the development of hyperglycemia and ketoacidosis result in an inflammatory state characterized by an elevation of proinflammatory cytokines and increased oxidative stress markers.[72,73] Severe hyperglycemia-induced macrophage production of proinflammatory cytokines such as tumor necrosis factor-alpha, interleukin (IL)-6 and IL-1β, and C-reactive protein, which in turn lead to impaired insulin secretion as well as reduced insulin sensitivity.[73–75] Increases in FFAs also increases insulin resistance as well as impaired nitric oxide production in endothelial cells and endothelial dysfunction.[76] The increased inflammatory response, oxidative stress and generation of reactive oxygen species can lead to capillary perturbation and cellular damage of lipids, membranes, proteins, and DNA.[73,77]

## DIAGNOSIS OF DIABETIC KETOACIDOSIS
### Signs and Symptoms

Patients with DKA often present following a short clinical course characterized by fatigue and classic symptoms of hyperglycemia: polyuria, polydipsia, and weight loss. Gastrointestinal complaints are common with diffuse abdominal pain reported in 46% of patients and nausea and vomiting in up to two-thirds of patients.[42] About one-half of patients present with lethargy and stupor, but less than 25% present with loss of consciousness.[1] On physical examination, patients often present with signs of dehydration with dry mucous membranes and poor skin turgor, tachycardia, or hypotension. Patients in DKA may exhibit Kussmaul respirations and a classic fruity (acetone) breath odor (**Table 2**).

### Laboratory Findings

The syndrome of DKA consists of the triad of hyperglycemia, ketonemia, and metabolic acidosis (**Table 3**). The American Diabetes Association classifies DKA by severity as mild, moderate, or severe depending on the degree of acidosis (along with decrease in bicarbonate) and altered sensorium.[1] Most patients with DKA present with mild to moderate DKA with a blood glucose greater than 250 mg/dL, bicarbonate between 10 and 18 mEq/L, arterial pH of greater than 7.3, high ketones in the urine or blood, and increased anion gap metabolic acidosis of greater than 12.

The anion gap is calculated with the following formula: sodium $[Na^+]$ – chloride $[Cl^-]$ + bicarbonate $[HCO_3^-]$. Although the majority of patients present with plasma glucose levels of greater than 250 mg/dL, some patients exhibit only mild elevations in plasma glucose levels (termed 'euglycemic DKA').[78] This phenomenon has been reported during pregnancy, in patients with prolonged starvation, alcohol intake, partially treated patients receiving insulin, and more recently in the setting of SGLT-2 inhibitor use.[57,79,80]

The key diagnostic criterion is an elevation in circulating total blood ketone and high anion gap metabolic acidosis of greater than 12. Assessment of ketonemia can be performed by the nitroprusside reaction in urine or serum, which provides a

---

**Table 2**
**Clinical features of hyperglycemic emergencies**

| Condition | Symptoms | Signs | Presentation |
|-----------|----------|-------|--------------|
| DKA | Polydipsia<br>Polyuria<br>Weakness<br>Weight loss<br>Nausea<br>Vomiting<br>Abdominal pain | Hypothermia<br>Tachycardia<br>Tachypnea<br>Kussmaul breathing<br>Ileus<br>Acetone breath<br>Altered sensorium | Acute onset (hours-days)<br>More common in T1D than T2D |
| HHS | Polydipsia<br>Polyuria<br>Weakness<br>Weight loss | Hypothermia<br>Hypotension<br>Tachycardia<br>Altered sensorium | Insidious onset (days-weeks)<br>Older age<br>More common in T2D than T1D |

*Abbreviations:* DKA, diabetic ketoacidosis; HHS, hyperglycemic hyperosmolar state; T1D, type 1 diabetes; T2D, type 2 diabetes.

**Table 3**
**Diagnostic criteria for DKA and HHS**

| Measure | DKA | | | HHS |
|---|---|---|---|---|
| | Mild | Moderate | Severe | |
| Plasma glucose (mg/dL) | >250 | >250 | >250 | >600 |
| Arterial pH | 7.25 to 7.30 | 7.00 to <7.24 | <7.00 | >7.30 |
| Serum bicarbonate (mEq/L) | 15 to 18 | 10 to < 15 | <10 | >18 |
| Urine or serum ketones[a] | Positive | Positive | Positive | Small |
| Urine or serum β-hydroxybutyrate (mmol/L) | >3.0 | >3.0 | >3.0 | <3.0 |
| Effective serum osmolality[b] | Variable | Variable | Variable | >320 mOsm/kg |
| Anion gap | >10 | >12 | >12 | Variable |
| Mental status | Alert | Alert/drowsy | Stupor/coma | Stupor/coma |

*Abbreviations:* DKA, diabetic ketoacidosis; HHS, hyperglycemic hyperosmolar state.
[a] Nitroprusside reaction.
[b] Effective serum osmolality: 2[measured $Na^+$ (mEq/L)] + glucose (mg/dL)/18.
*Adapted from* Kitabchi AE, Umpierrez GE, Miles JM, et al. Hyperglycemic crises in adult patients with diabetes. Diabetes Care 2009;32(7):1336; with permission.

semiquantitative estimation of acetoacetate and acetone levels. The nitroprusside test is highly sensitive, but it can underestimate the severity of ketoacidosis because this assay does not recognize the presence of β-hydroxybutyrate, the main metabolic product in ketoacidosis.[67,81] Therefore, direct measurement of serum β-hydroxybutyrate is preferred for diagnosis.[82]

## DIAGNOSIS OF HYPERGLYCEMIC HYPEROSMOLAR STATE
### Symptoms and Signs

The majority of patients with HHS present with a history of polyuria, polydipsia, weakness, blurred vision, and progressive decline in mental status.[50,83] The typical patient with HHS is older than 60 years of age with an infection or acute illness who has delayed seeking medical attention. On physical examination, similar to DKA, patients with HHS frequently have clear signs of dehydration, dry mucous membranes and poor skin turgor, or hypotension.[50]

### Laboratory Findings

The diagnostic criteria for HHS includes a plasma glucose of greater than 600 mg/dL, and effective osmolality of greater than 320 mOsm/kg, and the absence of ketoacidosis.[1] Effective osmolality is calculated with the following formula: sodium ion (mEq/L) × 2 + glucose (mg/dL)/18. Although by definition HHS is characterized by a pH of greater than 7.3, a bicarbonate of greater than 18 mEq/L, and negative ketone bodies, mild to moderate ketonemia may be present. Patients with HHS have an increased anion gap metabolic acidosis as the result of concomitant ketoacidosis and/or to an increase in serum lactate levels or renal failure.[21]

## COMMON LABORATORY PITFALLS

Patients with DKA frequently present with significant leukocytosis with white cell counts in the 10,000 to 15,000 $mm^3$ range. A leukocyte count of greater than 25,000 $mm^3$ or the presence of greater than 10% neutrophil bands is seldom seen in the absence of bacterial infection.[64,84] In ketoacidosis, leukocytosis is attributed to stress, dehydration, and demargination of leukocytes.

The admission serum sodium may be low because of the osmotic flux of water from the intracellular to the extracellular space in the presence of hyperglycemia. To assess the severity of sodium and water deficit, serum sodium may be corrected by adding 1.6 mg/dL to the measured serum sodium for each 100 mg/dL of glucose greater than 100 mg/dL.[1] An increase in serum sodium concentration in the presence of severe hyperglycemia indicates a profound degree of dehydration and water loss.

The admission serum potassium concentration is usually elevated in patients with DKA and HHS.[64] In a several studies,[1,39,85] the mean serum potassium in patients with DKA and HHS was 5.6 mEq/L and 5.7 mEq/L, respectively. These high levels occur because of a shift of potassium from the intracellular to the extracellular space owing to insulin deficiency and hypertonicity, as well as academia in DKA.[86] It is important to keep in mind that, during insulin treatment and fluid administration, potassium levels decrease owing to a shift back to the intracellular space, which may result in hypokalemia.

Similarly, serum phosphate levels in patients with DKA do not reflect the actual body deficit that uniformly exists, because phosphate shifts from the intracellular to the extracellular space owing to insulin deficiency, hypertonicity, and catabolic state. Dehydration also can lead to increases in total serum protein, albumin, amylase, and creatinine phosphokinase concentration in patients with hyperglycemic crises.

Not all patients who present with ketoacidosis have DKA. Patients with chronic ethanol abuse with a recent binge culminating in nausea, vomiting, and acute starvation may present with alcoholic ketoacidosis. The key diagnostic feature that differentiates diabetic and alcohol-induced ketoacidosis is the concentration of blood glucose.[87] The presence of ketoacidosis without hyperglycemia in an alcoholic patient is virtually diagnostic of alcoholic ketoacidosis. In addition, some patients with decreased food intake and caloric intake of lower than 500 calories per day for several days may present with starvation ketosis. Patients with starvation ketosis rarely present with a serum bicarbonate concentration of less than 18 mEq/L because of the slow onset of ketosis that allows increased ketone clearance by peripheral tissue (brain and muscle) and enhancement of the kidney's ability to excrete ammonia to compensate for the increased acid production.[88]

## MANAGEMENT OF HYPERGLYCEMIC CRISES

The American Diabetes Association algorithm for the management of hyperglycemic emergencies is shown in **Fig. 2**.[1] Similar therapeutic measures are recommended for the treatment of DKA and HHS. In general, treatment goals include correction of dehydration, hyperglycemia, hyperosmolality, electrolyte imbalance, and increased ketonemia, and the identification and treatment of precipitating event(s). The average time to resolution is between 10 and 18 hours for DKA[89,90] and approximately 9 and 11 hours for HHS.[4] During treatment, frequent monitoring of vital signs, volume, and rate of fluid administration, insulin dosage, and urine output are needed to assess response to medical treatment. In addition, laboratory measurements of glucose and electrolytes, venous pH, bicarbonate, and anion gap should be repeated every 2 to 4 hours.[91]

Most patients with uncomplicated DKA can be treated in the emergency department or in stepdown units if close nursing supervision and monitoring is available. Several studies have failed to demonstrate clear benefits in treating DKA patients in the intensive care unit (ICU) compared with stepdown units.[92–94] The mortality rate, duration of

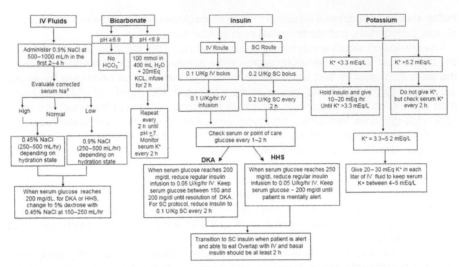

**Fig. 2.** Management of hyperglycemic emergencies. [a] Subcutaneous insulin protocol has not been validated for a hyperglycemic hyperosmolar state (HHS). [b] Correct serum sodium by adding 1.6 mg/dL to the measured serum sodium for each 100 mg/dL of glucose above 100 mg/dL. DKA, diabetic ketoacidosis; IV, intravenous; SC, subcutaneous. (*Adapted from* Kitabchi AE, Umpierrez GE, Miles JM, et al. Hyperglycemic crises in adult patients with diabetes. Diabetes Care 2009;32(7):1339; with permission.)

hospital stay, or time to resolve ketoacidosis are similar between patients treated in ICU and non-ICU settings. In addition, ICU admission has been associated with more laboratory testing and higher hospitalization cost in patients with DKA.[36,92] Patients with mild to moderate DKA can be managed safely in the emergency department or in stepdown units, and only patients with severe DKA or those with a critical illness as precipitating cause (ie, myocardial infarction, gastrointestinal bleeding, sepsis)[1,95] should be treated in the ICU. Because patients with HHS frequently present with altered mental status and have significantly higher mortality than patients with DKA, we recommend that patients with HHS be managed in the ICU.

## FLUID THERAPY

Intravenous (IV) fluids are a critical aspect of treatment of hyperglycemic emergencies. Treatment with IV fluids alone expands intravascular volume, restores renal perfusion, and reduces insulin resistance by decreasing circulating counterregulatory hormone levels.[62] Isotonic saline (0.9% NaCl) is the preferred solution and is given at an initial rate of 500 to 1000 mL/h during the first 2 to 4 hours. A study comparing 2 IV fluid regimens with sodium chloride and lactate ringers found no significant difference in time to resolution of DKA, but the time to correct hyperglycemia was significantly longer in the lactated Ringers' group.[96] After intravascular volume depletion has been corrected, the rate of normal saline infusion should be reduced to 250 mL/h or changed to 0.45% saline (250–500 mL/h) depending on the serum sodium concentration and state of hydration.[1] Once the plasma glucose level reaches approximately 200 mg/dL (11.1 mosm/L), replacement fluids should contain 5% to 10% of dextrose to allow continued insulin administration until ketonemia is corrected, while avoiding hypoglycemia.[97] Adequate fluid resuscitation is of particular importance in management of HHS, because many of these patients may see improvement in or resolution of mental status changes with correction of fluid deficits.[83]

## Potassium

Metabolic acidosis and insulin deficiency both lead to extracellular movement of potassium. Thus, although serum potassium levels may be normal or increased in DKA, patients are actually total body depleted. Similarly, HHS is associated with total body potassium depletion owing to lack of insulin and increased plasma osmolality.[20,86] The total body potassium deficit has been estimated to be approximately 3 to 5 mEq/kg.[85,98] Insulin therapy lowers serum potassium levels by promoting the movement of potassium back into the intracellular compartment. Thus, potassium replacement should be started when the serum concentration is less than 5.2 mEq/L to maintain a level of 4 to 5 mEq/L. The administration of 20 to 30 mEq of potassium per liter of fluids is sufficient for most patients; however, lower doses are required for patients with acute or chronic renal failure. Among patients with admission hypokalemia, with serum potassium levels of less than 3.3 mEq/L, insulin administration may result in severe symptomatic hypokalemia with muscle weakness and increased risk of cardiac arrhythmias. In such patients, potassium replacement should begin at a rate of 10 to 20 mEq/h and insulin therapy should be delayed until the potassium level increases to greater than 3.3 mEq/L.

## Bicarbonate

The routine administration of bicarbonate has not been shown to improve clinical outcomes, such as time to resolution, duration of hospital stay, or mortality in patients with DKA[99–102] and is generally only recommended in patients with life-threatening acidosis with a pH of less than 6.9. Bicarbonate therapy may increase the risk of hypokalemia and cerebral edema.[103,104] Although no studies have looked at the effect of bicarbonate therapy in patients with severe acidosis, because of the potential risk of reduced cardiac contractility and arrhythmias, clinical guidelines recommend the administration of 50 to 100 mmol of sodium bicarbonate as an isotonic solution (in 400 mL of water) until pH is greater than 6.9. In patients with mild DKA with pH of greater than 7.0 or with HHS, bicarbonate therapy is not indicated.

## Insulin Regimens

Insulin administration is the mainstay of DKA therapy because it lowers the serum glucose by inhibiting endogenous glucose production and increasing peripheral use. Insulin also inhibits lipolysis, ketogenesis, and glucagon secretion, thereby decreasing the production of ketoacidosis.

A continuous IV infusion of regular insulin is the treatment of choice. Most treatment protocols recommend the administration of 0.1 U/kg body weight bolus followed by continuous insulin infusion at 0.1 U/kg per hour until blood glucose is approximately 200 mg/dL (see **Fig. 2**). At this point, the dose is reduced by one-half (0.05 U/kg per hour) and rate is adjusted between 0.02 to 0.05 U/kg per hour, along with the addition of 5% dextrose, to maintain glucose concentrations between 140 and 200 mg/dL until resolution of ketoacidosis.[1]

Several studies have demonstrated that the administration of subcutaneous doses of rapid insulin analogs (Lispro and Aspart) every 1 to 2 hours is an effective alternative to the IV infusion of regular insulin in terms of time to resolution of DKA.[105–107] Patients are treated with an initial bolus of 0.2 to 0.3 U/kg followed by 0.1 to 0.2 U/kg every 1 to 2 hours, respectively until glucose is less than 250 mg/dL. The dose is then reduced by one-half to 0.05 U/kg every 1 hour or 0.01 U/kg every 2 hours until the resolution of DKA.[89,105] Using scheduled subcutaneous insulin allows for safe and effective treatment in the emergency room and stepdown units without the need for ICU care.

The use of intramuscular injections of rapid-acting insulin is also effective in the treatment of DKA, but this route tends to be more painful than subcutaneous injection and might increase the risk of bleeding among patients receiving anticoagulation therapy.[97,108] It is important to keep in mind that the use of rapid-acting subcutaneous insulin analogues is not recommended for patients with arterial hypotension, severe and complicated DKA, or with HHS.

## TRANSITION TO MAINTENANCE INSULIN REGIMEN

Resolution of DKA is defined when glucose levels are lower than 250 mg/dL, venous pH is greater than 7.30, there is a normal anion gap, and serum bicarbonate is 18 mEq/L or greater.[1] HHS resolution is achieved when effective serum osmolality is less than 310 mOsm/kg and the glucose level is 250 mg/dL or less (13.8 mmol/L) in a patient who has recovered mental alertness and regaining of mental status.[1,97]

Because of the short half-life of intravenous insulin (<10 minutes),[109] abrupt cessation of the insulin may result is rebound hyperglycemia, ketogenesis, and recurrent metabolic acidosis. Subcutaneous basal insulin (NPH, Glargine, Detemir, Degludec), should be given at least 2 hours before discontinuing the IV insulin infusion.[1] Earlier initiation, 3 to 4 hours before discontinuation of insulin drip, should be considered when using basal insulin analogues (Glargine, Determir, Degludec), which have a longer delay in onset of action than NPH insulin. One randomized controlled trial evaluated the effect of coadministration of IV insulin with subcutaneous Glargine shortly after the onset of treatment of DKA compared with IV insulin alone.[110] Patients who received Glargine had a trend towards shorter time to resolution of DKA (based on closure of anion gap) and shorter duration of hospital stay; however, these differences were not statistically significant.[110] Another study found that the administration of Glargine early in the course of treatment reduced the frequency of rebound hyperglycemia after transition off of insulin drip.[111]

For insulin-naïve patients, a starting total daily insulin dose of 0.5 to 0.6 U/kg may be started (one-half as basal and one-half as bolus).[1] Patients with poor oral intake should receive basal insulin alone or, alternatively, may be continued on an insulin drip until they are able to eat. Patients with known diabetes can be restarted on their previous insulin regimens; however, an adjustment of the previous regimen should be considered if there is a history of frequent hypoglycemia, or significantly uncontrolled hyperglycemia before admission, as indicated by admission HbA1c. Multidose insulin regimens with basal insulin and prandial rapid-acting insulin analogues are the preferred insulin regimen for patients with T1D and DKA, and for most patients with HHS. A randomized, controlled trial in DKA patients compared transition regimens of NPH and regular insulin twice daily versus Glargine once daily and Glulisine before meals found similar glycemic control between the 2 groups; however, the NPH/regular insulin group had more than double the rate of hypoglycemia (<70 mg/dL) compared with the Glargine/Glulisine group.[112]

## COMPLICATIONS

Hypoglycemia is the most common complication during treatment, reported in 5% to 25% of patients with DKA.[1,4,105] Lack of frequent monitoring and the failure to reduce insulin infusion rate and/or to use dextrose-containing solutions when blood glucose levels are less than 200 mg/dL are the most important risk factors associated with hypoglycemia during insulin treatment. Many patients with hypoglycemia do not experience adrenergic manifestations of sweating, nervousness, fatigue, hunger, and tachycardia, and thus frequent blood glucose monitoring (every 1 to 2 hours) is mandatory.[97] Acute adverse outcomes of hypoglycemia include seizures, arrhythmias, and cardiovascular events. Clinicians should be aware that recurrent episodes of hypoglycemia might be associated with a state of hypoglycemia unawareness (loss of perception of warning symptoms of developing hypoglycemia), which may complicate diabetes management after the resolution of hyperglycemic crises.

Hypokalemia is the second most common complication during DKA and HHS treatment.[4] Although the admission serum potassium concentration is commonly elevated, during insulin treatment, the plasma concentration of potassium will invariably decrease owing to increased cellular potassium uptake in peripheral tissues.[1] Thus, to prevent hypokalemia, replacement with IV potassium when concentration is less than 5.2 mEq/L is indicated. In patients admitted with reduced serum potassium less than 3.3 mEq/L, IV potassium replacement should begin immediately and insulin therapy should be held until serum potassium is 3.3 mEq/L or greater to avoid severe hypokalemia.

Cerebral edema is rare in adults, but is reported in approximately 1% of children with DKA with a mortality rate between 20% and 40%.[103,113] The pathogenesis of cerebral edema is incompletely understood. Evidence for disruption of the blood–brain barrier has been found in cases of fatal cerebral edema.[103,114] The degree of edema formation during DKA in children correlates with the degree of dehydration and hyperventilation at presentation, but it does not correlate with initial osmolality, osmotic changes during treatment, or rate of fluid or sodium administration.[115] Clinically significant cerebral edema usually develops 4 to 12 hours after treatment has started, but it can occur as late as 24 to 48 hours after the start of treatment. Clinical criteria include altered mentation or fluctuating level of consciousness, abnormal motor or verbal response to pain, decorticate or decerebrate posturing, cranial nerve palsy (especially III, IV, and VI), and an abnormal neurogenic respiratory pattern (eg, grunting, tachypnea, Cheyne–Stokes respiration). Recommended treatment includes the administration of mannitol 0.5 to 1 g/kg IV over 20 minutes and repeat if there is no initial response in 30 minutes.[116,117] Hypertonic saline (3%), 5 to 10 mL/kg over 30 minutes, may be an alternative to mannitol, especially if there is no initial response to mannitol.[118] After treatment for cerebral edema has been started, a cranial computed tomography scan should be obtained to rule out other possible intracerebral causes of neurologic deterioration (approximately 10% of cases), especially thrombosis and cerebral infarction, hemorrhage, or dural sinus thrombosis, which may benefit from specific therapy.[113,119–121] Corticosteroid and diuretic therapy are of no proven benefits in the treatment of cerebral edema in DKA patients.[122]

Rhabdomyolysis may occur in patients with DKA and more commonly with HHS resulting in increased risk of acute kidney failure. The classic symptom triad of rhabdomyolysis includes myalgia, weakness, and dark urine, and monitoring creatine kinase concentrations every 2 to 3 hours is recommended for early detection.

## PREVENTION

Medication noncompliance is a leading cause of DKA among both newly diagnosed and recurrent episodes of DKA.[39–41] The mean cost of hospitalization is about $7500.[40] In one-half of such episodes, patients report an inability to afford medication or to pay for transportation as the reason why medication was discontinued.[41] Development of system-wide changes such as assistance programs to provide insulin to patients and reduce lapses in treatment may be a cost-effective way to reduce the rate of hospitalization for hyperglycemic emergencies.

Multidisciplinary approaches with the use of clinical diabetes educators in close contact with and easily accessible to the patients has been shown to reduce the number of hospitalizations related to hyperglycemic emergencies.[123] Systems-based methods to reduce preventable causes of hyperglycemic emergencies may represent an important next step in reducing costs and improving patient care.

## REFERENCES

1. Kitabchi AE, Umpierrez GE, Miles JM, et al. Hyperglycemic crises in adult patients with diabetes. Diabetes Care 2009;32(7):1335–43.
2. Centers for Disease Control and Prevention. Mortality due to Hyperglycemic crises. 2013. Available at: http://www.cdc.gov/diabetes/statistics/complications_national.htm. Accessed September 2, 2016.
3. Ennis ED, Stahl EJVB, Kreisberg RA. The hyperosmolar hyperglycemic syndrome. Diabetes Rev 1994;2:115–26.
4. Umpierrez GE, Kelly JP, Navarrete JE, et al. Hyperglycemic crises in urban blacks. Arch Intern Med 1997;157(6):669–75.
5. von Stosch A. Versuch einer Pathologie und Therapie des Diabetes Mellitus. Berlin: Duncker und Humblot; 1828 [in German].
6. Parsons J. Case of infantile diabetes. Prov Med Surg J 1849;13(13):342–3.
7. Hindle R. Case of acute diabetes. Prov Med Surg J 1845;9(29):452–3.
8. Favell CF. Cases of diabetes. Prov Med J Retrosp Med Sci 1843;6(153):467–9.
9. Kussmaul A. Zur lehre vom diabetes mellitus. Dtsch Arch Klin Med 1874;14:1–46 [in German].
10. Adolf Kussmaul (1822-1902)–Country Doctor to Clinical Professor. JAMA 1964;189:58–9.
11. Stadelmann E. Ueber die Ursachen der pathologischen ammoniakausscheidung beim diabetes mellitus und des coma diabeticum. Arch Exp Pathol Pharmakol 1883;17:419–44 [in German].
12. Külz E. Ueber eine neue linksdrehende saure (pseudo-oxybuttersaure). Zeitschr f Biologie 1884;20:165–78 [in German].
13. Dreschfeld J. The Bradshawe lecture on diabetic coma. Br Med J 1886;2(1338):358–63.
14. Banting FG, Best CH, Collip JB, et al. Pancreatic extracts in the treatment of diabetes mellitus: preliminary report. Can Med Assoc J 1962;87(20):1062–7.
15. Rabinowitch IM. Diabetic coma and diabetic mortality rates. Can Med Assoc J 1929;21(5):583–6.
16. Clements RS Jr, Vourganti B. Fatal diabetic ketoacidosis: major causes and approaches to their prevention. Diabetes Care 1978;1(5):314–25.
17. Felig P. Diabetic ketoacidosis. N Engl J Med 1974;290(24):1360–3.
18. Graves EJ, Gillium BS. Detailed diagnosis and procedures: National Discharge Survey, 1995. National Center for Health Statistics. Vital Health Stat 13 1997;13(130):1–146.
19. Wagner A, Risse A, Brill HL, et al. Therapy of severe diabetic ketoacidosis. Zero-mortality under very-low-dose insulin application. Diabetes Care 1999;22(5):674–7.
20. Pasquel FJ, Umpierrez GE. Hyperosmolar hyperglycemic state: a historic review of the clinical presentation, diagnosis, and treatment. Diabetes Care 2014;07(11):3124–31.

21. Fadini GP, de Kreutzenberg SV, Rigato M, et al. Characteristics and outcomes of the hyperglycemic hyperosmolar non-ketotic syndrome in a cohort of 51 consecutive cases at a single center. Diabetes Res Clin Pract 2011;94(2):172–9.

22. Wang ZH, Kihl-Selstam E, Eriksson JW. Ketoacidosis occurs in both type 1 and type 2 diabetes–a population-based study from Northern Sweden. Diabet Med 2008;25(7):867–70.

23. Karges B, Rosenbauer J, Holterhus PM, et al. Hospital admission for diabetic ketoacidosis or severe hypoglycemia in 31,330 young patients with type 1 diabetes. Eur J Endocrinol 2015;173(3):341–50.

24. Maahs DM, Hermann JM, Holman N, et al. Rates of diabetic ketoacidosis: international comparison with 49,859 pediatric patients with type 1 diabetes from England, Wales, the U.S., Austria, and Germany. Diabetes Care 2015;38(10): 1876–82.

25. Miller KM, Foster NC, Beck RW, et al. Current state of type 1 diabetes treatment in the U.S.: updated data from the T1D Exchange clinic registry. Diabetes Care 2015;38(6):971–8.

26. Rosenbloom AL. Hyperglycemic hyperosmolar state: an emerging pediatric problem. J Pediatr 2010;156(2):180–4.

27. Savage MW, Dhatariya KK, Kilvert A, et al. Joint British Diabetes Societies guideline for the management of diabetic ketoacidosis. Diabet Med 2011; 28(5):508–15.

28. Otieno CF, Kayima JK, Omonge EO, et al. Diabetic ketoacidosis: risk factors, mechanisms and management strategies in sub-Saharan Africa: a review. East Afr Med J 2005;82(12 Suppl):S197–203.

29. Bhowmick SK, Levens KL, Rettig KR. Hyperosmolar hyperglycemic crisis: an acute life-threatening event in children and adolescents with type 2 diabetes mellitus. Endocr Pract 2005;11(1):23–9.

30. Wachtel TJ, Silliman RA, Lamberton P. Prognostic factors in the diabetic hyperosmolar state. J Am Geriatr Soc 1987;35(8):737–41.

31. Basu A, Close CF, Jenkins D, et al. Persisting mortality in diabetic ketoacidosis. Diabet Med 1993;10(3):282–4.

32. Malone ML, Gennis V, Goodwin JS. Characteristics of diabetic ketoacidosis in older versus younger adults. J Am Geriatr Soc 1992;40(11):1100–4.

33. Gibb FW, Teoh WL, Graham J, et al. Risk of death following admission to a UK hospital with diabetic ketoacidosis. Diabetologia 2016;59(10):2082–7.

34. Huang CC, Weng SF, Tsai KT, et al. Long-term mortality risk after hyperglycemic crisis episodes in geriatric patients with diabetes: a national population-based cohort study. Diabetes Care 2015;38(5):746–51.

35. Gregg EW, Williams DE, Geiss L. Changes in diabetes-related complications in the United States. N Engl J Med 2014;371(3):286–7.

36. Javor KA, Kotsanos JG, McDonald RC, et al. Diabetic ketoacidosis charges relative to medical charges of adult patients with type I diabetes. Diabetes Care 1997;20(3):349–54.

37. Klingensmith GJ, Tamborlane WV, Wood J, et al. Diabetic ketoacidosis at diabetes onset: still an all too common threat in youth. J Pediatr 2013;162(2): 330–4.e1.

38. Dabelea D, Rewers A, Stafford JM, et al. Trends in the prevalence of ketoacidosis at diabetes diagnosis: the SEARCH for diabetes in youth study. Pediatrics 2014;133(4):e938–45.

39. Randall L, Begovic J, Hudson M, et al. Recurrent diabetic ketoacidosis in inner-city minority patients: behavioral, socioeconomic, and psychosocial factors. Diabetes Care 2011;34(9):1891–6.

40. Maldonado MR, Chong ER, Oehl MA, et al. Economic impact of diabetic ketoacidosis in a multiethnic indigent population: analysis of costs based on the precipitating cause. Diabetes Care 2003;26(4):1265–9.

41. Musey VC, Lee JK, Crawford R, et al. Diabetes in urban African-Americans. I. Cessation of insulin therapy is the major precipitating cause of diabetic ketoacidosis. Diabetes Care 1995;18(4):483–9.

42. Umpierrez G, Freire AX. Abdominal pain in patients with hyperglycemic crises. J Crit Care 2002;17(1):63–7.

43. Barnard KD, Skinner TC, Peveler R. The prevalence of co-morbid depression in adults with type 1 diabetes: systematic literature review. Diabet Med 2006;23(4): 445–8.

44. Canadian Diabetes Association Clinical Practice Guidelines Expert Committee, Goguen J, Gilbert J. Hyperglycemic emergencies in adults. Can J Diabetes 2013;37(Suppl 1):S72–6.

45. Garg SK, Walker AJ, Hoff HK, et al. Glycemic parameters with multiple daily injections using insulin glargine versus insulin pump. Diabetes Technol Ther 2004; 6(1):9–15.

46. Implementation of treatment protocols in the Diabetes Control and Complications Trial. Diabetes Care 1995;18(3):361–76.

47. Ly TT, Nicholas JA, Retterath A, et al. Effect of sensor-augmented insulin pump therapy and automated insulin suspension vs standard insulin pump therapy on hypoglycemia in patients with type 1 diabetes: a randomized clinical trial. JAMA 2013;310(12):1240–7.

48. Johnson SR, Cooper MN, Jones TW, et al. Long-term outcome of insulin pump therapy in children with type 1 diabetes assessed in a large population-based case-control study. Diabetologia 2013;56(11):2392–400.

49. Wachtel TJ, Tetu-Mouradjian LM, Goldman DL, et al. Hyperosmolarity and acidosis in diabetes mellitus: a three-year experience in Rhode Island. J Gen Intern Med 1991;6(6):495–502.

50. Gerich JE, Martin MM, Recant L. Clinical and metabolic characteristics of hyperosmolar nonketotic coma. Diabetes. 1971;20(4):228–38.

51. Ben Salem C, Fathallah N, Hmouda H, et al. Drug-induced hypoglycaemia: an update. Drug Saf 2011;34(1):21–45.

52. Caro JJ, Ward A, Levinton C, et al. The risk of diabetes during olanzapine use compared with risperidone use: a retrospective database analysis. J Clin Psychiatry 2002;63(12):1135–9.

53. Buse JB, Cavazzoni P, Hornbuckle K, et al. A retrospective cohort study of diabetes mellitus and antipsychotic treatment in the United States. J Clin Epidemiol 2003;56(2):164–70.

54. Gianfrancesco F, Grogg A, Mahmoud R, et al. Differential effects of antipsychotic agents on the risk of development of type 2 diabetes mellitus in patients with mood disorders. Clin Ther 2003;25(4):1150–71.

55. Ananth J, Parameswaran S, Gunatilake S. Side effects of atypical antipsychotic drugs. Curr Pharm Des 2004;10(18):2219–29.

56. Lipscombe LL, Austin PC, Alessi-Severini S, et al. Atypical antipsychotics and hyperglycemic emergencies: multicentre, retrospective cohort study of administrative data. Schizophr Res 2014;154(1–3):54–60.

57. Peters AL, Buschur EO, Buse JB, et al. Euglycemic diabetic ketoacidosis: a potential complication of treatment with sodium-glucose cotransporter 2 inhibition. Diabetes Care 2015;38(9):1687–93.

58. Perspective Taylor SI, Blau JE, Rother KI. SGLT2 inhibitors may predispose to ketoacidosis. J Clin Endocrinol Metab 2015;100(8):2849–52.

59. Erondu N, Desai M, Ways K, et al. Diabetic ketoacidosis and related events in the canagliflozin type 2 diabetes clinical program. Diabetes Care 2015;38(9): 1680–6.

60. Tang H, Li D, Wang T, et al. Effect of sodium-glucose cotransporter 2 inhibitors on diabetic ketoacidosis among patients with type 2 diabetes: a meta-analysis of randomized controlled trials. Diabetes care 2016;39(8):e123–4.

61. Kibbey RG. SGLT-2 inhibition and glucagon: cause for alarm? Trends Endocrinol Metab 2015;26(7):337–8.

62. Waldhausl W, Kleinberger G, Korn A, et al. Severe hyperglycemia: effects of rehydration on endocrine derangements and blood glucose concentration. Diabetes. 1979;28(6):577–84.

63. Chupin M, Charbonnel B, Chupin F. C-peptide blood levels in keto-acidosis and in hyperosmolar non-ketotic diabetic coma. Acta Diabetol Lat 1981;18(2):123–8.

64. Kitabchi AE, Umpierrez GE, Murphy MB, et al. Management of hyperglycemic crises in patients with diabetes. Diabetes Care 2001;24(1):131–53.

65. Maldonado M, Hampe CS, Gaur LK, et al. Ketosis-prone diabetes: dissection of a heterogeneous syndrome using an immunogenetic and beta-cell functional classification, prospective analysis, and clinical outcomes. J Clin Endocrinol Metab 2003;88(11):5090–8.

66. Miles JM, Rizza RA, Haymond MW, et al. Effects of acute insulin deficiency on glucose and ketone body turnover in man: evidence for the primacy of overproduction of glucose and ketone bodies in the genesis of diabetic ketoacidosis. Diabetes 1980;29(11):926–30.

67. Foster DW, McGarry JD. The metabolic derangements and treatment of diabetic ketoacidosis. N Engl J Med 1983;309(3):159–69.

68. Laffel L. Ketone bodies: a review of physiology, pathophysiology and application of monitoring to diabetes. Diabetes Metab Res Rev 1999;15(6):412–26.

69. Miles JM, Haymond MW, Nissen SL, et al. Effects of free fatty acid availability, glucagon excess, and insulin deficiency on ketone body production in postabsorptive man. J Clin Invest 1983;71(6):1554–61.

70. McGarry JD, Foster DW. Effects of exogenous fatty acid concentration on glucagon-induced changes in hepatic fatty acid metabolism. Diabetes. 1980; 29(3):236–40.

71. McGarry JD, Foster DW. Regulation of hepatic fatty acid oxidation and ketone body production. Annu Rev Biochem 1980;49:395–420.

72. Rains JL, Jain SK. Oxidative stress, insulin signaling, and diabetes. Free Radic Biol Med 2011;50(5):567–75.

73. Li J, Huang M, Shen X. The association of oxidative stress and pro-inflammatory cytokines in diabetic patients with hyperglycemic crisis. J Diabetes Complications 2014;28(5):662–6.

74. Vaarala O, Yki-Jarvinen H. Diabetes: should we treat infection or inflammation to prevent T2DM? Nat Rev Endocrinol 2012;8(6):323–5.

75. Pickup JC. Inflammation and activated innate immunity in the pathogenesis of type 2 diabetes. Diabetes Care 2004;27(3):813–23.

76. Kim F, Tysseling KA, Rice J, et al. Free fatty acid impairment of nitric oxide production in endothelial cells is mediated by IKKbeta. Arterioscler Thromb Vasc Biol 2005;25(5):989–94.
77. Chaudhuri A, Umpierrez GE. Oxidative stress and inflammation in hyperglycemic crises and resolution with insulin: implications for the acute and chronic complications of hyperglycemia. J Diabetes Complications 2012;26(4):257–8.
78. Jenkins D, Close CF, Krentz AJ, et al. Euglycaemic diabetic ketoacidosis: does it exist? Acta Diabetol 1993;30(4):251–3.
79. Bas VN, Uytun S, Torun YA. Diabetic euglycemic ketoacidosis in newly diagnosed type 1 diabetes mellitus during Ramadan fasting. J Pediatr Endocrinol Metab 2015;28(3–4):333–5.
80. Guo RX, Yang LZ, Li LX, et al. Diabetic ketoacidosis in pregnancy tends to occur at lower blood glucose levels: case-control study and a case report of euglycemic diabetic ketoacidosis in pregnancy. J Obstet Gynaecol Res 2008;34(3):324–30.
81. Stephens JM, Sulway MJ, Watkins PJ. Relationship of blood acetoacetate and 3-hydroxybutyrate in diabetes. Diabetes. 1971;20(7):485–9.
82. Sheikh-Ali M, Karon BS, Basu A, et al. Can serum beta-hydroxybutyrate be used to diagnose diabetic ketoacidosis? Diabetes Care 2008;31(4):643–7.
83. Arieff AI, Carroll HJ. Nonketotic hyperosmolar coma with hyperglycemia: clinical features, pathophysiology, renal function, acid-base balance, plasma-cerebrospinal fluid equilibria and the effects of therapy in 37 cases. Medicine (Baltimore) 1972;51(2):73–94.
84. Slovis CM, Mork VG, Slovis RJ, et al. Diabetic ketoacidosis and infection: leukocyte count and differential as early predictors of serious infection. Am J Emerg Med 1987;5(1):1–5.
85. Beigelman PM. Potassium in severe diabetic ketoacidosis. Am J Med 1973;54(4):419–20.
86. Adrogue HJ, Lederer ED, Suki WN, et al. Determinants of plasma potassium levels in diabetic ketoacidosis. Medicine (Baltimore). 1986;65(3):163–72.
87. Umpierrez GE, DiGirolamo M, Tuvlin JA, et al. Differences in metabolic and hormonal milieu in diabetic- and alcohol-induced ketoacidosis. J Crit Care 2000;15(2):52–9.
88. Cahill GF Jr. Starvation in man. N Engl J Med 1970;282(12):668–75.
89. Umpierrez GE, Cuervo R, Karabell A, et al. Treatment of diabetic ketoacidosis with subcutaneous insulin aspart. Diabetes Care 2004;27(8):1873–8.
90. Hara JS, Rahbar AJ, Jeffres MN, et al. Impact of a hyperglycemic crises protocol. Endocr Pract 2013;19(6):953–62.
91. Kitabchi AE, Umpierrez GE, Murphy MB, et al. Hyperglycemic crises in diabetes. Diabetes Care 2004;27(Suppl 1):S94–102.
92. May ME, Young C, King J. Resource utilization in treatment of diabetic ketoacidosis in adults. Am J Med Sci 1993;306(5):287–94.
93. Moss JM. Diabetic ketoacidosis: effective low-cost treatment in a community hospital. South Med J 1987;80(7):875–81.
94. Umpierrez GE, Latif KA, Cuervo R, et al. Subcutaneous aspart insulin: a safe and cost effective treatment of diabetic ketoacidosis. Diabetes. 2003;52(Suppl 1):584A.
95. Glaser NS, Ghetti S, Casper TC, et al, Pediatric Emergency Care Applied Research Network DKAFSG. Pediatric diabetic ketoacidosis, fluid therapy, and cerebral injury: the design of a factorial randomized controlled trial. Pediatr Diabetes 2013;14(6):435–46.

96. Van Zyl DG, Rheeder P, Delport E. Fluid management in diabetic-acidosis–Ringer's lactate versus normal saline: a randomized controlled trial. QJM 2012;105(4):337–43.

97. Umpierrez G, Korytkowski M. Diabetic emergencies - ketoacidosis, hyperglycaemic hyperosmolar state and hypoglycaemia. Nat Rev Endocrinol 2016; 12(4):222–32.

98. Abramson E, Arky R. Diabetic acidosis with initial hypokalemia. Therapeutic implications. JAMA 1966;196(5):401–3.

99. Lever E, Jaspan JB. Sodium bicarbonate therapy in severe diabetic ketoacidosis. Am J Med 1983;75(2):263–8.

100. Green SM, Rothrock SG, Ho JD, et al. Failure of adjunctive bicarbonate to improve outcome in severe pediatric diabetic ketoacidosis. Ann Emerg Med 1998;31(1):41–8.

101. Latif KA, Freire AX, Kitabchi AE, et al. The use of alkali therapy in severe diabetic ketoacidosis. Diabetes Care 2002;25(11):2113–4.

102. Gamba G, Oseguera J, Castrejon M, et al. Bicarbonate therapy in severe diabetic ketoacidosis. A double blind, randomized, placebo controlled trial. Rev Invest Clin 1991;43(3):234–8.

103. Glaser N, Barnett P, McCaslin I, et al. Risk factors for cerebral edema in children with diabetic ketoacidosis. The Pediatric Emergency Medicine Collaborative Research Committee of the American Academy of Pediatrics. N Engl J Med 2001;344(4):264–9.

104. Fraley DS, Adler S. Correction of hyperkalemia by bicarbonate despite constant blood pH. Kidney Int 1977;12(5):354–60.

105. Umpierrez GE, Latif K, Stoever J, et al. Efficacy of subcutaneous insulin lispro versus continuous intravenous regular insulin for the treatment of patients with diabetic ketoacidosis. Am J Med 2004;117(5):291–6.

106. Ersoz HO, Ukinc K, Kose M, et al. Subcutaneous lispro and intravenous regular insulin treatments are equally effective and safe for the treatment of mild and moderate diabetic ketoacidosis in adult patients. Int J Clin Pract 2006;60(4): 429–33.

107. Karoli R, Fatima J, Salman T, et al. Managing diabetic ketoacidosis in non-intensive care unit setting: role of insulin analogs. Indian J Pharmacol 2011; 43(4):398–401.

108. Kitabchi AE, Ayyagari V, Guerra SM. The efficacy of low-dose versus conventional therapy of insulin for treatment of diabetic ketoacidosis. Ann Intern Med 1976;84(6):633–8.

109. Hipszer B, Joseph J, Kam M. Pharmacokinetics of intravenous insulin delivery in humans with type 1 diabetes. Diabetes Technol Ther 2005;7(1):83–93.

110. Doshi P, Potter AJ, De Los Santos D, et al. Prospective randomized trial of insulin glargine in acute management of diabetic ketoacidosis in the emergency department: a pilot study. Acad Emerg Med 2015;22(6):657–62.

111. Hsia E, Seggelke S, Gibbs J, et al. Subcutaneous administration of glargine to diabetic patients receiving insulin infusion prevents rebound hyperglycemia. J Clin Endocrinol Metab 2012;97(9):3132–7.

112. Umpierrez GE, Jones S, Smiley D, et al. Insulin analogs versus human insulin in the treatment of patients with diabetic ketoacidosis: a randomized controlled trial. Diabetes Care 2009;32(7):1164–9.

113. Wolfsdorf J, Glaser N, Sperling MA, American Diabetes Association. Diabetic ketoacidosis in infants, children, and adolescents: a consensus statement from the American Diabetes Association. Diabetes Care 2006;29(5):1150–9.

114. Hoffman WH, Stamatovic SM, Andjelkovic AV. Inflammatory mediators and blood brain barrier disruption in fatal brain edema of diabetic ketoacidosis. Brain Res 2009;1254:138–48.
115. Glaser NS, Wootton-Gorges SL, Buonocore MH, et al. Subclinical cerebral edema in children with diabetic ketoacidosis randomized to 2 different rehydration protocols. Pediatrics 2013;131(1):e73–80.
116. Shabbir N, Oberfield SE, Corrales R, et al. Recovery from symptomatic brain swelling in diabetic ketoacidosis. Clin Pediatr (Phila) 1992;31(9):570–3.
117. Roberts MD, Slover RH, Chase HP. Diabetic ketoacidosis with intracerebral complications. Pediatr Diabetes 2001;2(3):109–14.
118. Kamat P, Vats A, Gross M, et al. Use of hypertonic saline for the treatment of altered mental status associated with diabetic ketoacidosis. Pediatr Crit Care Med 2003;4(2):239–42.
119. Marcin JP, Glaser N, Barnett P, et al. Factors associated with adverse outcomes in children with diabetic ketoacidosis-related cerebral edema. J Pediatr 2002; 141(6):793–7.
120. Roe TF, Crawford TO, Huff KR, et al. Brain infarction in children with diabetic ketoacidosis. J Diabetes Complications 1996;10(2):100–8.
121. Keane S, Gallagher A, Ackroyd S, et al. Cerebral venous thrombosis during diabetic ketoacidosis. Arch Dis Child 2002;86(3):204–5.
122. Rosenbloom AL. Intracerebral crises during treatment of diabetic ketoacidosis. Diabetes Care 1990;13(1):22–33.
123. Deeb A, Yousef H, Abdelrahman L, et al. Implementation of a diabetes educator care model to reduce paediatric admission for diabetic ketoacidosis. J Diabetes Res 2016;2016:3917806.

# Monoarticular Arthritis

Namrata Singh, MD[a,b], Scott A. Vogelgesang, MD[a,b],*

## KEYWORDS

- Monoarticular arthritis • Gout • Calcium pyrophosphate • Arthrocentesis
- Septic joint

## KEY POINTS

- Crystalline arthritis (gout, calcium pyrophosphate) is a common cause of monoarticular arthritis.
- Septic arthritis is a medical emergency.
- Crystalline and septic arthritis can coexist. Identifying intracellular crystals does not automatically exclude septic arthritis.
- The first, most important, step in diagnosing monoarticular arthritis is often arthrocentesis.

## CASE

A 63-year-old man with a medical history of chronic stage 3 kidney disease from diabetes, congestive heart failure, hypertension, and atrial fibrillation presents to his primary care provider with an acute onset of pain and swelling of his right knee that started 2 days prior (**Box 1**).[1–3] It is very tender to touch and he has not been able to bear weight. He felt feverish without rigors or chills and denies similar episodes in the past. No other joints are bothering him currently. His medications include metformin, warfarin, metoprolol, aspirin, hydrochlorothiazide, simvastatin, ibuprofen (recently started for knee pain). He drinks beer on the weekends, is a nonsmoker, and uses no illicit drugs. He is not sure but thinks his grandfather might have had gout. His vitals are normal except for a temperature of 38.3°C. His right knee is moderately swollen, erythematous, and is tender to palpation. The remainder of the physical examination is unremarkable.

The authors have no conflicts of interest.
[a] Division of Immunology: Rheumatology and Allergy, Department of Internal Medicine, University of Iowa Carver College of Medicine, 200 Hawkins Drive, C 42 GH, Iowa City, IA 52242, USA; [b] Division of Immunology: Rheumatology and Allergy, Department of Internal Medicine, University of Iowa Carver College of Medicine, 200 Hawkins Drive, C 42 GH, Iowa City, IA 52242, USA
* Corresponding author. Division of Immunology: Rheumatology and Allergy, Department of Internal Medicine, University of Iowa Carver College of Medicine, 200 Hawkins Drive, C 42 GH, Iowa City, IA 52242.
*E-mail address:* scott-vogelgesang@uiowa.edu

> **Box 1**
> **Differential diagnosis of monoarticular arthritis**
>
> Crystalline arthritis
>   Gout
>   Calcium pyrophosphate arthritis
>   Others (eg, basic calcium phosphate)
>
> Septic arthritis
>
> Lyme arthritis
>
> Foreign body synovitis
>
> Pigmented villonodular synovitis
>
> Hemarthrosis
>
> Avascular necrosis
>
> Palindromic rheumatism
>
> Malignancy
>
> Initial presentation of systemic, polyarticular arthritis

## DIFFERENTIAL DIAGNOSIS

Crystalline arthritides are common causes of monoarticular arthritis and typically include gout, calcium pyrophosphate (CPP) arthropathy, and basic calcium phosphate disease. However, other crystals have also been rarely described as causes of inflammatory arthritis (eg, oxalate, corticosteroid, and lipid crystals). This article discusses gout and CPP arthritis in further detail because they are the most common.

Gout is the prototypical crystalline arthritis caused by uric acid deposition in and around the joints. It tends to affect men and postmenopausal women; it is rare in premenopausal women. The acute attacks of gout are characterized by intense pain, swelling, warmth and redness of the involved joint, and limited weight-bearing if lower extremities are involved. The involvement of the first metatarsal phalangeal joint is called podagra and is usually the initial presentation. Other joints frequently involved with gout attacks are the ankles and knees. Periarticular structures such as the olecranon bursa can be affected; rarely, the fingers and elbows may also be involved. Due to the cutaneous erythema associated with gouty attack, bacterial cellulitis is sometimes in the differential diagnosis. A definitive diagnosis of gout is made by aspirating synovial fluid from the affected joint and demonstrating the presence of intracellular, negatively birefringent monosodium urate crystals. The cell count usually ranges from 2000 to 80,000 cells per $mm^3$ but suspicion for coexisting infection should rise with synovial white blood cell (WBC) counts higher than 50,000 cells per $mm^3$.

Treatment of gout involves 2 components: (1) treating the acute episode of inflammation and (2) preventing future attacks using urate-lowering therapy (ULT). The treatments of choice for the control of an initial attack include nonsteroidal anti-inflammatory drugs (NSAIDs), systemic or intra-articular steroids (if infection is excluded), and colchicine. The choice between these options is best made by keeping in mind the patient's comorbidities, concurrent medications, and the severity of the attack. The gastrointestinal and renal toxicity of NSAIDs must be kept in mind when choosing these agents. Systemic steroids work well if the attack is polyarticular and severe but can worsen hyperglycemia in the diabetic patient. The American College of Rheumatology (ACR) 2012 guidelines recommend using 0.5 mg/kg/d of prednisone or methylprednisolone for 5 to 10 days and then stopping.[4,5]

The ACR guidelines have recommended 4 clinical situations that are appropriate to start chronic ULT: (1) presence of 1 or more tophi (a cutaneous collection of uric acid crystals), (2) frequent gout attacks defined as 2 or more attacks per year, (3) chronic kidney disease (CKD) stages 2 to 5, (4) or previous urolithiasis. Asymptomatic hyperuricemia not meeting these criteria does not usually need to be treated. Nonpharmacologic measures for preventing gouty arthritis should be discussed and emphasized to the patient. The ACR 2012 guidelines provide recommendations on the foods and drinks thought to increase serum urate levels and those with potential urate lowering effects. Diet and lifestyle choices for the prevention and optimal management of diabetes, obesity, and cardiovascular diseases need to be stressed as well. The use of medications that are known to increase serum urate levels (eg, diuretics, cyclosporine and tacrolimus, nicotinic acid, teriparatide) should be carefully evaluated for therapeutic benefits versus risk of gout exacerbations.

The 2 most common pharmacologic mechanisms used to lower urate levels are decreasing the synthesis of urate by inhibiting the enzyme xanthine oxidase (XO) and increased renal excretion of uric acid (uricosurics). These can be initiated during an acute attack once the medications for acute gouty arthritis have also been started. One of the XO inhibitors commonly used in practice is allopurinol. It should be started at low doses (eg, 100 mg; lower if CKD stage 4–5 is present) and titrated by 50 to 100 mg every 2 to 5 weeks until the desired uric acid levels are achieved. The ACR recommends the goal of ULT to achieve and maintain serum urate levels less than 6 mg/dL in most cases. Few common side-effects can be seen and include pruritus, rash, and elevated liver tests. Allopurinol hypersensitivity syndrome (AHS) is a rare but potentially life-threatening adverse effect. The presence of a variant allele, human leukocyte antigen (HLA)-B*5801, is associated with severe cutaneous reactions during allopurinol treatment and the ACR now recommends screening certain Asian populations considered to be at higher risk of AHS, including Koreans with stage 3 CKD or worse, Han Chinese and Thai individuals, independent of renal function. Febuxostat, another XO inhibitor, is typically used after intolerance or inefficacy of allopurinol has been demonstrated. The recommended starting dose is 40 mg daily with titration up to 80 mg daily based on serum uric acid levels. It has an advantage compared with allopurinol in that it does not require dosage adjustment when creatinine clearance is greater than 30 mL per minute.

Probenecid is a uricosuric agent used in the treatment of gout and is considered an alternative to XO inhibitors in cases in which they are not tolerated or are contraindicated. In addition, there are agents that are not specific gout medications but help in prevention of recurrent attacks through secondary uricosuric effects. The 2012 ACR guidelines recommend fenofibrate or losartan in refractory disease and these can be used in combination with XO inhibitors, if required. In refractory cases of gout, pegloticase can be used. It is a pegylated enzyme that converts uric acid to allantoin and thus lowers serum urate concentrations. However, frequent side effects limit its use. Another agent that was approved by the US Federal Food and Drug Administration in December 2015 for prevention of acute gouty arthritis in combination with an XO inhibitor is lesinurad. It works by inhibiting the transporter proteins URAT1 and OAT4 that reabsorb uric acid in the kidney.

CPP arthritis (formerly called CPPD or CPP deposition disease) results from inflammation caused by CPP crystals.[6,7] Acute CPP crystal arthritis (formerly called pseudogout) is the most commonly recognized form of CPP arthritis. A typical presentation of an acute CPP arthritis attack includes warmth, erythema, and swelling in and around the affected joint. It may be clinically indistinguishable from gout or septic arthritis. The knee is the most commonly involved joint, followed by the wrist. A rare presentation is involvement of the C2 vertebra with calcium deposits and manifests as acute, severe neck pain, fevers, and elevated inflammatory markers. This is referred to as the crowned dens syndrome.[8] The most accurate way to diagnose CPP arthritis is by aspiration of the affected joint and demonstrating positively birefringent, rhomboid-shaped crystals in the synovial fluid. In the absence of clinical arthritis, the radiographic finding of chondrocalcinosis (CPP deposition in the cartilaginous structure of a joint) should not be exclusively used to diagnose CPP arthritis. Risk factors for CPP arthritis include older age (rarely seen in patients younger than 60 years), osteoarthritis, and metabolic conditions such as hyperparathyroidism, hemochromatosis, and hypomagnesemia.

The management of acute episodes aims to reduce inflammation. If the affected joint is amenable to intra-articular corticosteroid injection (and infection is excluded), it is the treatment of choice. Another alternative for treatment of acute episodes is oral colchicine at doses of 0.6 mg once or twice daily, if no contraindications to its use exist. If these treatments are not feasible or indicated, systemic steroids can be used for a short course. Unlike gouty arthritis, no disease-modulating therapies are available for chronic CPP arthritis. Repeated intra-articular glucocorticoid injections can be considered in monoarticular large-joint involvement. Daily oral colchicine at 0.6 mg once or twice daily may be useful in reducing the frequency of acute attacks. If the patient can tolerate NSAIDs, they are another option for use to prevent recurrent attacks.

Septic arthritis[9] is the most important consideration in adults presenting with monoarticular arthritis. One important caution is that crystalline arthritides can sometimes coexist with septic arthritis.[10] Patients with septic arthritis present with acute joint swelling, erythema, warmth, and difficulty with range of motion. Hematogenous spread during bacteremia is the most common route of entry of infectious agents into the joint. Physical examination should differentiate whether the inflammation is periarticular or intra-articular. Usually septic arthritis is monoarticular but rarely can be oligoarticular. The knee is the most commonly affected joint. Laboratory evaluation typically shows elevated serum WBC counts and inflammatory markers (eg, erythrocyte sedimentation rate and C-reactive protein). Arthrocentesis is the key to help distinguish septic arthritis from other causes of monoarticular arthritis. Synovial fluid should be sent for WBC count, crystals, Gram stain, and culture. A synovial fluid WBC (White Blood Cell) count greater than 50,000 cells per mm$^3$ is very suspicious for septic arthritis. The range of pathogens causing septic arthritis is large. Bacterial causes include staphylococci, streptococci, gram-negative bacilli, mycobacteria, and anaerobes. Gonococcal arthritis, caused by *Neisseria gonorrhoeae*, can be seen in young, healthy, and sexually active adults and often has a coexistent rash that is frequently overlooked by the patient. The musculoskeletal presentation of disseminated gonococcal infection typically includes migratory arthralgias, tenosynovitis, and/or nonerosive arthritis. A few other unique but unusual causes of septic arthritis include infection with *Mycobacterium marinum* in people who clean fish tanks, *Pasteurella multocida* with a cat bite, ingestions of unpasteurized dairy products with *Brucella* species, and *Pseudomonas aeruginosa* or *Staphylococcus aureus* with intravenous drug use. Management involves prompt diagnosis and initiation of empiric intravenous antibiotics based on the organism found in the Gram stain of synovial fluid, or on clinical suspicion. Blood and synovial fluid cultures should be sent before starting antibiotics.

Lyme disease presents early with arthralgias and myalgias; however, Lyme arthritis is recognized later in the course of the infection (weeks to months after the initial infection) and typically presents with a monoarticular (or occasionally an oligoarticular) inflammatory arthritis, most commonly of the knee. Serologic diagnosis is made with the 2-tier approach using enzyme-linked immunosorbent assay as the initial step and, if positive, a western blot. Arthrocentesis reveals an inflammatory synovial fluid with no crystals and a negative Gram stain. Therapy is doxycycline 100 mg twice a day for 10 to 21 days.[11]

Foreign body synovitis occurs when a foreign body becomes lodged in the synovium of a joint. Plant thorn synovitis can be seen in gardeners who inadvertently impale a plant thorn into a joint, which can become inflamed with erythema and warmth. Plain radiographs are often normal but MRI may help identify the foreign material. Surgical removal of the foreign material is recommended.[12]

Pigmented villonodular synovitis is a rare tumor that, in its localized form, can affect a single joint such as the knee or ankle and presents with pain, locking, or catching; swelling and warmth can also be seen. Arthrocentesis reveals dark brown or frankly bloody fluid. Plain radiographs may be normal or nonspecific suggesting only a soft tissue density. MRI shows hyperplastic synovium and heterogeneous signal intensity. The hemosiderin in the tumor leads to low signal intensity and the congested synovium can show higher signal intensity. Surgical therapy is often required.[13]

Hemarthrosis can occur in several clinical settings, including in patients using anticoagulants or in those with bleeding diatheses such as hemophilia. Arthrocentesis often yields frankly bloody fluid. Blood is irritative and chronic hemarthroses can lead to advanced degenerative disease of the affected joint. Therapy is directed to evacuating the joint if there is a large effusion and reversing the reason for anticoagulation if possible.[14,15]

Avascular necrosis or osteonecrosis can be considered because it often affects a single joint or musculoskeletal area. It often occurs acutely and can be associated with severe pain but rarely with warmth or significant swelling of the joint. The pain is typically associated with weight-bearing and is much less symptomatic when not bearing weight. Risk factors for avascular necrosis include trauma, the use of corticosteroids, alcohol abuse, tobacco abuse, systemic diseases like systemic lupus erythematosus or renal failure, organ transplant recipients, sickle cell disease, use of chemotherapy or radiation, infection with human immunodeficiency virus, myeloproliferative disease, and Gaucher disease. Radiographs may be abnormal, showing subchondral collapse, but may only show advanced degenerative changes or, in some cases, no significant findings. Computed tomography or MRI may be necessary to make the diagnosis. Physical therapy and supportive therapy (analgesics and aids for ambulation) are often helpful but the secondary degenerative changes often progress, requiring surgical therapy.[16]

Palindromic rheumatism is a rare condition characterized by acute episodes of joint swelling, pain, warmth, and occasionally erythema in 1 or more joints. This condition resembles acute crystalline (eg, gout) arthritis but the inflammation resolves quicker (hours to days) than crystalline arthritis. Synovial fluid is inflammatory, sterile, and does not contain crystals. Many (perhaps as high as 30%) of patients who present with palindromic rheumatism evolve into what is later recognized as rheumatoid arthritis; however, some continue to have recurrent episodes of inflammatory arthritis and, for some, the joint inflammation remits.[17]

Although unusual, a polyarticular or systemic inflammatory disease (eg, rheumatoid arthritis or a spondyloarthritis) can present as a monoarticular arthritis. Rarely, malignancy can present as monoarticular arthritis. Examples include leukemic arthritis, in which leukemia cells infiltrate the joint space, or paraneoplastic arthritis, with direct involvement of the joint by metastatic cancer (eg, lung or breast cancer). Leukemic arthritis is more common in children than in adults.[18] Osteoarthritis can sometimes be confused with inflammatory monoarticular arthritis when it becomes significantly more symptomatic and associated with an effusion that is somewhat warm. Normal inflammatory markers, finding typical degenerative changes on radiographs, and noninflammatory joint fluid (synovial WBC counts <2000) all support the diagnosis.[19]

Arthrocentesis[20] is an important diagnostic tool in a patient with an inflammatory monoarticular arthritis. Evaluating the characteristics of joint fluid can confirm the clinical suspicion of inflammatory monoarticular arthritis and help identify the cause (eg, intracellular gout crystals in a typical clinical setting). Arthrocentesis is necessary in the clinical setting in which an infected joint is suspected. The procedure for doing arthrocentesis is relatively straight-forward: review the anatomy of the joint to be aspirated, prepare the area using betadine or chlorhexidine, anesthetize the skin using a topical anesthetic or local anesthetic (eg, bupivacaine or lidocaine without epinephrine), anesthetize the anticipated track of the needle, and use a larger bore needle (18–20 gauge for a larger joint, 20–23 for a smaller joint) to aspirate the joint fluid; smaller gauge needles can be more comfortable for the patient. Synovial fluid should be examined promptly because WBCs can become difficult to identify with time and CPP crystals resolubilize. Monosodium urate crystals, however, may continue to precipitate as the joint fluid sits on the microscope slide. Synovial fluid should be sent for cell count (WBCs, red blood cells), Gram stain, and culture; other tests have not proven to be helpful. Crystal analysis should be done in a timely fashion as well, either by the laboratory technician or by the clinician, depending on his or her experience in using a polarized microscope.

Monoarticular arthritis is not uncommon in the ambulatory setting and requires a careful clinical evaluation to arrive at the appropriate diagnosis and to initiate appropriate therapy. Septic arthritis is potentially dangerous and needs to be considered in a patient with monoarticular arthritis. Crystalline arthritis is a common cause of monoarticular arthritis but there are other potential causes that need to be considered. Often, the first and most important step in diagnosing a patient with monoarticular arthritis is arthrocentesis.

## REFERENCES

1. Genes N, Chisolm-Straker M. Monoarticular arthritis update: current evidence for diagnosis and treatment in the emergency department. Emerg Med Pract 2012; 14(5):1–19 [quiz: 19–20].
2. Siva C, Velazquez C, Mody A, et al. Diagnosing acute monoarthritis in adults: a practical approach for the family physician. Am Fam Physician 2003;68(1):83–90.
3. Umberhandt R, Isaacs J. Diagnostic considerations for monoarticular arthritis of the hand and wrist. J Hand Surg Am 2012;37(7):1480–5.
4. Khanna D, Fitzgerald JD, Khanna PP, et al. 2012 American College of Rheumatology guidelines for management of gout. Part 1: systematic nonpharmacologic and pharmacologic therapeutic approaches to hyperuricemia. Arthritis Care Res (Hoboken) 2012;64(10):1431–46.
5. Khanna D, Khanna PP, Fitzgerald JD, et al. 2012 American College of Rheumatology guidelines for management of gout. Part 2: therapy and antiinflammatory prophylaxis of acute gouty arthritis. Arthritis Care Res (Hoboken) 2012;64(10): 1447–61.
6. Zhang W, Doherty M, Bardin T, et al. European league against rheumatism recommendations for calcium pyrophosphate deposition. Part I: terminology and diagnosis. Ann Rheum Dis 2011;70(4):563–70.

7. Zhang W, Doherty M, Pascual E, et al. EULAR recommendations for calcium pyrophosphate deposition. Part II: management. Ann Rheum Dis 2011;70(4):571–5.

8. Uh M, Dewar C, Spouge D, et al. Crowned dens syndrome: a rare cause of acute neck pain. Clin Rheumatol 2013;32(5):711–4.

9. Mathews CJ, Weston VC, Jones A, et al. Bacterial septic arthritis in adults. Lancet 2010;375(9717):846–55.

10. Papanicolas LE, Hakendorf P, Gordon DL. Concomitant septic arthritis in crystal monoarthritis. J Rheumatol 2012;39(1):157–60.

11. Shapiro ED. Clinical practice. Lyme disease. N Engl J Med 2014;370(18): 1724–31.

12. Baskar S, Mann JS, Thomas AP, et al. Plant thorn tenosynovitis. J Clin Rheumatol 2006;12(3):137–8.

13. Ofluoglu O. Pigmented villonodular synovitis. Orthop Clin North Am 2006;37(1): 23–33.

14. Lobet S, Hermans C, Lambert C. Optimal management of hemophilic arthropathy and hematomas. J Blood Med 2014;5:207–18.

15. Wyseure T, Mosnier LO, von Drygalski A. Advances and challenges in hemophilic arthropathy. Semin Hematol 2016;53(1):10–9.

16. Mont MA, Cherian JJ, Sierra RJ, et al. Nontraumatic osteonecrosis of the femoral head: where do we stand today? A ten-year update. J Bone Joint Surg Am 2015; 97(19):1604–27.

17. Sanmarti R, Canete JD, Salvador G. Palindromic rheumatism and other relapsing arthritis. Best Pract Res Clin Rheumatol 2004;18(5):647–61.

18. Ashouri JF, Daikh DI. Rheumatic manifestations of cancer. Rheum Dis Clin North Am 2011;37(4):489–505.

19. Gelber AC. In the clinic. Osteoarthritis. Ann Intern Med 2014;161(1):ITC1–16.

20. Bettencourt RB, Linder MM. Arthrocentesis and therapeutic joint injection: an overview for the primary care physician. Prim Care 2010;37(4):691–702, v.

# Ocular Emergencies: Red Eye

Andreina Tarff, MD[a], Ashley Behrens, MD[b],*

## KEYWORDS

- Red eye • Conjunctiva • Conjunctivitis • Allergic • Ocular inflammation
- Ocular trauma

## KEY POINTS

- Red eye is one of the most common indicators that something in the eye is not going well.
- Different disorders can cause conjunctival injection, leading patients to seek emergency care.
- Because the eye is a visible organ, it may show the first signs of either local or systemic problems at early stages of the disease.
- It is important for general practitioners to identify the various causes of red eye to evaluate when to comfortably manage a particular case or consult with an eye specialist to provide adequate patient care.

Eye emergencies are part of a significant proportion of general visits to the emergency room. Some of these can be managed safely by general practitioners, but some more serious conditions require specialized treatment. Red eye is one of the most common indicators that something in the eye is not going well. Different disorders can cause conjunctival injection, leading patients to seek emergency care. Because the eye is a visible organ, it may show the first signs of either local or systemic problems at early stages of the disease. It is important for general practitioners to identify the various causes of red eye to evaluate when to comfortably manage a particular case or consult with an eye specialist to provide adequate patient care.

Most of the following eye conditions involve various degrees of ocular inflammation, which is the necessary condition to cause conjunctival injection and, therefore, visible redness in the eye.

## COMMON CAUSES OF RED EYE

Various events may cause dilation or exposure of the conjunctival vessel network, resulting in red eye. A short list of the most common problems associated with redness is shown here:

1. Dry eye syndrome (dysfunctional tear syndrome [DTS])
2. Conjunctivitis

[a] The Wilmer Eye Institute, Johns Hopkins University School of Medicine, 400 North Broadway, Suite 4001, Baltimore, MD 21231, USA; [b] Division of Comprehensive Eye Care, Wilmer Institute, Johns Hopkins University School of Medicine, 400 North Broadway, Suite 4001, Baltimore, MD 21231, USA
* Corresponding author.
E-mail address: abehrens@jhmi.edu

Med Clin N Am 101 (2017) 615–639
http://dx.doi.org/10.1016/j.mcna.2016.12.013
0025-7125/17/© 2017 Elsevier Inc. All rights reserved.

medical.theclinics.com

3. Keratitis and corneal ulcers
4. Corneal abrasions
5. Foreign body in the ocular surface
6. Blepharitis
7. Episcleritis and scleritis
8. Distichiasis
9. Uveitis
10. Endophthalmitis
11. Subconjunctival hemorrhage
12. Corneal graft rejection
13. Acute glaucoma
14. Chemical burns
15. Drug induced disorders

## DRY EYE SYNDROME (DYSFUNCTIONAL TEAR SYNDROME)

DTS is one of the most common conditions in ophthalmology, and is often unrecognized and underestimated. DTS is a cause of recurrent patient visits to health providers in the United States and a very frequent disease leading to chronic red eye. DTS may significantly affect visual acuity and impair daily activities, becoming a public health issue.[1–3] The prevalence of DTS increases with age and has been estimated to range from 5% to 34% of the adult population globally, affecting 18% of women and 11% of men in the United States.[4–7]

### Pathophysiology

There is an underlying inflammation of the ocular surface with an altered morphology in the corneal sub-basal nerve plexus affects the epithelial resurfacing. Inflammatory mediators and hypersensitivity generate hyperosmolarity of the tear film as a consequence of systemic (hormonal and autoimmune) or localized (mechanical) processes affecting the tear film.[8,9]

### Classification

#### Decreased tear production
Decreased tear production can be caused by any form of lacrimal gland dysfunction. The causes include autoimmune and infiltrative conditions affecting the ocular surface, such as Sjögren, sarcoidosis, graft-versus-host disease, mucous membrane pemphigoid, diabetes, and lymphomas; and localized mechanical conditions leading to a decreased reflex of tear secretion, including contact lens–related and age-related lacrimal gland impairment with ductal obstruction, and ocular burns.[10]

#### Increased evaporative loss
This condition is caused by dysfunctional meibomian glands, which are responsible for generating the lipid component that provides a barrier and minimizes evaporation. In addition, evaporative loss may be caused by a decreased blink function, use of certain preserved eye drops, contact lens wear, and ocular allergies.[11]

### Clinical Diagnosis and Primary Care Evaluation

#### Symptoms
This condition is commonly related to long working hours in a low-humidity environment, and the use of computers for a long time may exacerbate the symptoms. General irritation, red eye, burning, foreign body sensation, fatigue, light sensitivity, and blurred vision are common, usually at the end of the day. Paradoxically, epiphora or

excessive tearing is always present as a result of the reactive stimulation of the lacrimal gland and the lack or decrease in one of the components of the tear film. In severe cases, the degenerative inflammatory changes can lead to severe pain and visual impairment.[12]

### Signs

Signs can vary considerably in intensity over time and under different environmental conditions. Conjunctival injection, blepharitis, entropion, or ectropion may be present.

Because of the variability of findings on clinical evaluation, clinicians base their assessment of dry eye on the results of validated questionnaires.[13,14]

### Ophthalmologic Evaluation

#### Ocular surface staining
Fluorescein and lissamine green delineate areas of discontinuity on the corneal epithelial surface, and rose bengal is used to stain areas of devitalized epithelium in the cornea and conjunctiva.

#### Tear break-up time
Applying a fluorescein strip to the inferior cul-de-sac, the patient is instructed not to blink and the tear film is observed through the slit lamp. The appearance of dark spots between 1 and 10 seconds indicates rapid tear film break-up, which is considered abnormal (**Fig. 1**).

#### Tear hyperosmolarity
Tear hyperosmolarity is potentially useful as a marker for disease severity, and is commercially available in the clinical setting.[15,16]

#### Tear protein analysis
Enzyme-linked immunosorbent assay is a good method for measuring lactoferrin, aquaporin 5, epidermal growth factor, lipocalin, and immunoglobulin A levels. A lysozyme diffusion test by van Bijsterveld[19] is used to measure lysozyme levels in tears.[17–19]

### Treatment

Depending on the severity and the cause of DTS, the treatment should first focus on the primary cause. The first-line therapy includes nourishment with artificial tears

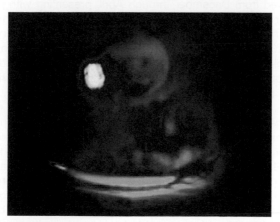

**Fig. 1.** Dysfunctional tear syndrome and rapid tear break-up time. Because of meibomian gland dysfunction, areas of yellow staining of fluorescein dye denote an irregular tear film causing ocular surface damage.

supplements and environmental coping strategies. The patient should discontinue any unnecessary systemic or ocular medications that can contribute to dryness. Topical cyclosporine has been shown to enhance the stability of the tear film in patients with even severe disease, by addressing immune-mediated inflammatory processes. It has been shown to decrease levels of interleukin-6 and activated lymphocytes in the conjunctiva, reducing the turnover of epithelial cells and increasing goblet cell numbers. More recently, lifitegrast has been US Food and Drug Administration approved for the treatment of DTS. This drug inhibits an integrin, lymphocyte function–associated antigen 1 (LFA-1), from binding to intercellular adhesion molecule 1 (ICAM-1). The mechanism downregulates inflammation mediated by T lymphocytes.[20] Additional novel drug formulations are currently under investigation to improve tolerance and bioavailability.[21,22]

## CONJUNCTIVITIS

A common patient complaint and the most likely diagnosis in a patient with unilateral or bilateral red eye and discharge, conjunctivitis is often associated with morning crusting. Most types are self-limiting, but some may progress and cause serious complications. There is low clinical accuracy at differentiating the various causes of acute conjunctivitis. Its prevalence varies according to the cause, which may be influenced by the patient's age, as well as the season of the year. The economic impact of the disease in terms of lost work time, cost of medical visits, diagnostic testing, and medications is considerable.[23,24] The disease can be classified into acute, hyperacute, and chronic according to the mode of onset and the severity of the clinical response.

### Acute Conjunctivitis

Acute conjunctivitis is inflammation of the bulbar and tarsal conjunctiva, being present for less than 3 to 4 weeks, and potentially causing the conjunctiva to become scarred.

### Infectious conjunctivitis

Predisposing factors include ocular conditions with a disruption of the conjunctival epithelial barrier, trauma, compromised tear production, abnormality of adnexal structures, and immune-compromised status.[25]

**Bacterial** The second most common cause of infectious conjunctivitis, which is frequently observed from December through April, presenting with profuse purulent thick and globular discharge within 12 to 24 hours of inoculation, with more discharge appearing within minutes after wiping the lids.[23,26] Its annual incidence rate has been estimated to be 135 per 10,000 people in the United States. Common routes of transmission include direct contact with infected individuals, contaminated fingers and fomites, and oculogenital spread. The most common microorganisms for bacterial conjunctivitis in adults are staphylococcal species, followed by *Streptococcus pneumoniae* and *Haemophilus influenzae*. In children, the disease is often caused by *H influenzae*, *S pneumoniae*, and *Moraxella catarrhalis*. Ophthalmia neonatorum, mainly caused by *Chlamydia trachomatis*, *Neisseria gonorrhoeae*, and *Escherichia coli*, is known to be associated with systemic complications and severe visual loss in newborns born vaginally.[27] Bacterial conjunctivitis is more common in neonates and children than in adults, although clinical experience suggests that most infectious conjunctivitis is viral in both adults and children. Contact lens wearers are at highest risk for gram-negative infections such as *Pseudomonas aeruginosa*.[28] In particular, some bacteria, such *N gonorrhoeae*, cause severe hyperacute bacterial conjunctivitis that is sight threatening, presenting with severe purulent discharge and requiring immediate ophthalmologic evaluation, preventing severe keratitis and corneal melting with perforation.[29]

**Viral** The most common form of infectious conjunctivitis in both adult and children overall, with a rate of 80%, more prevalent during summer, and frequently misdiagnosed as bacterial conjunctivitis (**Fig. 2**).[30] Most cases are caused by adenovirus (90%), with its many serotypes being implicated,[31] generally presenting as a bilateral, nonpurulent conjunctivitis with watery discharge and a mild mucus component. Symptoms include grittiness, burning or irritation, and photophobia. This type of ocular infection is highly contagious and usually accompanied by prodromal upper respiratory symptoms. Adenovirus serotypes 8, 19, and 37 can be particularly fulminant because of variation in host immune factors leading to epidemic keratoconjunctivitis.[32] Other causes include herpes simplex (1.3%–4.8%), which is usually unilateral and associated with vesicular lip lesions (cold sores); herpes zoster, responsible for shingles, involving the first and second branches of the trigeminal nerve and potentially causing corneal complications and uveitis; and molluscum contagiosum. Those patients should be referred for evaluation by an ophthalmologist, because potentially severe ocular complications may occur.[33,34]

**Fungal and protozoan** Related to keratitis, often caused by filamentous fungi (*Fusarium*, *Alternaria*, and *Aspergillus* spp) and yeasts (*Candida* spp). These fungi almost always present in previously abnormal eyes. Worldwide contact lens–related epidemics of the filamentous fungus *Fusarium* and protozoan *Acanthamoeba* were reported in 2006 and 2007.[35]

## Noninfectious Conjunctivitis

### Allergic

Allergic conjunctivitis is the most prevalent form of acute and chronic conjunctivitis, affecting at least 20% of the population on an annual basis. This type of conjunctivitis is seasonal, more frequently occurring during spring and summer. It is predominantly a disease of young adults, with an average age of onset of 20 years; symptoms tend to decrease with age, but older adults can continue to have severe symptoms. It typically presents as bilateral redness of the tarsal conjunctiva with papillae, mucoserous discharge, and ocular pruritus as a cardinal symptom. Patients often have a history

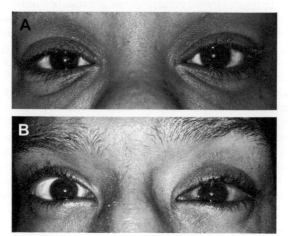

**Fig. 2.** Viral conjunctivitis. Conjunctival injection on the temporal side bilaterally with minimal discharge, usually watery type (*A*). More commonly, viral conjunctivitis starts as a unilateral disease with localized symptoms only in the involved eye (*B*).

of atopy, or seasonal or specific allergies.[36] In severe cases, marked chemosis with bulging edematous conjunctiva may be seen. These conditions are relatively benign ocular diseases that cause significant suffering and use of health care resources, although they typically do not threaten vision.[37]

### Systemic immune-mediated diseases associated with conjunctivitis

These conditions present with an abrupt onset or acute flares, affecting the mucous ocular membranes. Stevens-Johnson, ocular mucous membrane pemphigoid, graft-versus-host diseases, Kawasaki, and carotid cavernous fistula, among others, are characterized by nonpurulent conjunctivitis, uveitis, rash, changes in labial area and oral cavity, changes in peripheral extremities, and cervical lymphadenopathy. Patients with low-grade carotid cavernous fistula may present with chronic conjunctivitis not responding to medical therapy, which, if left untreated, can lead to death. Supplementary laboratory criteria can aid in the diagnosis.[38,39]

## Chronic Conjunctivitis

These conditions are inflammatory processes of gradual onset that persist for more than 4 weeks. Most cases of allergic conjunctivitis belong to this group: seasonal allergic conjunctivitis, perennial allergic conjunctivitis, vernal keratoconjunctivitis, and atopic keratoconjunctivitis. Giant papillary keratoconjunctivitis presenting with cobble-stoning and giant papillae are typically seen in contact lens wearers. This type of reaction may persist for several months, and even years. Follicles may also be present in chronic long-standing T cell–mediated conditions.

Ocular neoplasias, such as squamous carcinoma, malignant melanoma–primary acquired melanosis, and lymphomas, do not cause significant symptoms; however, conjunctival injection might be the first sign of presentation. Conjunctival involvement of lymphoma typically looks like a salmon-colored patch and is the first sign of systemic disease.[40]

## Diagnosis

It is important to differentiate conjunctivitis from other sight-threatening eye conditions that have similar clinical presentation and make appropriate decisions about further testing, treatment, or referral based on algorithmic approaches using a focused ocular history along with an eye examination.[41] Conjunctivitis is a diagnosis of exclusion. Conjunctival injection is usually diffuse, involving the bulbar conjunctiva as well as the tarsal conjunctiva. More serious conditions, such keratitis, iritis, and angle-closure glaucoma, usually present with a 360° ciliary flush pattern in the bulbar conjunctiva around the cornea. Cultures are usually inconclusive, being reserved for cases of suspected neonatal infectious conjunctivitis, recurrent conjunctivitis, conjunctivitis recalcitrant to therapy, conjunctivitis presenting with copious purulent discharge, and cases suspicious for gonococcal or chlamydial infection. Cultures may be also recommended in contact lens wearers, who are subject to myriad types of secondary chronic conjunctivitis.[25] Red flags of more serious ocular disorder (infectious keratitis, iritis, angle-closure glaucoma) should always be considered, because these require an immediate ophthalmology referral: reduction of visual acuity, ciliary flush, photophobia, foreign body sensation, corneal opacity, fixed pupil, and severe headache with nausea/vomiting.

## Treatment

Large meta-analyses have shown that at least 60% of cases of culture-proven acute bacterial conjunctivitis are self-limiting, with no differences observed in outcomes between treatment and placebo groups.[42,43] However, some bacteria, such as

*S pneumoniae, N gonorrhoeae*, and *H influenzae*, can penetrate an intact host defense more easily and cause more serious damage, probably because of bacteria mechanisms in acquiring resistance genes.[44] Bacterial conjunctivitis should be treated with broad-spectrum antibiotics, with no significant difference observed between types. Benefits of antibiotic treatment include quicker recovery, decrease in transmissibility, and early return to daily activities.[30] Fluoroquinolones are the preferred agents in contact lens wearers because of the high incidence of pseudomonas infection. Up to 64% of staphylococcal infections are caused by methicillin-resistant *Staphylococcus aureus* (MRSA), requiring an immediate ophthalmic evaluation and treatment with vancomycin.[45,46] Factors influencing antibiotic election include patient allergies, resistance patterns, and cost. In general, ointments are preferred rather than drops for children, patients with poor compliance, and those in whom it is difficult to administer eye medications. Conjunctivitis secondary to sexually transmitted diseases such as chlamydia requires systemic treatment in addition to topical antibiotic therapy. Treatment of hyperacute conjunctivitis secondary to *N gonorrhoeae* consists of intramuscular ceftriaxone with concurrent oral azithromycin for chlamydial co-infection.[47] Patients with bacterial conjunctivitis should respond in 1 to 2 days with a decrease in discharge, redness, and irritation. Patients who do not improve should be referred to an ophthalmologist.[25]

Viral conjunctivitis is a self-limited process; the symptoms frequently get worse for the first 3 to 5 days, with gradual resolution over the following weeks.

There is no specific therapy for viral conjunctivitis, although patients may receive symptomatic benefit from topical antihistamine/decongestants or from lubricating agents like those used for noninfectious conjunctivitis. Herpes simplex and herpes zoster treatment consists of a combination of oral and topical antivirals. In cases of severe inflammation (uveitis), steroids may be considered once antiviral treatment has been established.

The management of allergic conjunctivitis in mainly based on avoidance of the offending agent and artificial tears to physically dilute or remove the antigen. In large systemic reviews, antihistamines were superior to mast cell stabilizers in providing short-term benefits. Long-term use of the antihistamine antazoline and the vasoconstrictor naphazoline should be avoided because they both can cause rebound hyperemia. Steroids should be used with caution because they are associated with cataract formation and glaucoma.[48]

## KERATITIS AND CORNEAL ULCERS
### General Aspects of Infectious Keratitis

Keratitis is an active inflammatory corneal process characterized by red eye, purulent or nonpurulent discharge, considerable foreign body sensation, photophobia, and corneal opacity or infiltrate. It remains an important cause of ocular morbidity and blindness worldwide warranting an immediate ophthalmologic examination. It is caused by a variety of organisms, notably bacterial, but can also include amoebic, fungal, and viral agents invading the epithelium, stroma, and, in more severe disease, endothelium, anterior chamber of the eye, and sclera. Emergence of resistant pathogen strains has been reported in the literature. An ulcer larger than 0.5 mm can be distinguished with a penlight, not requiring the slit lamp for identification; fulminant cases may present with an associated hypopyon.

Predisposing factors such a disruption of the innate corneal immunity (ocular trauma, vegetative or soil-contaminated objects, corneal surgery, or chronic ocular surface disease), contact lens wear, and immunosuppressive conditions or treatments (diabetes, human immunodeficiency virus, corticosteroid use) have been identified.

Improper and overnight contact lens wear is the largest risk factor contributing to the local breakdown of the host defense mechanisms.[49,50]

Treatment requires prompt initiation of therapy, ideally after obtaining cultures; however corneal scrapings sometimes are required for faster microbiology identification.[51] Antimicrobial therapy is usually compounded in fortified concentrations, not in commercially available eye drops. The role of topical glucocorticoids and topical drug combinations containing topical steroids is controversial and best left to the discretion of the consulting ophthalmologist.

Despite systematic reviews including randomized control trials, the gold standard for the treatment of infectious keratitis remains elusive.[52] Current therapies rely on empiric, broad-spectrum medical (topical, intraocular, or systemic therapy, commonly vancomycin, amphotericin B, natamycin, and voriconazole) or surgical means (necrotic tissue debridement, conjunctival flap, lamellar or penetrating keratoplasty or enucleation, following primary medical failure). Corneal collagen cross-linking has been reported as an emerging treatment of infectious keratitis to reduce the parasite load and restore vision. However, it has variable outcomes in the setting of fungal and protozoan keratitis.[53–56]

### Acanthamoeba Keratitis

Acanthamoeba keratitis is an increasing public health problem affecting immune-competent young adults that has captured much attention because of an emerging trend in the United States.[57] Of considerations are the complexity of the pathogen's morphologic forms, and the lack of an acceptable treatment; treatments mainly consist of highly toxic, non–commercially available biocides usually prescribed hourly during weeks or months. Associated sequels include corneal melting, iris atrophy, persistent mydriasis, cataract, glaucoma, and loss of the eye.[58,59] Acanthamoeba keratitis (AK) is highly associated with direct exposure of contact lenses to infected water. The extracellular proteins secreted by the virulent *Acanthamoeba* spp digest corneal tissue, optimizing drug resistance and cyst formation.[60] The presence of pseudodendritic lesions often causes AK to be misdiagnosed as herpetic keratitis. A ring-shaped corneal infiltrate, punctate epithelial erosions, and subepithelial stromal and perineural infiltrates may be seen on slit-lamp examination. However, these can also be seen in other forms of keratitis. The corneal smear is a rapid and specific detection method; visualization of double-walled cellular structures are characteristic of *Acanthamoeba* cysts.[61] However, these are not always identifiable and special cultures are necessary.[62]

### Fungal Keratitis

Fungal keratitis is most frequently associated with filamentous fungi (*Fusarium* and *Aspergillus* spp) in tropical latitudes and yeast (*Candida* spp) in temperate climates. Despite its lower incidence, the diagnosis and treatment remain challenging because of its insidious and delayed clinical presentation, capability of corneal invasion, extended laboratory incubation periods, and a weak response to therapy compared with the bacterial analog.[63]

### Viral Keratitis

Adenovirus is typically associated with conjunctivitis, but some viral strains in predisposed individuals can cause epidemic keratoconjunctivitis. These patients start with the classic viral conjunctivitis, progressing to an active corneal process; the penlight examination of cornea is unremarkable, but fluorescein staining reveals multiple punctate keratopathy. Subepithelial infiltrates are also common in adenoviral keratitis. Other common viruses, such hepatitis B, have been implicated as rare causal agents (**Fig. 3**).[64]

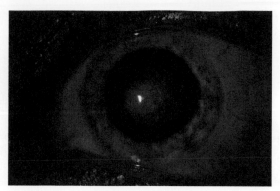

**Fig. 3.** Viral keratitis caused by herpes simplex virus. This condition is another cause of redness in the eye that persists for several days as long as there is viral activity. Note the central scar remaining after disciform herpes simplex virus keratitis occurred.

## CORNEAL ABRASIONS

Corneal abrasion is a frequently encountered condition in the emergency department, typically resulting from mechanical injuries leading to superficial scratches and micro-trauma involving the corneal epithelium. The condition typically presents with unilateral severe painful red eye (because the superficial cornea is replete of sensory nerve endings) and photophobia, and is often associated with retained foreign bodies. Traumatic corneal abrasions pose the highest risk for corneal infections, and treatment should be focused on prophylaxis and careful monitoring for progression to nonhealing states.[65] Key aspects of clinical management include exclusion of an open globe rupture on pen light examination, and suspicion for penetrating trauma in any patient with extruded ocular contents, or in whom the pupil is dilated, nonreactive, or irregular. These findings indicate severe injury and require immediate referral. After inspection, measurement of visual acuity should be documented; vision loss of more than 20/40 requires immediate ophthalmologic attention. Most small abrasions heal fully within 24 hours. Follow-up may not be necessary for patients with small (4 mm or less) uncomplicated abrasions, normal vision, and resolution of symptoms. Follow-up in 24 hours is indicated for other patients, including those with larger abrasions, contact lens–related abrasions, and diminished vision. Preventive antibiotic therapy against *Pseudomonas* is indicated. Meta-analysis of randomized trials and systematic reviews found that patching did not hasten the epithelialization process or reduce pain, and seems to worsen contact lens–related corneal abrasions.[66,67]

## FOREIGN BODIES

Foreign bodies represent the second most common cause of visual loss, accounting for approximately 30.8% of all eye injuries.[68,69] Clinical manifestations depend on the nature of the inert substance embedded in the cornea or conjunctiva. In general, sand and glass produce a nonsevere reaction; metals account for a major proportion of corneal foreign bodies, and organic matter is poorly tolerated, causing not only a localized inflammatory corneal edema with opacification but vascularization and stromal necrosis.[70] In all cases, the foreign body must be promptly removed, especially if it is in the visual axis or reduces visual acuity (**Fig. 4**). Slit-lamp examination sometimes fails to reveal the foreign substance because of the presence of edema, and anterior segment optical coherence tomography may be a valuable tool for the early diagnosis and progress of treatment.[71]

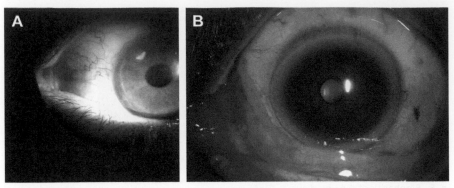

**Fig. 4.** (*A*) Foreign body located in the cornea. If not removed promptly, this may cause a keratitis with severe pain and redness. (*B*) Redundant conjunctiva (conjunctivochalasis) may cause foreign body sensation and ocular redness as well. (*Courtesy of* [*A*] Maria Carolina Marquezan, MD, Cuiabá, Mato Grosso, Brazil)

Contact lenses, the most commonly worn superficial foreign bodies, cause a constant chronic breakdown of the corneal epithelium. Cell damage and death occur through different mechanisms, including ocular surface microtrauma, nutrient deprivation, metabolic injury caused by tissue oxygen starvation/drying, and even chemical toxicity or hypersensitivity. Mild staining of the epithelium is common, usually asymptomatic, and of little clinical consequence. However, poorly fitting lenses may cause superficial punctate staining of the epithelium. Larger defects may cause pain, tearing, red eyes, photophobia, and blurred vision, with microcysts in the epithelial layer resulting from pockets of dead cellular debris associated with stromal edema.[72,73] Chronic hypoxia may lead to superficial, and rarely deep, corneal neovascularization, especially at the superior limbus. Patients who experience contact lens–related hypoxia may benefit from switching to a more oxygen-permeable lens material.[74] A condition resembling superior limbic keratoconjunctivitis may be seen in some contact lens wearers. Giant papillary conjunctivitis is the inflammatory disorder that represents a reaction to lid movement over a foreign substance.

## BLEPHARITIS

Blepharitis is one of the most common chronic ocular disorders in clinical practice, estimated to be the reason for referral in 12% to 15% of cases,[75] and mainly affecting the young and pediatric population, especially people of Asian descent.[76,77] However, a significant proportion of the US adult population is also affected (**Fig. 5**).[75] Blepharitis constitutes a diagnostic and therapeutic enigma because of the complexity underlying its pathogenesis, mainly involving interactions between abnormalities in the lid margin with meibomian gland dysfunction (chalazion, telangiectasia, thickening, and scarring), changes in the tear film dynamics, microbial colonization, and dermatologic conditions affecting the periocular area, such as seborrheic dermatitis, rosacea, and eczema. In addition, blepharokeratoconjunctivitis also involves inflammatory changes at the conjunctiva and cornea. Clinical manifestations include itching, foreign body and burning sensation, conjunctival hyperemia, excessive tearing, swelling of the eyelids, crusting and scaling of the eyelid skin, and photophobia, potentially leading to punctate epithelial keratitis, vascularization, corneal opacities, and ulceration.[78] Common associated conditions include dry eye, contact lens intolerance, chalazion, and hordeolum. At present there is no long-term cure for this condition because patients are likely to be susceptible

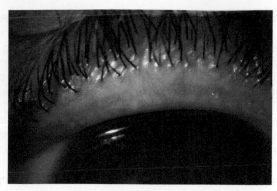

**Fig. 5.** Blepharitis of the upper eye lid. Note the presence of abnormal droplets in the surface of the lid margin, which are a sign of thickening of the secretions of meibomian glands. The opening of the glands becomes inspissated. Telangiectasias are also observed on the lid margin.

to the causative organisms. A prolonged therapeutic regimen directed toward preventing meibomian gland obstruction, such as lid hygiene, artificial tear supplementation, and topical antibiotics, is intended to alleviate symptoms and bring the disease under control. Topical corticosteroids may be helpful in patients with marked inflammation. A systematic review of 34 studies, including clinical trials and case control studies, regarding the treatment of chronic anterior or posterior blepharitis found topical antibiotics to be effective in eradicating bacteria at the lid margin but did not find effectiveness for oral antibiotics or topical glucocorticoids.[79,80]

## EPISCLERITIS AND SCLERITIS

Scleral inflammatory disease includes a spectrum from episcleritis, a more superficial inflammation generally idiopathic and self-limited in nature, to scleritis, a deeper and more destructive inflammation.[81,82] These conditions result from a heterogeneous group of local or systemic diseases that may be caused by local or systemic infections or immune-mediated diseases, or may be the primary manifestation of an acquired connective tissue disorder or vasculitis, which is a life-threatening condition.[83,84] Episcleritis usually poses no threat to visual acuity, and systemic autoimmune conditions are present in up to one-third of patients.[85] Previous studies have suggested that scleritis is more often associated with systemic autoimmune diseases; most commonly rheumatoid arthritis or granulomatosis with polyangiitis (formerly Wegener granulomatosis).[86,87] Postoperative necrotizing scleral inflammation at the surgical trauma site is a rare cause of scleritis and its risk seems to be increased in patients with an underlying inflammatory disease who undergo cataract extraction, trabeculectomy, strabismus, retinal detachment, and pterygium surgeries. There have been estimated to be up to 120,000 and 10,500 new-onset cases of episcleritis and scleritis, respectively, each year in the United States.[88] Both tend to affect the middle aged, between 43 and 60 years of age, being of rare occurrence in children, especially those younger than 5 years of age. Women are affected in most cases (70%–74% of total cases).[89]

Episcleritis is most commonly seen as a diffuse pattern with mild to moderate inflammation that usually subsides within 3 weeks, with possible recurrences. Nodular episcleritis presents with prolonged and more painful attacks.[82] Anatomically, scleritis can be anterior or posterior. Anterior scleritis can be classified as diffuse, nodular, necrotizing with inflammation, and necrotizing without inflammation (scleromalacia perforans).[90,91] The most prominent feature in patients presenting with anterior scleritis is red eye, usually accompanied by severe eye pain that radiates to the forehead and jaw, usually awakening the patient at night. Scleromalacia perforans may have minimal symptoms. Patients with posterior scleritis may present with reduced vision, with or without pain. Posterior scleritis is most often associated with systemic diseases and vision loss, requiring systemic immunosuppressants for the management of the inflammatory process.[92] However, pediatric posterior scleritis has not been associated with systemic disorders; it is often the result of typical childhood infectious diseases such as pharyngoamygdalitis caused by *Streptococcus pyogenes*, diagnosed by increased antistreptolysin O titer.[93]

Ocular complications commonly occur with scleritis and include interstitial keratitis, marginal corneal ulcer with limbal involvement, uveitis, glaucoma with anterior scleritis, and exudative detachments or other posterior segment complications with posterior disease.[94,95]

Patients with episcleritis usually do not require an extensive laboratory evaluation, unless there is persistence despite topical corticosteroid therapy. The differential diagnosis for scleritis is broad and often challenging. Diagnostic tests are selected based on history and physical examination, but basically include chest radiograph, renal function tests, and screening antibodies such as antineutrophil cytoplasmic antibody, FTA-abs (Fluorescent Treponemal Antibody absorption test), rheumatic factor and anticitrullinated antibody, antinuclear antibodies, and Lyme antibody in patients with a history of tick exposure.

Episcleritis usually responds to topical immunomodulatory agents, such as corticosteroids, whereas scleritis typically requires systemic medications to achieve rapid remission and restore vision, such as oral nonsteroidal antiinflammatory drugs, oral corticosteroids, and in some cases immunosuppressive drugs. Immunosuppressive agents include cyclophosphamide, azathioprine, tacrolimus, and high-dose pulse methylprednisolone. Other biologic agents can be used, particularly for the treatment of necrotizing scleritis, which potentially represents vasculitis; rituximab is generally recommended for the treatment of systemic vasculitis.[96,97] Treatment with immunosuppressive patch graft or amniotic membrane graft has been implemented.[98] Necrotizing scleritis has been treated successfully with implantation of multiple trabecular microbypass stents.[99]

## DISTICHIASIS

Distichiasis involves a double row of eyelashes as a consequence of the rare acquired or hereditary aberrant differentiation of meibomian glands at the eyelids, and is seen in all ethnic backgrounds. These supernumerary eyelashes often lean back, abrading the cornea, resulting in corneal irritation, recurrent conjunctivitis, styes, epithelial defects, photophobia, ectropion, corneal ulceration, and opacification. It typically presents sporadically or in association with lymphedema-distichiasis (LD) syndrome. Hereditary distichiasis is rarely observed; the LD syndrome is a dominant autosomal genetic disorder caused by mutations in *FOXC2*, with characteristics including distichiasis at birth, strabismus, ptosis, lower extremity lymphedema around puberty, congenital cardiac defects, cleft palate, and renal anomalies.[100,101] Lubricants temporarily relieve symptoms, but definitive treatment is removal of the redundant eyelashes; lid splitting, cryotherapy, and direct surgical excision by different approaches have been described.[102,103]

## UVEITIS

Uveitis is a wide spectrum of inflammatory processes characterized by the presence of leukocytes in the anterior uveal track causing iritis or iridocyclitis, and/or in the posterior uvea inducing vitritis, choroiditis, retinitis, chorioretinitis, and retinochoroiditis. In general, it is classified as anterior, intermediate, or posterior uveitis, or, in the case of involvement of the whole uvea, panuveitis.

## Cause

### Infectious

The cause of infectious uveitis include those of keratitis, with viruses playing a prominent role. Herpes simplex and herpes zoster can cause keratouveitis, which manifests with cutaneous vesicles, corneal changes, increased intraocular pressure, and iris atrophy potentially leading to retinitis and acute retinal necrosis.[104] Cytomegalovirus uveitis is found almost exclusively in immune-compromised hosts and Asian people who are not immune compromised. Fuchs heterochromic iridocyclitis, a form of chronic unilateral primarily anterior uveitis, is now considered to be most often secondary to a rubella infection.[105] Toxoplasmosis is a common cause of uveitis in immune-competent patients, presumed to be a reactivation of a congenitally acquired infection. Serologic evidence for previous infection by toxoplasmosis is extremely common in the healthy US population.[106] Tuberculosis is rare in North America, but should be considered when uveitis worsens despite glucocorticoid therapy. Cat-scratch disease is increasingly recognized as a cause of unilateral uveitis, with macular and optic nerve edema especially characteristic. West Nile viral infection may cause asymptomatic chorioretinitis and retinal vasculitis. Ebola convalescent phase is also related to uveitis. Zika virus exposure in utero results in scarring of the uveal tract, which leads to chorioretinal atrophy, pigmentary mottling in the retina, and optic nerve disease.[107]

### Systemic inflammatory diseases

Systemic inflammatory diseases include immune-mediated diseases such as multiple sclerosis, spondyloarthritis, sarcoidosis, juvenile idiopathic arthritis, psoriatic arthritis, inflammatory bowel disease, Kawasaki, relapsing polychondritis, systemic lupus erythematosus, systemic vasculitis, Behçet, Vogt-Koyanagi-Harada syndrome, and Sjögren syndrome.[108]

### Post-operative uveitis

Hyper-inflammatory reaction state occurring after ophthalmic surgeries such as cataract or Lasik surgery, generating a toxic anterior segment syndrome leading to a decreased visual acuity, ocular pain, photophobia, corneal edema, and glaucoma (**Fig. 6**). Postoperative uveitis may be accompanied with diffuse lamellar keratitis.[109] Individual susceptibility is unpredictable, even with the most advanced surgical

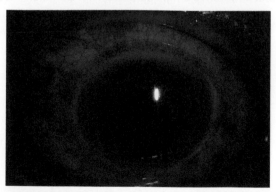

**Fig. 6.** Anterior uveitis as a result of quick tapering of topical steroids after cataract surgery. Steroid eye drops must be reinstated in these patients and a more prolonged tapering schedule planned. Note the limbal injection in uveitis as opposed to a more generalized injection of conjunctivitis.

techniques. Preoperative eye-drops of high-dose steroids are recommended for down regulating the activity of the inflammatory cascade, with nonsteroidal anti-inflammatory drugs (NSAIDs) working synergistically. Intraoperatively, a single intracameral steroid injection has also been implemented successfully in children with surgeries for traumatic cataract.[110] Steroids could lead to steroid-induced cataract formation, but the lack or improper dose-regimen and incorrect steroid-tapering after surgery could lead to a irreversible cicatricial damage such leukoma, endothelial depletion, synechiae, trabecular insufficiency, ciliary body fibrosis, and maculopathy.[111]

### Idiopathic

Uveitis without extraocular or infectious involvement is the most common diagnosis, accounting for about 30% of all patients.[112]

### Diagnosis and Management

A detailed medical history is the most important step to diagnose an associated systemic disease. Referral to an ophthalmologist for slit-lamp examination and a dilated fundus examination is required in patients suspected of uveal tract inflammation to establish the diagnosis. Ideally, therapy should be initiated promptly within 24 hours of the onset of acute infectious anterior uveitis. Antiviral therapy is especially important to limit retinal damage.

## ENDOPHTHALMITIS

Endophthalmitis is a serious paninflammatory ocular condition and a medical emergency for which prompt recognition and timely treatment can greatly affect the final outcome, preventing a severe visual loss or even eye enucleation. Hence, if the diagnosis is suspected, immediate referral is mandatory.[113]

### Classification and Etiology

Endophthalmitis, whether endogenous (5%–15%) or exogenous, involves the anterior and posterior segments and typically results from an infectious process (**Fig. 7**). Endogenous endophthalmitis mainly caused by fungi (50%, with *Candida* and *Aspergillus* spp being isolated most commonly) and bacteria (streptococcal species) usually begins as a focal right chorioretinal lesion that breaks into and seeds the vitreous because of the direct flow from the right carotid artery. Common infective foci include

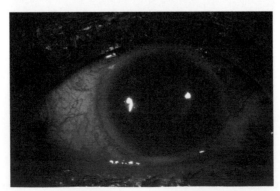

**Fig. 7.** Early postoperative endophthalmitis starting on day 3 after uneventful cataract surgery. Note the hazy view of the anterior chamber and a small level of purulent material in the anterior chamber (hypopyon).

endocarditis, and gastrointestinal and urinary tract infections. Risk factors include immunosuppression states, long-term indwelling catheters, recent abdominal surgery, and intravenous drug use.[114]

The exogenous form occurs by direct inoculation of the eye from outside via trauma; endophthalmitis following cataract extraction is the most studied presentation of exogenous endophthalmitis and has an increasing incidence.[115] In acute cases the presentation occurs within 6 weeks; *Propionibacterium acnes* is related to chronic or late-onset endophthalmitis after cataract surgery, causing a more indolent infection requiring surgical removal of the capsular bag and intraocular lens. Overall, 75% of post–cataract surgery endophthalmitis presents within 1 week of surgery.[116] Viral infections typically present differently, often leading to uveitis.

### Evaluation and Treatment

History should be focused on recent ocular trauma or ophthalmic intervention such as surgery or injection. Symptoms vary based on the cause but commonly include severe eye pain, decreased visual acuity, mild irritation, redness, and foreign body sensation for 24 to 72 hours following an ocular procedure. After intravitreal cultures are obtained, antimicrobial agents are delivered into the vitreous cavity, but in severe cases immediate vitrectomy is required. Empirically, intravitreal vancomycin and ceftazidime are indicated but insufficient and the role of systemic antibiotics as supplemental therapy remains elusive. Intravitreal dexamethasone is still controversial and its use should be determined by the ophthalmologist. In cases of fungal endophthalmitis, intravenous fluconazole has a better penetrance into the vitreous compared with other antifungals.[117,118]

### SUBCONJUNCTIVAL HEMORRHAGE

Frequently encountered at the emergency department, subconjunctival hemorrhage represents a collection of blood between the sclera and the conjunctiva and appears as a focal, flat, red region on the ocular surface where a conjunctival laceration and intraocular blood can leak creating a bullous, elevated subconjunctival hemorrhage with foreign body sensation. Common in the elderly with no history of trauma, the hemorrhage is noticed after waking from sleep, most often associated with systemic diseases and primary hypertension. In patients less than 40 years of age, ocular rather than systemic conditions, such as minor trauma and complications from removing a contact lens, are usually seen.[119] Other causes at any age include diabetes mellitus, coagulopathy, and increased venous pressure through Valsalva maneuver. Unilateral subconjunctival hemorrhage is usually related to warfarin, acetylsalicylic acid or nonsteroidal antiinflammatory drugs, and antihistamines. A bilateral subconjunctival hemorrhage has been associated with more serious disorders such as scurvy, hematological dyscrasias, and ocular or systemic malignancies.[120,121] Spontaneous, nontraumatic causes of subconjunctival hemorrhage are self-resolving over weeks without any ocular sequelae and require no treatment. In elderly patients, a complete history and assessment of blood pressure control and coagulation studies should be performed.

### CORNEAL GRAFT REJECTION

Keratoplasty is performed to restore vision, eliminate infection, or prevent perforation in the setting of corneal melting. Corneal transplant is the most common tissue transplant performed in the United States,[122] and, according the Eye Banking Statistical

Report (2013), 20,954 penetrating keratoplasty (for keratoconus, repeat corneal transplant, and postcataract corneal edema) and 24,987 endothelial keratoplasty (for Fuchs dystrophy, postcataract corneal edema, and other causes of endothelial dysfunction) procedures were performed.[123] Graft transparency, absence of rejection reactions, and good visual acuity have long been indicators of a successful corneal transplant. However, graft rejection, which occurs with grafts that have remained clear for at least 2 weeks postoperatively, has been observed as late as 20 years after transplant (**Fig. 8**). The highest incidence of rejection happens during the first year and endothelial failure is the most frequent indication for reintervention.[124] Despite the good overall outcome, the graft survival rate varies and some risk factors for graft rejection, such as age, preoperative diagnosis, corneal vascularization, donor and recipient factors, and type of procedure, have been identified. Ophthalmologic evaluation and prompt treatment are needed to maximize the likelihood of graft survival.[125] If clinical signs of rejection persist after 2 months of appropriate treatment, or endothelial decompensation occurs, graft failure is irreversible. It is important to instruct keratoplasty patients that rejection of the corneal transplant can occur at any time and it can come gradually or suddenly, with redness, decreased visual acuity, mild pain, irritation, and photophobia. Careful slit-lamp examination may show subepithelial infiltrates indicating an early rejection, or keratic precipitates localized at the endothelium, associated with graft failure.[126]

## ACUTE ANGLE-CLOSURE GLAUCOMA

Acute angle-closure glaucoma is the second leading cause of irreversible blindness worldwide according to the World Health Organization, and a sight-threatening emergency that manifests as a sudden increase of intraocular pressure (IOP) usually accompanied by extreme ocular pain, headache, blurred vision, semidilated and fixed pupil with no reaction to light, nausea, and vomiting.[127] The anatomic block of the aqueous humor outflow leads to optic nerve damage with accompanying retinal ganglion cell loss and glaucomatous optic neuropathy, ultimately resulting in blindness if the patient remains untreated.[128] Pupillary block, plateau iris syndrome, and other anatomic factors related to the iris, lens, and ciliary body configuration have been proposed as the mechanisms of the pathogenesis of primary angle-closure disease. Well-established ocular biometric factors have been associated, including a shorter axial length, shallower anterior chamber, thicker peripheral iris, and a thicker more anteriorly positioned lens. Angle-closure disease is classified into different

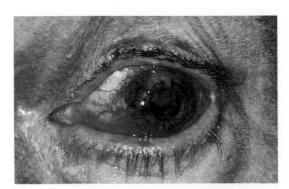

**Fig. 8.** Corneal graft rejection. Observe the ciliary injection, very typical of a rejection reaction.

subtypes, including primary angle-closure suspect, acute angle-closure, and primary angle-closure glaucoma.[129] Secondary causes include inflammation; intraocular hemorrhage; trauma; neovascularization; drug-induced glaucoma; and glaucoma associated with tumors, retinal detachment, and chemical burns. IOP measurements are not sensitive enough for screening; many normal individuals have an increased IOP consistently more than 21mmHg and never develop optic disc atrophy. Silent onset and asymptomatic progression of visual field narrowing are typical properties of the disease, with most visual field alterations detected when almost 20% to 40% of retinal ganglion cells are irreversibly damaged. Detailed mechanisms of the physiopathology remain unknown, with not all cases of retinal ganglion cell loss being related to an increased IOP. However, it still remains as the main risk factor for the development of glaucomatous optic neuropathy.[130] People at risk for closed-angle glaucoma should avoid over-the-counter decongestants, although these products are safe to use once the narrow angle has been treated with laser iridotomy. First-line treatment is drug-mediated IOP reduction followed by laser iridotomy or surgical therapy to restore normal aqueous drainage. Intravenous acetazolamide plus topical miotic analogs are indicated.[131]

## CHEMICAL BURNS

Chemical burns to the eye and adnexa are a serious problem in the United States, with great economic impact and loss of productivity, being responsible for approximately 90% of accidental industrial workplace exposures in which safety glasses are not an effective defense (**Fig. 9**).[132] Although most literature emphasizes an increased risk for ocular chemical burns among men aged between 18 and 64 years, the age-specific risk for chemical ocular injuries is highest among children 1 to 2 years old exposed to alkaline household cleaning chemicals.[133] Chemical injuries to the eye represent one of the true ophthalmic emergencies, in which time is also critical. Although almost any chemical can cause ocular irritation, serious damage generally results from either strongly alkaline compounds or strongly acidic compounds. Alkaline substances are lipophilic and can penetrate all cell membranes and therefore can be more clinically challenging with a significant potential for long-term morbidity. Acids cause protein denaturation, precipitation, and coagulation, creating a barrier and thus preventing its deeper penetration.[134] Chemical injuries present as burning pain, red eye, foreign body sensation, excessive tearing,

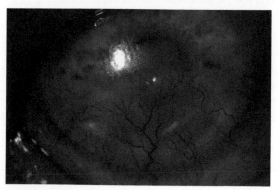

**Fig. 9.** Inferior neovascularization of the cornea caused by chemical burn. Limbal stem cell deficiency is a common potential result of these events.

and photophobia.[135] Immediate, prolonged irrigation followed by aggressive early management suppressing inflammation are essential in the acute phase, whereas close long-term monitoring is essential to promote ocular surface healing and provide the best opportunity for visual rehabilitation in the chronic phase.[136] A thorough eye examination should be performed with special attention to the clarity and integrity of the cornea, the degree of limbal ischemia, concomitant retained foreign bodies, conjunctival and lid trauma, and IOP. The degree of limbal ischemia is the most significant prognostic indicator for future corneal healing because the limbal stem cells are responsible for repopulating the corneal epithelium. The elicited inflammatory conjunctival response can be exuberant and must be aggressively treated for appropriate healing. In the treatment of corneal burns, amniotic membrane transplant (AMT) is used in the acute or chronic phase to reconstruct and protect the conjunctival surface, reduce limbal stromal inflammation, and provide pain control. AMT reduces perilimbal inflammation, creating a healthy corneal epithelium, reducing corneal neovascularization, and enhancing the success of subsequent limbal stem cell transplants and/or penetrating keratoplasty.[137,138]

## DRUG-INDUCED KERATOCONJUNCTIVAL DISORDERS

Ocular structures may show the earliest sensitivities to drug toxicity. Even at appropriate dosing and while being therapeutically beneficial, various drugs have shown ocular adverse effects, generating superficial corneal changes of little clinical significance or more profound alterations threatening eyesight; knowledge about the potential of drugs for ocular adverse effects is essential.

Hyperemia with or without corneal involvement is possible with all ophthalmic medications containing preservatives. Sulfa-based drugs cause swelling of the ciliary body and risk for development of angle-closure glaucoma. Also, beta2-adrenergic agonists and anticholinergic agents inducing pupillary dilation may precipitate acute angle-closure glaucoma in susceptible patients. Glucocorticoids are a well-known cause of increased IOP.[139] Anticholinergics are also associated with dry eye, potentially leading to a plethora of corneal inflammatory processes related to conjunctival injection. Antihistamines, antidepressants, and antipsychotics are related to dry eye as well. Bisphosphonates and tumor necrosis factor alpha inhibitors are known to cause anterior uveitis. In many cases withdrawal of the drug resolves the eye condition, but if treatment needs to be continued the use of palliative therapies such preservative-free lubricants may be indicated in minor irritating adverse effects. In those drugs affecting IOP, appropriate monitoring and warning to the patients should be addressed.[140]

## REFERENCES

1. Behrens A, Doyle JJ, Stern L, et al. Dysfunctional tear syndrome study group. Dysfunctional tear syndrome: a Delphi approach to treatment recommendations. Cornea 2006;25(8):900–7.
2. Pflugfelder SC. Prevalence, burden, and pharmacoeconomics of dry eye disease. Am J Manag Care 2008;14(3):102–6.
3. Haji-Ali-Nili N, Khoshzaban F, Karimi M. Lifestyle determinants on prevention and improvement of dry eye disease from the perspective of Iranian traditional medicine. Iran J Med Sci 2016;41(3):S39.
4. Olaniyan SI, Fasina O, Bekibele CO, et al. Dry eye disease in an adult population in south-west Nigeria. Cont Lens Anterior Eye 2016;39:359–64.

5. Maychuk DY, Anisimova S, Kapkova S, et al. Prevalence and severity of dry eye in candidates for laser in situ keratomileusis for myopia in Russia. J Cataract Refract Surg 2016;42:427–34.

6. Tan LL, Morgan P, Cai ZQ, et al. Prevalence of and risk factors for symptomatic dry eye disease in Singapore. Clin Exp Optom 2015;98:45–53.

7. Paulsen AJ, Cruickshanks KJ, Fischer ME, et al. Dry eye in the beaver dam offspring study: prevalence, risk factors, and health-related quality of life. Am J Ophthalmol 2014;157:799–806.

8. Sabatino F, Di Zazzo A, De Simone L, et al. The intriguing role of neuropeptides at the ocular surface. Ocul Surf 2016;15(1):2–14.

9. Dietrich J, Massie I, Roth M, et al. Development of causative treatment strategies for lacrimal gland insufficiency by tissue engineering and cell therapy, 2016 engineering and cell therapy. Part 1: regeneration of lacrimal gland tissue: can we stimulate lacrimal gland renewal in vivo? Curr Eye Res 2016;41(9):1131–42.

10. Li DQ, Chen Z, Song XJ, et al. Stimulation of matrix metalloproteinases by hyperosmolarity via a JNK pathway in human corneal epithelial cells. Invest Ophthalmol Vis Sci 2004;45(12):4302–11.

11. Bron AJ, Tiffany JM, Gouveia SM, et al. Functional aspects of the tear film lipid layer. Exp Eye Res 2004;78(3):347–60.

12. Rosenthal P, Borsook D. Ocular neuropathic pain. Br J Ophthalmol 2016;100(1):128–34.

13. Begley CG, Caffery B, Chalmers RL, et al, Dry Eye Investigation Study Group. Use of the dry eye questionnaire to measure symptoms of ocular irritation in patients with aqueous tear deficient dry eye. Cornea 2002;21(7):664–70.

14. Zhao H, Chen JY, Wang YQ, et al. In vivo confocal microscopy evaluation of meibomian gland dysfunction in dry eye patients with different symptoms. Chin Med J 2016;129(21):2617–22.

15. Sullivan BD, Whitmer D, Nichols KK, et al. An objective approach to dry eye disease severity. Invest Ophthalmol Vis Sci 2010;51(12):6125–30.

16. Lemp MA, Bron AJ, Baudouin C, et al. Tear osmolarity in the diagnosis and management of dry eye disease. Am J Ophthalmol 2011;151(5):792.

17. Aluru SV, Shweta A, Bhaskar S, et al. Tear fluid protein changes in dry eye syndrome associated with rheumatoid arthritis: a proteomic approach. Ocul Surf 2016;15(1):112–29.

18. Peral A, Loma P, Yerxa B, et al. Topical application of nucleotides increase lysozyme levels in tears. Clin Ophthalmol 2008;2(2):261–7.

19. van Bijsterveld OP. Standardization of the lysozyme test for a commercially available medium. Its use for the diagnosis of the sicca syndrome. Arch Ophthalmol 1974;91(6):432–4.

20. Tauber J, Karpecki P, Latkany R, et al, OPUS-2 Investigators. Lifitegrast ophthalmic solution 5.0% versus placebo for treatment of dry eye disease: results of the randomized phase III OPUS-2 study. Ophthalmology 2015;122(12):2423–31.

21. Al-Saedi Z, Zimmerman A, Bachu RD, et al. Dry eye disease: present challenges in the management and future trends. Curr Pharm Des 2016;22(28):4470–90.

22. Stonecipher KG, Torkildsen GL, Ousler GW III, et al. The IMPACT study: a prospective evaluation of the effects of cyclosporine ophthalmic emulsion 0.05% on ocular surface staining and visual performance in patients with dry eye. Clin Ophthalmol 2016;10:887–95.

23. Smith AF, Waycaster C. Estimate of the direct and indirect annual cost of bacterial conjunctivitis in the United States. BMC Ophthalmol 2009;9:13.

24. Zegans ME, Sanchez PA, Likosky DS, et al. Clinical features, outcomes, and costs of a conjunctivitis outbreak caused by the ST448 strain of *Streptococcus pneumoniae*. Cornea 2009;28:503–9.

25. American Academy of Ophthalmology. Cornea/external disease panel. Preferred practice pattern guidelines: conjunctivitis-limited revision. San Francisco (CA): American Academy of Ophthalmology; 2011.

26. Wan WL, Farkas GC, May WN, et al. The clinical characteristics and course of adult gonococcal conjunctivitis. Am J Ophthalmol 1986;102(5):575.

27. Dey AC, Hossain MI, Dey SK, et al. Neonatal conjunctivitis leading to neonatal sepsis–a case report. Mymensingh Med J 2016;25(1):161–2.

28. Hutnik C, Mohammad-Shahi MH. Bacterial conjunctivitis. Clin Ophthalmol 2010; 4:1451–7.

29. Ullman S, Roussel TJ, Culbertson WW, et al. *Neisseria gonorrhoeae* keratoconjunctivitis. Ophthalmology 1987;94(5):525.

30. O'Brien TP, Jeng BH, McDonald M, et al. Acute conjunctivitis: truth and misconceptions. Curr Med Res Opin 2009;25(8):1953–61.

31. Roba LA, Kowalski RP, Gordon AT, et al. Adenoviral ocular isolates demonstrate serotype-dependent differences in in vitro infectivity titers and clinical course. Cornea 1995;14(4):388.

32. Jernigan JA, Lowry BS, Hayden FG, et al. Adenovirus type 8 epidemic keratoconjunctivitis in an eye clinic: risk factors and control. J Infect Dis 1993;167(6):1307.

33. Puri LR, Shrestha GB, Shah DN, et al. Ocular manifestations in herpes zoster ophthalmicus. Nepal J Ophthalmol 2011;3(2):165–71.

34. Falzon K, Scotcher S, Parulekar M. Primary epibulbar molluscum contagiosum in an immunocompetent child. J Pediatr 2016;167(4):936.

35. Klotz SA, Penn CC, Negvesky GJ, et al. Fungal and parasitic infections of the eye. Clin Microbiol Rev 2000;13(4):662–85.

36. Shaker M, Salcone E. An update on ocular allergy. Curr Opin Allergy Clin Immunol 2016;16(5):505–10.

37. Bielory L, Syed BA. Pharmacoeconomics of anterior ocular inflammatory disease. Curr Opin Allergy Clin Immunol 2013;13:537–42.

38. Gregory DG. The ophthalmologic management of acute Stevens-Johnson syndrome. Ocul Surf 2008;6(2):87–95.

39. Miller NR. Diagnosis and management of dural carotid-cavernous sinus fistulas. Neurosurg Focus 2007;23(5):13.

40. Shields CL, Alset AE, Boal NS, et al. Conjunctival tumors in 5002 cases. Comparative analysis of benign versus malignant counterparts. The 2016 James D. Allen Lecture. Am J Ophthalmol 2016. http://dx.doi.org/10.1016/j.ajo.2016.09.034.

41. Azari AA, Barney NP. Conjunctivitis: a systematic review of diagnosis and treatment. JAMA 2013;310(16):1721–9.

42. Høvding G. Acute bacterial conjunctivitis. Acta Ophthalmol 2008;86(1):5–17.

43. Sheikh A, Hurwitz B, van Schayck CP, et al. Antibiotics versus placebo for acute bacterial conjunctivitis. Cochrane Database Syst Rev 2012;(9):CD001211.

44. Szaflik J, Szaflik JP, Kaminska A, Levofloxacin Bacterial Conjunctivitis Dosage Study Group. Clinical and microbiological efficacy of levofloxacin administered three times a day for the treatment of bacterial conjunctivitis. Eur J Ophthalmol 2009;19(1):1–9.

45. Shanmuganathan VA, Armstrong M, Buller A, et al. External ocular infections due to methicillin-resistant *Staphylococcus aureus* (MRSA). Eye 2005;19(3):284–91.

46. Freidlin J, Acharya N, Lietman TM, et al. Spectrum of eye disease caused by methicillin-resistant *Staphylococcus aureus*. Am J Ophthalmol 2007;144(2): 313–5.

47. Tarabishy AB, Jeng BH. Bacterial conjunctivitis: a review for internists. Cleve Clin J Med 2008;75(7):507–12.

48. Shaker M, Salcone E. An update on ocular allergy. Curr Opin Allergy Clin Immunol 2016;16(5):505–10.

49. Keay L, Edwards K, Naduvilath T, et al. Microbial keratitis predisposing factors and morbidity. Ophthalmology 2006;113(1):109–16.

50. Liesegang TJ. Contact lens-related microbial keratitis: part I: epidemiology. Cornea 1997;16(2):125–31.

51. Zhang W, Yang H, Jiang L, et al. Use of potassium hydroxide, Giemsa and cal-cofluor white staining techniques in the microscopic evaluation of corneal scrapings for diagnosis of fungal keratitis. J Int Med Res 2010;38:1961–7.

52. Karsten E, Watson SL, Foster LJR. Diversity of microbial species implicated in keratitis: a review. Open Ophthalmol J 2012;6:110–24.

53. Tabibian D, Mazzotta C, Hafezi F. PACK-CXL: corneal cross-linking in infectious keratitis. Eye Vis (Lond) 2016;3:11.

54. Khandelwal SS, Randleman JB. Current and future applications of corneal cross-linking. Curr Opin Ophthalmol 2015;26(3):206–13.

55. Abbouda A, Abicca I, Alió JL. Current and future applications of photoactivated chromophore for keratitis-corneal collagen cross-linking (PACK-CXL): an overview of the different treatments proposed. Semin Ophthalmol 2016. [Epub ahead of print].

56. Price MO, Price FW Jr. Corneal cross-linking in the treatment of corneal ulcers. Curr Opin Ophthalmol 2016;27(3):250–5.

57. Thebpatiphat N, Hammersmith KM, Rocha FN, et al. *Acanthamoeba* keratitis: a parasite on the rise. Cornea 2007;26(6):701–6.

58. Carvalho FR, Foronda AS, Mannis MJ, et al. Twenty years of *Acanthamoeba* keratitis. Cornea 2009;28:516–9.

59. Khairnar K, Tamber GS, Ralevski F, et al. Comparison of molecular diagnostic methods for the detection of *Acanthamoeba* spp. from clinical specimens submitted for keratitis. Diagn Microbiol Infect Dis 2011;70:499–506.

60. Lorenzo-Morales J, Martín-Navarro CM, López-Arencibia A, et al. *Acanthamoeba* keratitis: an emerging disease gathering importance worldwide? Trends Parasitol 2013;29:181–7.

61. Dart JK, Saw VP, Kilvington S. *Acanthamoeba* keratitis: diagnosis and treatment. Update 2009. Am J Ophthalmol 2009;148:487–99.

62. Kwok PW, Kam KW, Jhanji V, et al. Painless *Acanthamoeba* keratitis with normal vision. Optom Vis Sci 2016. [Epub ahead of print].

63. Zbiba W, Baba A, Bouayed E, et al. A 5-year retrospective review of fungal keratitis in the region of Cap Bon. J Fr Ophtalmol 2016;39(10):843–8.

64. Wei DW, Pagnoux C, Chan CC. Peripheral ulcerative keratitis secondary to chronic hepatitis B infection. Cornea 2016. [Epub ahead of print].

65. Jeng BH. Abrasions, planned defects, and persistent epithelial defects in corneal epithelial wound healing. JAMA Ophthalmol 2016;134(10):1176–7.

66. Lim CH, Turner A, Lim BX. Patching for corneal abrasion. Cochrane Database Syst Rev 2016;(7):CD004764.

67. Wipperman JL, Dorsch JN. Evaluation and management of corneal abrasions. Am Fam Physician 2013;87(2):114–20.

68. McGwin G Jr, Owsley C. Incidence of emergency department treated eye injury in the United States. Arch Ophthalmol 2005;123:662–6.
69. Nash EA, Margo CE. Patterns of emergency department visits for disorders of the eye and ocular adnexa. Arch Ophthalmol 1998;116:1222–6.
70. Arora T, Arora S, Sinha R. Management of intrastromal glass foreign body based on anterior segment optical coherence tomography and Pentacam analysis. Int Ophthalmol 2015;35:1.
71. Celebi AR, Kilavuzoglu AE, Altiparmak UE, et al. The role of anterior segment optical coherence tomography in the management of an intra-corneal foreign body. Springerplus 2016;5(1):1559.
72. Zantos SG. Cystic formation in the corneal epithelium during extended wear of contact lenses. Int Contact Lens Clin 1983;10:128.
73. Catania LJ. Management of corneal abrasions in an extended-wear patient population. Optom Clin 1991;1:123.
74. Sweeney DF. Have silicone hydrogel lenses eliminated hypoxia? Eye Contact Lens 2013;39(1):53–60.
75. Lemp MA, Nichols KK. Blepharitis in the United States 2009: a survey-based perspective on prevalence and treatment. Ocul Surf 2009;7(2):S1–14.
76. Hammersmith KM, Cohen EJ, Blake TD, et al. Blepharokeratoconjunctivitis in children. Arch Ophthalmol 2005;123(12):1667–70.
77. Viswalingam M, Rauz S, Morlet N, et al. Blepharokeratoconjunctivitis in children: diagnosis and treatment. Br J Ophthalmol 2005;89(4):400–3.
78. Hamada S, Nischal K, Evans J. The activity and damage of blepharokeratoconjunctivitis in children. J AAPOS 2013;17(1):e16.
79. Jackson WB. Blepharitis: current strategies for diagnosis and management. Can J Ophthalmol 2008;43(2):170–9.
80. O'Gallagher M, Banteka M, Bunce C, et al. Systemic treatment for blepharokeratoconjunctivitis in children. Cochrane Database Syst Rev 2016;(5):CD011750.
81. Wakefield D, Di Girolamo N, Thurau S, et al. Scleritis: immunopathogenesis and molecular basis for therapy. Prog Retin Eye Res 2013;35:44–62.
82. Daniel Diaz J, Sobol EK, Gritz DC. Treatment and management of scleral disorders. Surv Ophthalmol 2016;61(6):702–17.
83. Abbey AM, Shah NV, Forster RK, et al. Infectious pseudomonas and *Bipolaris* scleritis following history of pterygium surgery. Indian J Ophthalmol 2016; 64(9):674–6.
84. Diaz-Valle D, Gomez-Gomez A, Pascual-Martin A. Bilateral scleritis and retinal vasculitis in microscopic polyangiitis. Ophthalmology 2016;123(12):2553.
85. Akpek EK, Uy HS, Christen W, et al. Severity of episcleritis and systemic disease association. Ophthalmology 1999;106(4):729–31.
86. McGavin DDM, Williamson J, Forrester JV, et al. Episcleritis and scleritis. A study of their clinical manifestation and association with rheumatoid arthritis. Br J Ophthalmol 1976;60:192–226.
87. Tuft SJ, Watson PG. Progression of scleral disease. Ophthalmology 1991;98(4): 467–71.
88. Honik G, Wong IG, Gritz DC. Incidence and prevalence of episcleritis and scleritis in northern California. Cornea 2013;32(12):1562–6.
89. Homayounfar G, Nardone N, Borkar DS, et al. Incidence of scleritis and episcleritis results from the pacific ocular inflammation study. Am J Ophthalmol 2013; 156(4):752–8.
90. Watson PG, Hayreh SS. Scleritis and episcleritis. Br J Ophthalmol 1976;60(3): 163–91.

91. Al Barqi M, Behrens A, Alfawaz AM. Clinical features and visual outcomes of scleritis patients presented to tertiary care eye centers in Saudi Arabia. Int J Ophthalmol 2015;8(6):1215–9.
92. Murray PI, Rauz S. The eye and inflammatory rheumatic diseases: the eye and rheumatoid arthritis, ankylosing spondylitis, psoriatic arthritis. Best Pract Res Clin Rheumatol 2016;30(5):802–25.
93. Hilkert SM, Koreishi AF, Pyatetsky D. Poststreptococcal syndrome presenting as posterior scleritis in a child. J AAPOS 2016. http://dx.doi.org/10.1016/j.jaapos.2016.09.019.
94. McCluskey PJ, Watson PG, Lightman S, et al. Posterior scleritis. Clinical features, systemic associations, and outcome in a large series of patients. Ophthalmology 1999;106:2380–6.
95. Sainz de la Maza M, Jabbur NS, Foster CS. Severity of scleritis and episcleritis. Ophthalmology 1994;101:389–96.
96. Stone JH, Merkel PA, Spiera R, et al, RAVE-ITN Research Group. Rituximab versus cyclophosphamide for ANCA-associated vasculitis. N Engl J Med 2010;363(3):221–32.
97. Fidelix TS, Vieira LA, Trevisani VF. Management of necrotizing scleritis after pterygium surgery with rituximab. Arq Bras Oftalmol 2016;79(5):339–41.
98. Beardsley RM, Suhler EB, Rosenbaum JT, et al. Pharmacotherapy of scleritis: current paradigms and future directions. Expert Opin Pharmacother 2013;14(4):411–24.
99. Sandhu S, Heckler L, Mah D, et al. Trabecular micro-bypass stent use in necrotizing scleritis. J Glaucoma 2016. [Epub ahead of print].
100. Vreeburg M, Heitink MV, Damstra RJ, et al. Lymphedema-distichiasis syndrome: a distinct type of primary lymphedema caused by mutations in the FOXC2 gene. Int J Dermatol 2008;47(1):52–5.
101. Zhang L, He J, Han B, et al. Novel FOXC2 mutation in hereditary distichiasis impairs DNA-binding activity and transcriptional activation. Int J Biol Sci 2016;12(9):1114–20.
102. Moosavi AH, Mollan SP, Berry-Brincat A, et al. Simple surgery for severe trichiasis. Ophthal Plast Reconstr Surg 2007;23(4):296–7.
103. Aziz S, Bhatt PR, Lavy T, et al. A simple correction for congenital tarsal kink associated with distichiasis. J AAPOS 2006;10(3):281–2.
104. Schwartzman S. Advancements in the management of uveitis. Best Pract Res Clin Rheumatol 2016;30(2):304–15.
105. Quentin CD, Reiber H. Fuchs heterochromic cyclitis: rubella virus antibodies and genome in aqueous humor. Am J Ophthalmol 2004;138(1):46.
106. Weiss MJ, Velazquez N, Hofeldt AJ. Serologic tests in the diagnosis of presumed toxoplasmic retinochoroiditis. Am J Ophthalmol 1990;109(4):407.
107. Furtado JM, Espósito DL, Klein TM, et al. Uveitis associated with Zika virus infection. N Engl J Med 2016;375(4):394.
108. Amin RM, Goweida M, Bedda A, et al. Clinical patterns and causes of intraocular inflammation in a uveitis patient cohort from Egypt. Ocul Immunol Inflamm 2016;1–9 [Epub ahead of print].
109. Mora P Gonzales S, Ghirardini S, Rubino P, et al. Perioperative prophylaxis to prevent recurrence following cataract surgery in uveitic patients: a two-centre, prospective, randomized trial. Acta Ophthalmol 2016;94(6):e390–4.
110. Mohamed TA, Soliman W, Fathalla AM. Effect of intracameral triamcinolone acetonide on postoperative intraocular inflammation in pediatric traumatic cataract. Eur J Ophthalmol 2016;26(2):114–7.

111. American Acedemy of Ophthalmology. Savvy steroid use. EyeNet Magazine February 2013. Available at: https://www.aao.org/eyenet/article/savvy-steroid-use.
112. Rosenbaum JT. Nibbling away at the diagnosis of idiopathic uveitis. JAMA Ophthalmol 2015;133(2):146–7.
113. Schubert HD, Bobrow JC. Basic clinical science course, section 11/12, lens and cataract/retina and vitreous. 2014–2015. Chicago, IL: American Academy of Ophthalmology; 2014.
114. Vaziri K, Schwartz SG, Kishor K, et al. Endophthalmitis: state of the art. Clin Ophthalmol 2015;9:95–108.
115. Gower E, Keay L, Stare D, et al. Characteristics of endophthalmitis after cataract surgery in the United States Medicare population. Ophthalmology 2015;122(8):1625–32.
116. Meyer JJ, Polkinghorne PJ, McGhee CN. Cataract surgery practices and endophthalmitis prophylaxis by New Zealand ophthalmologists. Clin Exp Ophthalmol 2016;44(7):643–5.
117. Results of the Endophthalmitis Vitrectomy Study. A randomized trial of immediate vitrectomy and of intravenous antibiotics for the treatment of postoperative bacterial endophthalmitis. Endophthalmitis Vitrectomy Study Group. Arch Ophthalmol 1995;113(12):149.
118. Cunningham C, Raiji V. Endophthalmitis. Dis Mon 2016. http://dx.doi.org/10.1016/j.disamonth.2016.09.005.
119. Mimura T, Usui T, Yamagami S, et al. Recent causes of subconjunctival hemorrhage. Ophthalmologica 2010;224(3):133.
120. Taamallah-Malek I, Chebbi A, Bouladi M, et al. Massive bilateral subconjunctival hemorrhage revealing acute lymphoblastic leukemia. J Fr Ophtalmol 2013;36:45–8.
121. Huynh N, Wang J, Vavvas D. Dilated fundus exam and associated findings in spontaneous subconjunctival haemorrhage. Acta Ophthalmol 2016. http://dx.doi.org/10.1111/aos.13309.
122. Bentley TS. U.S. organ and tissue transplant cost estimates and discussion. Milliman research report. Brookfield (WI): Milliman; 2014.
123. Woodford VM. 2013 eye banking statistical report. Eye Bank Association of America. Washington, DC: Eye Bank Association of America; 2014.
124. Tan DT, Dart JK, Holland EJ, et al. Corneal transplantation. Lancet 2012;379(9827):1749–61.
125. Panda A, Vanathi M, Kumar A, et al. Corneal graft rejection. Surv Ophthalmol 2007;52(4):375–96.
126. Ling JD, Mehta V, Fathy C, et al. Racial disparities in corneal transplantation rates, complications, and outcomes. Semin Ophthalmol 2016;31(4):337–44.
127. Tham YC, Li X, Wong TY, et al. Global prevalence of glaucoma and projections of glaucoma burden through 2040: a systematic review and meta-analysis. Ophthalmology 2014;121(11):2081–90.
128. Akal A, Kucuk A, Yalcin F, et al. Do we really need to panic in all acute vision loss in ICU? Acute angle-closure glaucoma. J Pakistan Med Assoc 2014;64(8):960–2.
129. Moghimi S, Chen R, Hamzeh N, et al. Qualitative evaluation of anterior segment in angle closure disease using anterior segment optical coherence tomography. J Curr Ophthalmol 2016;28(4):170–5.
130. Casson RJ, Chidlow G, Wood JP, et al. Definition of glaucoma: clinical and experimental concepts. Clin Exp Ophthalmol 2012;40(4):341–9.

131. Lorenz K, Beck S, Keilani MM, et al. Course of serum autoantibodies in patients after acute angle closure glaucoma attack. Clin Exp Ophthalmol 2016. http://dx.doi.org/10.1111/ceo.12864.
132. Morgan SJ. Chemical burns of the eye: causes and management. Br J Ophthalmol 1987;71(11):854–7.
133. Haring R, Sheffield ID, Channa R, et al. Epidemiologic trends of chemical ocular burns in the United States. JAMA Ophthalmol 2016;134(10):1119–24.
134. Bunker DJL, George RJ, Kleinschmidt A, et al. Alkali-related ocular burns: a case series and review. J Burn Care Res 2014;35(3):261–8.
135. Eslani M, Baradaran-Rafii A, Movahedan A, et al. The ocular surface chemical burns. J Ophthalmol 2014;2014:196827.
136. Cabalag MS, Wasiak J, Syed Q, et al. Early and late complications of ocular burn injuries. J Plast Reconstr Aesthet Surg 2015;68(3):356–61.
137. Meller D, Pires RT, Mack RJ, et al. Amniotic membrane transplantation for acute chemical or thermal burns. Ophthalmology 2000;107(5):980–9.
138. Tseng SC, Prabhasawat P, Barton K, et al. Amniotic membrane transplantation with or without limbal allografts for corneal surface reconstruction in patients with limbal stem cell deficiency. Arch Ophthalmol 1998;116(4):431–41.
139. Li J, Tripathi RC, Tripathi BJ. Drug-induced ocular disorders. Drug Saf 2008;31(2):127–41.
140. Tripathi RC, Tripathi BJ, Haggerty C. Drug-induced glaucomas: mechanism and management. Drug Saf 2003;26:749–67.

# Otolaryngologic Emergencies in the Primary Care Setting

Kendall K. Tasche, MD, Kristi E. Chang, MD*

## KEYWORDS

- Otolaryngologic emergencies • Sinusitis • Foreign bodies • Trauma

## KEY POINTS

- The vast majority of otolaryngology-related complaints are straightforward and easily recognized and treated. However, given the proximity of the ears, nose, and throat to numerous vital structures in the head and neck, the potential for serious consequences exists if disease processes go unrecognized and untreated.
- This article serves to familiarize the primary care provider with the clinical presentation of various complications associated with common otolaryngologic complaints.
- Clinicians who care for patients presenting with otolaryngologic complaints should keep these entities in mind and attempt to rule out any serious complication.
- Patients with suspected complications should be promptly referred to an emergency department at a facility with subspecialist support.
- Many of these complications are thankfully rare, and continued diligence and familiarization with these disease processes will serve to maintain them as such.

## INTRODUCTION

It is not uncommon for the primary care provider to encounter otolaryngologic conditions on a daily basis. Most practitioners are familiar with the vast majority of these conditions, and they can be readily treated in an outpatient setting without requiring subspecialist involvement. Many serious complications or sequelae of untreated disease, such as mastoiditis following AOM, are significantly less common than in past years as a result of improvement in antimicrobial therapies and general medical treatment. As an unintended consequence, however, clinicians are less familiar with and may be less adept at recognizing such complications. These now rare complications, in conjunction with less common although still serious conditions, can present with subtle clinical findings, which may result in misdiagnosis and delays in appropriate referral and subsequent treatment. In addition, their proximity to numerous vital

University of Iowa, Iowa City, IA, USA
* Corresponding author.
*E-mail address:* kristi-chang@uiowa.edu

Med Clin N Am 101 (2017) 641–656
http://dx.doi.org/10.1016/j.mcna.2016.12.009
medical.theclinics.com

neurologic, vascular, and airway structures renders otolaryngologic disease processes and their complications prone to rapid and potentially devastating consequences if not recognized early.

The purpose of this article is to familiarize the primary care practitioner with the clinical presentation of several potentially serious otolaryngologic disease processes. Although most patients with obvious or severe illness generally present to the emergency department, some patients may initially present to primary care practitioners in the outpatient setting. Others with less severe or obvious illness may be less likely to present to an emergency setting; however, the subtlety of the disease and potential for missed diagnoses as well as the potential to develop into life-threatening conditions supports the need for primary care providers to have some level of familiarity with these disease processes.

## COMPLICATIONS OF EAR INFECTIONS

Acute otitis media (AOM) and otitis externa are both very common infections that virtually all primary care providers have encountered. It has been estimated that up to 85% of children have had at least one episode of AOM by the age of 3, and AOM is the most common condition for which children are prescribed antibiotics in the United States.[1,2] Despite the widespread use of antibiotics, otitis media can still lead to a variety of complications with significant morbidity. Infectious complications include mastoiditis and intracranial infection, and noninfectious complications include tympanic membrane perforation, ossicular erosion, and tympanosclerosis leading to hearing loss. Complications may also be stratified by location: intracranial or extracranial. Although less widespread and typically uncomplicated, otitis externa is still a relatively common condition that can have serious consequences in certain patient populations.

### Mastoiditis and Petrous Apicitis

AOM that does not resolve can result in the development of acute mastoiditis. The incidence of mastoiditis has generally decreased with increased availability and use of antibiotics in addition to pneumococcal vaccination in the twentieth century, although some investigators have reported an increase in incidence in recent years.[3,4] Generally, mastoiditis is defined by findings of AOM on otoscopic examination in conjunction with inflammatory changes over the mastoid process (eg, swelling, erythema, tenderness, and auricular protrusion), or these inflammatory changes as well as radiologic findings supportive of mastoiditis.

A subtype of mastoiditis is coalescent mastoiditis, which may occur if an AOM and mastoiditis persist unabated, generally for 2 or more weeks. The term "coalescent" refers to the appearance of the mastoid on computed tomography (CT) imaging, in which the mastoid is filled with fluid and with loss of the bony septations between individual air cells. Patients with coalescent mastoiditis present with similar symptoms as acute mastoiditis and may have a preceding history of AOM, although in general they appear more toxic and systemically ill. Diagnosis requires CT imaging of the bone, and if there is any concern for intracranial abnormality, a contrasted MRI should be obtained as well. Patients with coalescent mastoiditis require surgical management, including cortical mastoidectomy, tympanostomy tube placement, and drainage of any associated abscess.

Another infection of the temporal bone that occurs rarely is petrous apicitis, which occurs with spread of infection to the petrous apex and is analogous to mastoiditis. The petrous apex may be partially pneumatized in some individuals, which increases the likelihood of an infection spreading there. Classically, patients present with a triad of symptoms, including retro-orbital pain, cranial nerve VI palsy, and otorrhea, that was first described by Gradenigo in 1904 and is termed Gradenigo's syndrome, although patients do not always present with all 3 of these symptoms.[3] Treatment requires intravenous antibiotics with or without surgical drainage. Because of the location of the petrous apex and necessity to work around the labyrinth and internal carotid artery, surgical management can be challenging.

### Intracranial Complications

Given the proximity of the inner and middle ear spaces to the intracranial cavity, several intracranial complications may occur as a result of infection in these spaces. Similar to mastoiditis, the availability and use of antibiotics and vaccination led to a dramatic decline in the incidence of intracranial complications; however, they are still reported. The incidence of otogenic intracranial complications is estimated to be up to 2%, and most patients are in the first 2 decades of life, with mortalities as high as 16%.[5,6] The most common complication is meningitis followed by intraparenchymal abscess (most commonly in the temporal lobe or cerebellum), with other intracranial complications, including subdural empyema and epidural abscess, occurring less frequently.[7]

Common presenting symptoms include fever, headache, purulent otorrhea, hearing loss, vomiting, and lethargy as well as symptoms attributable to the specific intracranial process (eg, nuchal rigidity and photophobia with meningitis, focal neurologic deficits with intraparenchymal abscess). In general, subdural empyema and meningitis present more acutely and have a more fulminant course, whereas epidural and intraparenchymal abscesses may be more indolent. The most commonly reported cultured pathogens include *Proteus mirabilis*, in addition to gram-negative and streptococcal species, although frequently no organisms are able to be cultured, likely owing to prior antibiotic administration.[5,6] Diagnosis of intracranial complications requires imaging with CT or MRI with contrast. Lumbar puncture should be performed if there is concern for meningitis. Treatment generally requires at least 6 weeks of broad-spectrum intravenous antibiotics with or without surgical drainage of the abscess depending on the type of complication or complications present, and with mastoidectomy required for all patients.

### Lateral Sinus Thrombosis

Lateral sinus thrombosis generally forms as an extension of a perisinus infection that occurs following mastoid bone erosion from cholesteatoma or coalescence, or septic thrombophlebitis disseminated through emissary veins. Damage to the tunica intima of the sinus leads to an inflammatory process and formation of fibrin and aggregation of platelets and other blood components, leading to mural thrombosis. Untreated, the thrombus may propagate in both retrograde (ie, toward the sagittal sinus) and anterograde (ie, toward the internal jugular vein) fashion. Lateral sinus thrombosis may occur as a complication of acute infection as well as chronic otitis media and cholesteatoma. As the sinus is an extension of cerebellar dura mater, infection may spread and result in meningitis, epidural abscess, subdural empyema, and cerebritis or cerebellar abscess as well.[3]

Classically, patients will present with "picket-fence" fevers, headache (often with acute worsening), neck pain, and evidence of increased intracranial pressure in conjunction with signs and symptoms of mastoiditis/ear infection, although these signs are not always present.[7] Contrast-enhanced CT or MRI is required for definitive diagnosis. All patients require urgent mastoidectomy with drainage of perisinus infection to prevent further intravascular thrombosis and intracranial complications.

Management of the actual thrombus may involve opening of the sinus and evacuation of the infected clot, and less commonly, ligation of the jugular vein in the neck and/or anticoagulation.[3]

## Malignant Otitis Externa

Necrotizing otitis externa is classically known as malignant otitis externa (MOE) and is characterized by an aggressive infection of the external auditory canal (EAC) with involvement of the mastoid and skull base. Spread of this disease occurs through the fissures of Santorini, a set of channels through the cartilaginous EAC, as well as through the tympanomastoid suture to gain access to the lateral skull base, jugular foramen, and stylomastoid foramen. Most cases occur in diabetics, and virtually all cases occur in patients with some underlying immunosuppression. *Pseudomonas aeruginosa* can be isolated from aural drainage in more than 90% of patients.[8]

The most common presenting symptom in MOE is severe pain, classically worse at night, with associated otorrhea. Later signs include neuropathies of the lower cranial nerves VII-XII, with the facial nerve the most commonly affected. Classically, on otoscopic examination, there is granulation tissue present at the bony-cartilaginous junction. A high index of suspicion for this disease process is required in any immunosuppressed patient presenting with an external otitis with unresolving otorrhea and/or pain out of proportion to the examination findings, because patients may not always present with classic findings.

Diagnosis and workup of MOE generally requires imaging studies. A CT scan will provide the most useful anatomic information, whereas nuclear studies such as technetium bone scan and radioisotope scans are more sensitive than CT for detecting early infection, although they are not very specific. Technetium scans in particular will remain positive for an extended period of time after an infection and are not useful for following a patient's clinical course. MOE is typically treated with a 4- to 6-week course of broad-spectrum antibiotics with *Pseudomonas* coverage; early infections may be treated with oral antibiotics and close follow-up; however, more severe infections require admission with intravenous antibiotics initially.

## COMPLICATIONS OF SINUSITIS

Sinusitis affects roughly 1 in 8 adults in the United States each year and is one of the most common diagnoses responsible for antibiotic usage.[9,10] Most cases of sinusitis are uncomplicated and resolve with conservative management or simple antibiotic therapy. When complications do occur, it is typically via 2 main mechanisms: direct extension following loss of an anatomic barrier and/or hematologic spread. Because of the proximity of the sinuses to the orbit and the anterior cranial fossa, the most common complications generally involve these structures.

### Orbital Complications

A useful distinction for orbital complications of sinusitis is the location of the infectious process with regard to the orbital septum. The orbital septum is a fascial layer that is continuous with the periosteum of the superior and inferior edges of the orbit and extends to the edges of each eyelid. It forms a barrier between the orbit posteriorly and periorbital soft tissues more anteriorly. Infections that are preseptal or anterior to the septum tend to be less severe and less complicated, whereas the reverse is true for postseptal processes. The most commonly used classification of orbital infections was described by Chandler and colleagues[11] in 1970 and is known as the Chandler classification (**Table 1**).

| Table 1 Chandler classification of orbital infections | | |
|---|---|---|
| Group I | Preseptal/periorbital cellulitis | Inflammatory edema of the eyelids secondary to impaired venous drainage |
| Group II | Orbital cellulitis | Diffuse edema and inflammation of orbital adipose tissue, although without discrete abscess formation |
| Group III | Subperiosteal abscess | Collection of pus between the periorbita and bony wall of the orbit |
| Group IV | Orbital abscess | Discrete collection of pus within the orbital tissues |
| Group V | Cavernous sinus thrombosis | Extension of inflammation/phlebitis intracranially into the cavernous sinus |

*Data from* Chandler JR, Langenbrunner DJ, Stevens ER. The pathogenesis of orbital complications in acute sinusitis. Laryngoscope 1970;80:1414–28.

Generally, all patients with orbital and periorbital infections will present with some degree of inflammation and swelling around the orbit, pain, and fever, making clinical determination of the degree of infection somewhat difficult. However, the presence of other ocular signs or symptoms, including chemosis, proptosis, ophthalmoplegia, and visual disturbance, are helpful in distinguishing preseptal cellulitis from intraorbital processes, generally being absent in the former. Further distinguishing intraorbital processes from one another, such as subperiosteal abscess from orbital abscess, is difficult without the use of CT imaging. Most patients will require inpatient admission, with the exception of patients with limited upper lid edema, a normal eye examination, and reliability for medical compliance and close follow-up. Patients with visual changes, abnormal eye examination, cranial nerve deficits, signs or symptoms of central dysfunction (including lethargy, headache, vomiting, or seizures), or those who are systemically ill require admission to a facility with ophthalmologic and otolaryngologic capabilities.[12]

The most common organisms mirror those involved in upper respiratory infections/sinusitis and include *Streptococcus* species, *Staphylococcus aureus*, and *Haemophilus influenzae*, as well as anaerobic bacteria.[12] The mainstay of treatment is intravenous antibiotics, typically with broad-spectrum coverage that includes anaerobes, such as a broad-spectrum cephalosporin and metronidazole. A CT scan should be obtained in any patient in whom there are signs or symptoms of central involvement; ocular symptoms including proptosis, ophthalmoplegia, or decreased visual acuity; or lack of improvement or clinical deterioration after 24 hours of appropriate treatment.[12] Surgical therapy is required if an abscess is present.

Alternative causes of periorbital/orbital inflammation and swelling to be considered are conjunctivitis, dacryocystitis, trauma, contact allergy, neoplasm, or insect bites.

## Cavernous Sinus Thrombosis

Group V in the Chandler classification is cavernous sinus thrombosis, an extension of infection and inflammation intracranially into the cavernous sinus. Historically, before the widespread availability of antimicrobial agents, cavernous sinus thrombosis was uniformly fatal. Although much improved in the present day, the morbidity and mortality associated with this condition are significant enough that early diagnosis and treatment are crucial.

Cranial nerves III, IV, V, and VI, in addition to the horizontal segment of the internal carotid artery, either pass through or are in close proximity to the cavernous sinus, and therefore, patients with cavernous sinus thrombosis can present with ophthalmoplegia in addition to sensory disturbance, proptosis, chemosis, and fever. Other signs and symptoms include lethargy, headache, visual loss, papilledema, and pupillary defects. Extension of infection into other intracranial structures may result in meningitis or subdural empyema.[13] The clinical course of the disease generally develops within 1 week from the onset of the infectious process. Diagnosis requires either high-resolution CT with 3 mm or less slices or MR angiography. The primary modality of treatment is aggressive intravenous antibiotic therapy. The use of anticoagulation is controversial, and there is no role for surgical management of cavernous sinus thrombosis with the exception of addressing the primary site of infection (ie, sinusitis, odontogenic source).

### Frontal Osteomyelitis

Also known as Pott's puffy tumor, frontal osteomyelitis is a rare complication of frontal sinusitis that classically occurs in the pediatric population. Patients will present with a fluctuant, well-circumscribed swelling over the forehead, typically that has developed over the course of several weeks. Infection can extend to involve adjacent structures, leading to epidural abscess, subdural empyema, or brain abscess. Diagnosis can be confirmed with CT or MRI, and treatment involves surgical drainage and debridement in conjunction with antibiotic therapy.

### Intracranial Complications

The most serious complications of sinusitis are those that extend to involve intracranial structures. Cavernous sinus thrombosis is one such complication; however, more common complications include meningitis, epidural abscess, intracerebral abscess, and subdural empyema. Infection extending into the intracranial cavity generally does so by direct extension through either anatomic or traumatically induced pathways, or via retrograde thrombophlebitis. The clinical presentation of these complications may vary; bacterial meningitis, cavernous sinus thrombosis, and subdural empyema tend to be acute and fulminant, with symptoms including systemic toxicity, seizures, photophobia, nuchal rigidity, and encephalopathy, whereas brain abscess and epidural abscess may present more indolently with symptoms not dissimilar to uncomplicated sinusitis before progressing to more obvious symptoms of intracranial abnormality.[12]

The most common pathogens isolated in subdural empyema, which is the most common intracranial complication of sinusitis, include the *Streptococcus milleri* group (*Streptococcus anginosus*, *Streptococcus intermedius*, *Streptococcus constellatus*), other streptococcal species, enterococci, anaerobes, and gram-negative bacilli, most infections are polymicrobial.[14] Diagnosis of most intracranial complications requires imaging, ideally MRI with gadolinium contrast. Treatment invariably requires early and aggressive intravenous antibiotics in conjunction with surgical decompression and/or drainage of the infected sinuses, and potential drainage of any suppurative intracranial process.

## COMPLICATED ORAL CAVITY AND PHARYNGEAL INFECTIONS

Like ear and sinus disease, most cases of pharyngeal infection are mild and self-limited, or easily treated with oral antibiotics. As outlined in later discussion, the head and neck has numerous communicating potential spaces between fascial planes, some of which contain important neurovascular structures or lead to other parts of the body, and the upper airway is in close proximity to most of these spaces. Because of these anatomic features, infections that gain access to these spaces have the potential to cause rapid and serious complications.

### Epiglottitis

Acute epiglottitis is characterized by cellulitis and inflammation of the supraglottis, which may lead to rapid and potentially fatal airway compromise. Classically, this disease was associated with *H influenzae* infections; however, the introduction of a vaccine for *H influenzae* type B in 1985 resulted in a declining prevalence of the disease, shifting microbiology, and a trend toward fewer pediatric and more adult cases.[15,16] In the post–vaccination era, beta-hemolytic streptococcal species account for a higher number of cases in addition to other serotypes of *H influenzae*.

The classic features of acute epiglottitis are fever, dysphagia/odynophagia, drooling, stridor, and respiratory distress that are rapidly progressive over hours, although this particular clinical presentation is more common in children, whereas adults may present with fewer symptoms over a more protracted time course.[17] Patients generally prefer minimal movement or speaking and may prefer to sit in the "tripod" position to maximize airflow. Laryngospasm resulting in respiratory arrest may occur with aspiration of secretions into the narrowed airway. Because of the tenuous nature of the airway and rapidity in which it can decompensate, a high index of suspicion is required for prompt diagnosis. In patients who are stable, mildly symptomatic, not distressed and cooperative, and for whom a broader differential diagnosis is being considered, cervical plain films may be considered; patients with acute epiglottitis will have swelling and rounding of the epiglottis ("thumbprint sign") on lateral films. Patients with more moderate or severe symptoms should forego imaging, and particularly in children, interventions that may cause pain or discontent, such as placing lines or a separation from parents, should be avoided. Definitive diagnosis is made with visualization of the supraglottis, although in general this should only be attempted in the operating room at a facility with appropriate otolaryngology, anesthesia, and pediatric intensivist support and the capability to secure a surgical airway if necessary.

### Deep Neck Space Infections

The neck can be anatomically divided into several spaces that are invested in fibrous fascial layers. These fascial planes form potential spaces and provide limitations to the spread of infection as well as direct infectious spread once they are eroded. A useful anatomic landmark for classification of deep space infections is the hyoid bone, because there are strong fascial attachments to this bone anteriorly, making downward spread difficult. As such, deep space infections may be classified into 3 groups based on this: those above the level of the hyoid (eg, peritonsillar, parapharyngeal, temporal fossa, infratemporal fossa, pterygomaxillary fossa, masticator, submandibular, and parotid spaces); those involving the entire length of the neck (eg, retropharyngeal, prevertebral, carotid sheath, and danger spaces); and those involving the visceral or pretracheal space inferior to the hyoid.[18] Notably, some of these spaces extend outside of the neck, such as the retropharyngeal and danger spaces, which can allow infections to spread to the mediastinum. Other potential complications of deep neck infections include Lemierre's syndrome (thrombophlebitis of the internal jugular vein), cavernous sinus thrombosis, and carotid artery pseudoaneurysm or rupture; however, a major source of mortality associated with deep neck infections is respiratory distress due to airway obstruction. In adults, odontogenic infections are the most common source of deep neck infections, whereas in children, oropharyngeal infections are usually the cause.[19] Unsurprisingly, the organisms involved in deep neck infections are typically a mixture of aerobic and anaerobic species that are part of normal oropharyngeal flora, such as *Streptococcus*, *Staphylococcus*, *Bacteroides*, and *Prevotella*. Some of the more commonly encountered deep space abscesses are discussed later.

### Peritonsillar Abscess

The peritonsillar space lies between the palatine tonsil medially and superior pharyngeal constrictor muscle laterally and is bound anteriorly and posteriorly by the tonsillar pillars. It contains loose connective tissue and vasculature to the tonsil and communicates with the parapharyngeal space. A collection of pus in this space is what is called a peritonsillar abscess (PTA), and it is the most common deep neck space infection.[20] It most commonly affects young adults, and incidence peaks in winter and spring, coinciding with the highest incidences of streptococcal pharyngitis. PTAs have classically been thought to be a complication of acute tonsillitis, typically untreated, with spread of bacteria to peritonsillar tissue leading to peritonsillar inflammation and ultimately abscess formation, although an alternate theory that has gained support recently is that PTAs are the result of blockage of Weber's glands: salivary glands located in the supratonsillar fossa.[21]

Patients with PTA will typically present with fever, sore throat (often following an upper respiratory illness), dysphagia/odynophagia, trismus, and a muffled or garbled "hot potato voice." On examination, the oropharynx appears erythematous; the uvula is deviated to the contralateral side, and there is an underlying fullness of the soft palate and displacement of the anterior tonsillar pillar. Diagnosis may be made clinically and confirmed with needle aspiration of pus from the peritonsillar space. There is debate over the best method of surgical management (aspiration vs incision and drainage vs tonsillectomy); however, any patient with a confirmed or suspected PTA should be referred to the emergency room, ideally at a facility with otolaryngology support given potential for airway compromise.[22] In addition to surgical drainage of the abscess, patients should be treated with a course of broad-spectrum antibiotics with coverage of oral flora. There is also evidence that a course of oral steroids leads to quicker resolution of symptoms.[22]

### Ludwig's Angina

Ludwig's angina is characterized by rapidly progressive cellulitis of the submandibular, sublingual, and submental spaces.[19] Infectious spread tends to occur posteriorly because these spaces have open posterior borders, and this generally causes swelling of the floor of mouth and elevation/displacement of the tongue with the potential for rapid airway compromise. Nearly all cases are caused by an odontogenic infection, most commonly associated with a mandibular molar. Infections are usually polymicrobial with both aerobic and anaerobic organisms. Patients may have a preceding history of recent dental work. They will present with severe trismus, dysphagia/odynophagia, and drooling, often in conjunction with fever and general malaise. Patients may complain of dyspnea, and marked anxiety may preclude impending airway obstruction. On examination, the tongue will be pushed superiorly in the oral cavity due to swelling and induration of the floor of mouth, and patients will have brawny neck swelling. Treatment requires broad-spectrum intravenous antibiotics and potentially surgical drainage or debridement, although airway management is often the most pressing issue. Given the propensity for rapid clinical decline, patients with suspected Ludwig's angina should be promptly transported to a facility with the ability to manage a difficult airway and obtain a surgical airway if need be.

## Parapharyngeal Space Infection

The parapharyngeal, or lateral pharyngeal, space is an inverted pyramid-shaped space that is bounded superiorly by the skull base, inferiorly by the hyoid bone, medially by the superior constrictor muscle, and laterally by the parotid and medial pterygoid muscle. It is separated into 2 subdivisions, the pre–styloid space, which contains mainly adipose and connective tissue, and the post–styloid space, which notably contains the common carotid and internal jugular vessels as well as cranial nerves IX, X, and XII and the cervical sympathetic chain. This space communicates with several other neck spaces, and infections here may stem from a variety of sources, including the pharynx, teeth, tonsils/adenoids, parotid gland, and submandibular, retropharyngeal, and masticator spaces.

Depending on which compartment is involved, patients will present with differing symptoms, although in general all patients will present with fever and signs of toxicity. Patients with pre–styloid involvement will typically present with pain, dysphagia, and severe trismus due to inflammation of the pterygoid muscles, and swelling of the lateral pharyngeal wall and over the angle of the mandible. Patients with post–styloid involvement generally will have less pain and will present without trismus, and they may lack obvious intraoral or neck swelling. Because of the important neurovascular contents of the post–styloid space, patients with infections here may present with neurologic deficits, such as hoarseness, unilateral tongue weakness, or Horner's syndrome, and the potential for serious complications exists, such as suppurative jugular thrombophlebitis, Lemierre's syndrome, or carotid artery erosion.[23,24] A contrasted CT scan can be used to determine the extent and location of involvement. Definitive treatment requires broad-spectrum intravenous antibiotics, and in most cases, surgical drainage.

## Retropharyngeal Space Infection

The retropharyngeal space is located between the pharynx and esophagus and the alar fascia over the spine, and it extends vertically from the skull base to the mediastinum. It communicates with the parapharyngeal space as well as the danger space, a potential space found posterior to the retropharyngeal space that extends from the skull base all the way to the diaphragm. Causes of retropharyngeal space infection include extension from communicating spaces, trauma from pharyngeal instrumentation (eg, endoscopy, intubation, nasogastric tube placement), and foreign bodies. In children, there are 2 paramedian deep cervical lymph node chains found in the retropharyngeal space that involute around the age of 5 years; because of this, suppurative adenitis can be the underlying cause of retropharyngeal infections in children, although rarely in adults.[23]

Patients with retropharyngeal space infections may present with fever, dysphagia, odynophagia, and neck stiffness. There may be swelling of the posterior pharyngeal wall seen on examination. Potential serious complications include loss of airway patency as well as spread of infection to the mediastinum. When mediastinitis occurs as a result of infectious spread from the head and neck, it is known as descending necrotizing mediastinitis, which is a particularly aggressive type that has mortalities reported as high as 30% to 40%.[25] Lateral soft tissue radiographs may show thickening of the retropharyngeal tissue that is suggestive of infection here; however, contrasted CT scan should be obtained in any patient with suspected retropharyngeal space infection for confirmation as well as delineation of the extent of infection. As with all deep neck space infections, management includes intravenous antibiotics in conjunction with surgical drainage in the case of abscess formation. The presence of mediastinal involvement necessitates involvement by cardiothoracic surgery.

## FOREIGN BODIES

Foreign bodies in the airway or alimentary tract are most commonly encountered in the pediatric population, although they may be encountered in any age group. Clinical history is important in this subset of patients, because patient presentation may vary from life-threatening airway compromise to subtle respiratory symptoms to asymptomatic.

### Airway Foreign Bodies

The highest incidence of airway foreign bodies occurs in boys under the age of 3 years, and commonly aspirated materials include organic material, such as nuts, seeds, popcorn, and vegetable matter, although nonfood items, such as small toys and jewelry, are also encountered.[26] When aspirated, foreign bodies tend to lodge in the right main stem bronchus given its wider diameter and more vertical positioning compared with the left.

Depending on the location of the aspirated object, clinical presentation may vary, with objects lodged high in the airway (such as the trachea or larynx) typically causing more significant airway compromise and respiratory distress, and objects that are situated lower down causing less severe symptoms. Because of this, obtaining a good history is vital in evaluating a patient for an upper airway foreign body. In neurologically normal individuals with an intact cough reflex, aspiration will always elicit an episode of choking, coughing, or gagging as the object passes the glottic structures. Eventually, as the object comes to rest, these symptoms will start to wane and the patient may be relatively asymptomatic. This asymptomatic period may last hours to days and is followed later on by complications from continued presence of the foreign body in the respiratory tree, such as localized inflammation, obstruction, and infection.[27] Physical examination findings include decreased or asymmetric lung sounds, prolonged expiratory phase, and wheezing, and in later stages, patients may present with recurrent pneumonias.

Frontal and lateral plain films may be helpful in diagnosing an upper airway foreign body, especially if the object is radiopaque; however, a normal imaging study does not rule out the presence of a foreign body. More subtle findings, such as unilateral hyperinflation or localized atelectasis or infiltrates, may suggest a bronchial foreign body. Definitive diagnosis is made on bronchoscopy with visualization of the object. Any patient with a history of a witnessed aspiration and/or clinical suspicion of an airway foreign body should be taken to the operating room for rigid bronchoscopy and removal, as the risk of complications is too high if left untreated.[27]

### Esophageal Foreign Bodies

Esophageal foreign bodies are more common than airway foreign bodies, and in general, are more common in children. The most commonly ingested items include coins, pins, toy parts, jewelry, and batteries. In the pediatric population, food bolus impactions are rare, although they may occur in the setting of eosinophilic esophagitis or esophageal strictures from prior surgical intervention (eg, esophageal atresia repair). Most ingested foreign bodies are located in the stomach (60%), with about 20% becoming stuck in the esophagus and 5% to 10% in the oropharynx.[28]

Presenting symptoms may include drooling, dysphagia, emesis, chest discomfort, and anorexia; however, a large proportion of patients may be completely asymptomatic, which highlights the importance of the history because there is often a preceding history of witnessed ingestion. In severe cases, small children in particular may present with respiratory symptoms as a result of swelling of and pressure on the common wall between trachea and esophagus and the more compressible pediatric trachea.

More often than not, patients with esophageal foreign bodies will not have any specific physical examination findings.

Plain films may be helpful in determining the location of radiopaque objects; with esophageal foreign bodies, a lateral film is also required to ensure that the foreign body is not in the airway. In general, there are 4 areas of physiologic narrowing in the esophagus where foreign bodies often become trapped: at the upper esophageal sphincter, over the aortic arch, over the mainstem bronchus, and at the lower esophageal sphincter. The decision to remove an esophageal foreign body depends on several different factors. In general, urgent endoscopy should be considered for young children; foreign bodies present for more than 24 hours; sharp, metallic, or caustic foreign bodies; or symptomatic patients.[27] A sharp or caustic foreign body, such as a pin or button battery, or a foreign body that has been stuck for a prolonged period of time has a much higher risk of causing localized esophageal injury and eventually perforation. Spontaneous passage of coins from the esophagus is reported at around 25% to 30%, and in asymptomatic patients with recent ingestion of a low-risk object, a period of waiting up to 16 hours before repeating another radiograph may be appropriate.[29] If the object passes in to the stomach, generally it is allowed to pass through the gastrointestinal tract.

## TRAUMA

Most patients with significant facial trauma will present to the emergency department; however, patients with less severe injuries or those with delayed presentations may present to primary care providers in the outpatient setting. In any patient presenting with a history of trauma, the basic ABCs (airway, breathing, circulation) of trauma management should be followed. Patients with a derangement of any of those 3 categories are more appropriately managed in an emergency department or trauma center and should be expeditiously transferred for further care. In a stable patient with subtle findings, attention should be paid to the mechanism of trauma, because this may direct the care provider toward likely injuries. Given the increased likelihood of their involvement as victims of domestic violence, this is particularly important in women and children.

Physical examination of the head and face can reveal areas of concern. Visual inspection of the face may reveal subtle asymmetry or deformity. Palpation of the orbital rims and nasal bones should be performed to evaluate for any bony step-offs, suggesting an underlying fracture. Otoscopy can be used to detect the presence of hemotympanum, which may indicate a temporal bone fracture. A full cranial nerve examination should be performed. Visual acuity and pupillary reflexes should be tested. The presence of clear watery rhinorrhea may represent cerebrospinal fluid (CSF) leak from skull base fractures. Loss of normal occlusion or report of malocclusion by the patient may accompany both mandibular and mid-facial fractures; in addition, the presence of maxillary mobility on examination suggests mid-facial fractures. The patient's neck should also be examined for bruising, swelling, or crepitus, which may indicate underlying laryngeal injury.

When operative repair is indicated, the timing of repair is an issue that generates some debate. Some early studies on mandibular fractures suggested a higher infection rate when repair was delayed, although more recent data do not fully support this. Some surgeons argue that delayed repair results in less satisfactory healing and overall outcomes, while others think that delaying surgery until after the acute swelling has resolved allows for more accurate assessment of facial asymmetry and subsequent reconstruction. In many circumstances, the patient may have other critical injuries or issues that take precedence over his/her maxillofacial injuries.[30]

### Orbital Fractures

Orbital wall fractures are not uncommon in facial trauma. In adults, they typically result from motor vehicle collisions or assault; however, in children, they more often stem from athletic injuries and falls. The medial wall and orbital floor tend to be most commonly involved.[31] Because ocular injuries may occur in up to 13% of patients with orbital fractures, it is imperative for the patient to have an eye examination.[32] Proptosis, enophthalmos, periocular swelling and/or ecchymosis, and chemosis are potential clinical findings in a patient with an orbital wall fracture. The presence of disrupted ocular motility suggests entrapment of the extraocular muscles. Patients with suspected orbital wall fractures should be further evaluated with a CT scan and will require consultation with ophthalmology and otolaryngology services as well.

### Nasal Fractures

Nasal fractures are another common type of facial fracture encountered in the trauma setting. They may occur in isolation or in conjunction with other injuries. Most nasal fractures generally do not require immediate intervention and can be safely addressed within 1 to 2 weeks of injury. Displaced nasal fractures may be reduced shortly after injury; however, if there is enough swelling as to make landmarks and normal anatomy difficult to determine, closed nasal reduction may be more easily performed 5 to 7 days later when swelling has improved or resolved. When there is concern for a septal fracture, a septal hematoma, which is a collection of blood between the perichondrium and cartilage of the septum, must be ruled out. Untreated, a septal hematoma can result in necrosis of the underlying septum followed by septal perforation. This is treated by incision and drainage with packing of the space to ensure that blood does not reaccumulate. In general, inspection and palpation of the nose are the best way to diagnose a nasal fracture, and imaging is not always helpful or necessary.

### Mid-face Fractures

There are several classification schema used for mid-face fractures. One of the most commonly used is the Le Fort classification, a system developed more than 100 years ago by analyzing the fracture patterns of cadavers dropped from heights. This system spans from maxillary separation from the rest of the craniofacial skeleton (Le Fort I) to complete craniofacial separation (Le Fort III). Clinically, maxillary mobility to suggest a Le Fort–type fracture can be assessed by gently tugging on the maxilla. Zygomaticomaxillary complex fractures, or ZMC fractures, are commonly encountered fractures in the trauma setting that can significantly alter the appearance of the face. The ZMC functions as a buttress for the face and has 4 points of articulation with the frontal bone, temporal bone, maxilla, and greater wing of the sphenoid bone, and fractures may be complex and occur in multiple locations. Importantly, the lateral wall of the orbit may be involved in ZMC fractures, and so a prompt ophthalmologic examination should be obtained.[33] Naso-orbital-ethmoid fractures are another subset of midfacial fractures that refer to injuries involving the intersection of the nose, orbit, ethmoids, frontal sinus, and floor of the anterior cranial base. This area includes the insertion of the medial canthal tendon of the eye, and injuries here often result in telecanthus.

Diagnosis of mid-face fractures is confirmed by CT imaging. Although some simple and nondisplaced zygomatic fractures may be managed conservatively, many midface fractures will ultimately require operative reduction and fixation for optimal facial cosmetic and functional outcomes.

## Mandibular Fractures

Fractures of the mandible are the most common type of maxillofacial fracture that occurs after motor vehicle accident or following physical altercation. Patients are typically young, in the third decade of life, and most are men.[34] They are classified based on the anatomic location of the fracture (eg, parasymphysis, subcondylar), as well. Patients with mandibular fractures may complain of malocclusion and/or trismus. There may be associated intraoral communication and dental injuries present. CT imaging and orthopantogram are diagnostic of mandibular fractures. Most patients will require operative reduction and fixation, although this does in part depend on the anatomic location of the fracture.[30,34]

## Temporal Bone Fractures

A large amount of force is required to fracture the temporal bone; because of this, fractures here most commonly result from high-energy mechanisms such as motor vehicle accidents. With improving vehicle safety measures over time, assault and falls are accounting for a larger proportion of cases. Given the high-energy impacts required for temporal bone fractures to occur, patients often will sustain other skull fractures or intracranial injuries, maxillofacial injuries, and other orthopedic injuries, and as such, will generally present to emergency departments or trauma centers. Historically, temporal bone fractures have been classified based on the axis of the fracture: longitudinal (occurring parallel to the petrous ridge of the temporal bone) or transverse (occurring perpendicular to the petrous ridge). When classified as such, approximately 70% to 90% of fractures are longitudinal and 10% to 30% are transverse. A more useful clinical classification, however, pertains to involvement of the otic capsule as either otic capsule–violating or otic capsule–sparing.[35,36] Fractures disrupting the otic capsule almost always result in sensorineural hearing loss (whereas otic capsule–sparing fractures generally result in a conductive loss), are significantly more likely to result in facial paralysis and CSF otorrhea, and carry a higher risk of delayed meningitis.

Patients will present with a history of a high-energy injury mechanism. With specific attention to the ear, they may have external ear lacerations or hematomas. It is not uncommon for patients to have lacerations of the ear canal on otoscopic examination stemming from underlying fracture. Hemotympanum or bloody otorrhea is invariably present; the ear canal should be inspected for the presence of CSF otorrhea. Patients will have a conductive hearing loss on tuning fork examination due to the presence of hemotympanum, although ossicular chain disruption may also contribute if present. A sensorineural loss may also be present. A cranial nerve examination should be performed, with particular attention to the facial nerve function on the ipsilateral side. If facial nerve weakness is present, if possible, it should be determined whether its onset was immediate after the injury or delayed.

CT imaging with thin slices through the temporal bone is helpful for diagnosis, although patients will often already have had a head CT with thicker slices to evaluate for intracranial injuries, and this is often enough to make the diagnosis of temporal bone fracture. Attention should be paid to the carotid canal, because this may be injured in temporal bone trauma. The presence of immediate onset facial paralysis often warrants surgical exploration. Traumatic CSF leaks often resolve spontaneously, although may require CSF diversion with lumbar drain or surgical intervention. In the absence of these complications, temporal bone fractures are generally managed conservatively, with formal audiogram testing occurring in 6 or more weeks following resolution of hemotympanum.[35,36]

## SUDDEN SENSORINEURAL HEARING LOSS

Although many adults develop sensorineural hearing loss from of variety of causes, a subset will develop hearing loss acutely and without an obvious underlying cause. Sudden sensorineural hearing loss is poorly understood and is not truly a diagnosis but rather a syndrome. There have been numerous causes proposed for it, principally of which include viral infection, vascular event, intracochlear membrane rupture, and autoimmune process. Most commonly, patients will notice a unilateral hearing loss on awakening; the hearing loss is usually stable and not fluctuating. Aural fullness, tinnitus, and vertigo may be present. In general, the more severe the loss and the older the patient, the less likely hearing will recover, and it is reported that 65% of patients overall will recover hearing.[37,38]

Patients presenting with a sudden hearing loss should have a formal audiogram for characterization of the loss and for comparison in the future. Sudden hearing loss may be the initial presentation of a retrocochlear lesion such as acoustic neuroma; as such, a contrasted MRI is recommended for further evaluation. If a specific cause is uncovered during workup (such as pharmacologic ototoxicity or acoustic neuroma), treatment is directed at the underlying cause. For idiopathic cases, steroids are currently the most widely accepted treatment option: typically patients are treated with a 7- to 10-day course of 1 mg/kg/d of oral prednisone, with a repeat audiogram obtained after this is completed. Intratympanic steroid injections may be used in patients in whom oral steroids are contraindicated or who have failed to benefit from oral steroids.[39] Because of its potential to have a significant impact on a patient's quality of life, sudden sensorineural hearing loss should be treated as an otologic emergency and prompt early treatment and referral to an otolaryngologist.

## SUMMARY

Each year primary care providers evaluate and treat countless patients with otolaryngology-related complaints. The vast majority are straightforward and easily recognized and treated; however, given the proximity of the ears, nose, and throat to numerous vital structures in the head and neck, the potential for serious consequences exists if disease processes go unrecognized and untreated. This article serves to familiarize the primary care provider with the clinical presentation of various complications associated with common otolaryngologic complaints. Clinicians who care for patients presenting with otolaryngologic complaints should keep these entities in mind and attempt to rule out any serious complication. Patients with suspected complications should be promptly referred to an emergency department at a facility with subspecialist support. Many of these complications are thankfully rare, and continued diligence and familiarization with these disease processes will serve to maintain them as such.

## REFERENCES

1. Chole RA. Chronic otitis media, mastoiditis, and petrositis. In: Flint PW, Haughey BH, Lund V, et al, editors. Cummings otolaryngology. 6th edition. Philadelphia: Saunders Elsevier; 2015.
2. Grijalva CG, Nuorti JP, Griffin MR. Antibiotic prescription rates for acute respiratory tract infections in US ambulatory settings. JAMA 2009;302(7):758–66.
3. Budenz CL, El-Kashlan HK, Shelton C, et al. Complications of temporal bone infections. In: Flint PW, Haughey BH, Lund V, et al, editors. Cummings otolaryngology. 6th edition. Philadelphia: Saunders Elsevier; 2015.

4. Luntz M, Brodsky A, Nusem S, et al. Acute mastoiditis–the antibiotic era: a multi-center study. Int J Pediatr Otorhinolaryngol 2001;57(1):1–9.

5. de Oliveira Penido N, Borin A, Iha LCN, et al. Intracranial complications of otitis media: 15 years of experience in 33 patients. Otolaryngol Head Neck Surg 2005;132(1):37–42.

6. Osma U, Cureoglu S, Hosoglu S. The complications of chronic otitis media: report of 93 cases. J Laryngol Otol 2000;11(2):97–100.

7. Wanna GB, Dharamsi LM, Moss JR, et al. Contemporary management of intracra-nial complications of otitis media. Otol Neurotol 2010;31(1):111–7.

8. Rubin Grandis J, Branstetter BF 4th, Yu VL. The changing face of malignant (ne-crotising) external otitis: clinical, radiological, and anatomic correlations. Lancet Infect Dis 2004;4(1):34–9.

9. Blackwell DL, Lucas JW, Clarke TC. Summary health statistics for U.S. adults: Na-tional Health Interview Survey, 2012. Vital Health Stat 10 2014;260:1–161.

10. Rosenfeld RM, Riccirillo JF, Chandrasekhar SS, et al. Clinical practice guideline (update): adult sinusitis. Otolaryngol Head Neck Surg 2015;152(2):S1–39.

11. Chandler JR, Langenbrunner DJ, Stevens ER. The pathogenesis of orbital com-plications in acute sinusitis. Laryngoscope 1970;80:1414–28.

12. Howe L, Jones NS. Guidelines for the management of periorbital cellulitis/ab-scess. Clin Otolaryngol 2004;29(6):725–8.

13. Ebright JR, Pace MT, Niazi AF. Septic thrombosis of the cavernous sinuses. Arch Intern Med 2001;161(22):2671–6.

14. Osborn MK, Steinberg JP. Subdural empyema and other suppurative complica-tions of paranasal sinusitis. Lancet Infect Dis 2007;7(1):62–7.

15. Senior BA, Radkowski D, MacArthur C, et al. Changing patterns in pediatric supraglottitis: a multi-institutional review, 1980 to 1992. Laryngoscope 1994; 104(11):1314–22.

16. Shah RK, Stocks C. Epiglottitis in the United States: national trends, variances, prognosis, and management. Laryngoscope 2010;120(6):1256–62.

17. Meyer A. Pediatric infectious disease. In: Flint PW, Haughey BH, Lund V, et al, editors. Cummings otolaryngology. 6th edition. Philadelphia: Saunders Elsevier; 2015.

18. Vieira F, Allen SM, Stocks RM, et al. Deep neck infection. Otolaryngol Clin North Am 2008;41(3):459–83.

19. Christian JM, Goddard AC, Gillespie MB. Deep neck and odontogenic infections. In: Flint PW, Haughey BH, Lund V, et al, editors. Cummings otolaryngology. 6th edition. Philadelphia: Saunders Elsevier; 2015.

20. Rusan M, Klug TE, Ovesen T. An overview of the microbiology of acute ear, nose and throat infections requiring hospitalization. Eur J Clin Microbiol Infect Dis 2009;28(3):243–51.

21. Klug TE, Rusan M, Fuursted K, et al. Peritonsillar abscess: complication of acute tonsillitis or Weber's glands infection? Otolaryngol Head Neck Surg 2016;155(2): 199–207.

22. Johnson RF, Stewart MG. The contemporary approach to diagnosis and manage-ment of peritonsillar abscess. Curr Opin Otolaryngol Head Neck Surg 2005;13(3): 157–60.

23. Marra S, Hotaling AJ. Deep neck infections. Am J Otolaryngol 1996;17(5): 287–98.

24. Reynolds SC, Chow AW. Severe soft tissue infections of the head and neck: a primer for critical care physicians. Lung 2009;187(5):271–9.

25. Estrera AS, Landay MJ, Grisham JM, et al. Descending necrotizing mediastinitis. Surg Gynecol Obstet 1983;157(6):545–52.
26. Foltran F, Ballali S, Rodriguez H, et al. Inhaled foreign bodies in children: a global perspective on their epidemiological, clinical, and preventive aspects. Pediatr Pulmonol 2013;48(4):344–51.
27. Schoem SR, Rosbe KW, Bearelly S. Aerodigestive foreign bodies and caustic ingestions. In: Flint PW, Haughey BH, Lund V, et al, editors. Cummings otolaryngology. 6th edition. Philadelphia: Saunders Elsevier; 2015.
28. Yalcin S, Karnak I, Ciftci AO, et al. Foreign body ingestion in children: an analysis of pediatric surgical practice. Pediatr Surg Int 2007;23(8):755–61.
29. Waltzman ML, Baskin M, Wypii D, et al. A randomized clinical trial of the management of esophageal coins in children. Pediatrics 2005;116(3):614–9.
30. Kellman RM. Maxillofacial trauma. In: Flint PW, Haughey BH, Lund V, et al, editors. Cummings otolaryngology. 6th edition. Philadelphia: Saunders Elsevier; 2015.
31. Boyette JR, Pemberton JD, Bonilla-Valez J. Management of orbital fractures: challenges and solutions. Clin Ophthalmol 2015;9:2127–37.
32. Kreidl KO, Kim DY, Mansour SE. Prevalence of significant intraocular sequelae in blunt orbital trauma. Am J Emerg Med 2003;21(7):525–8.
33. Jamal BT, Pfahler SM, Lane KA, et al. Ophthalmic injuries in patients with zygomaticomaxillary complex fractures requiring surgical repair. J Oral Maxillofac Surg 2009;67(5):986–9.
34. Motamedi MH, Dadgar E, Ebrahimi A, et al. Pattern of maxillofacial fractures: a 5-year analysis of 8,818 patients. J Trauma Acute Care Surg 2014;77(4):630–4.
35. Brodie HA, Wilkerson BJ. Management of temporal bone trauma. In: Flint PW, Haughey BH, Lund V, et al, editors. Cummings otolaryngology. 6th edition. Philadelphia: Saunders Elsevier; 2015.
36. Johnson F, Semaan MT, Megerian CA. Temporal bone fracture: evaluation and management in the modern era. Otolaryngol Clin North Am 2008;41(3):597–618.
37. Arts HA. Sensorineural hearing loss in adults. In: Flint PW, Haughey BH, Lund V, et al, editors. Cummings otolaryngology. 6th edition. Philadelphia: Saunders Elsevier; 2015.
38. Mattox DE, Simmons FB. Natural history of sudden sensorineural hearing loss. Ann Otol Rhinol Laryngol 1977;86(4 Pt 1):463–80.
39. Lawrence R, Thevasagayam R. Controversies in the management of sudden sensorineural hearing loss: an evidence-based review. Clin Otolaryngol 2015; 40(3):176–82.

# Index

*Note:* Page numbers of article titles are in **boldface** type.

### A

ABCD2 score, 485
Abrasions, corneal, 623
Abscess
   in ear infections, 643
   in sinusitis, 646
   peritonsillar, 648
*Acanthamoeba* keratitis, 622
Acids, eye burns from, 631–632
Acoustic neuroma, 654
Acute coronary syndrome, in hypertension, 472
Adenosine, for tachyarrhythmias, 498–499
Adenovirus
   in conjunctivitis, 619
   in keratitis, 622
AFFIRM (Atrial Fibrillation Follow-Up Investigation of Rhythm Management) trial, 500
Airway
   foreign bodies in, 650
   obstruction of, in anaphylaxis, 522
Albuterol
   for anaphylaxis, 526
   for asthma, 541–542
   for COPD, 545–546
Alcohol intoxication, 574–575, 578–583
Alkaline compounds, eye burns from, 631–632
Allantoin, for crystalline arthritis, 609
Allergy
   anaphylaxis in, **521–536**
   conjunctivitis in, 619–620
Allopurinol, for crystalline arthritis, 609
Amniotic membrane transplant, for corneal burns, 632
Anaphylaxis, **521–536**
   definition of, 522
   follow-up education for, 533–534
   forms of, 523
   imitators of, 521
   pathophysiology of, 522–523
   population at risk for, 522
   symptoms of, 522–523
   treatment of, 523–533
Angina, Ludwig, 648
Angioedema, in anaphylaxis, 522

Med Clin N Am 101 (2017) 657–671
http://dx.doi.org/10.1016/S0025-7125(17)30045-7
0025-7125/17

# Moving?

## Make sure your subscription moves with you!

To notify us of your new address, find your **Clinics Account Number** (located on your mailing label above your name), and contact customer service at:

**Email: journalscustomerservice-usa@elsevier.com**

**800-654-2452** (subscribers in the U.S. & Canada)
**314-447-8871** (subscribers outside of the U.S. & Canada)

**Fax number: 314-447-8029**

**Elsevier Health Sciences Division**
**Subscription Customer Service**
**3251 Riverport Lane**
**Maryland Heights, MO 63043**

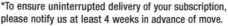

*To ensure uninterrupted delivery of your subscription, please notify us at least 4 weeks in advance of move.